ILLUSTRATED TEXTBOOK OF

OBSTETRICS

A slide Atlas of *Illustrated Textbook of Obstetrics,* based on
the contents of this book, is available. In the slide atlas format,
the material is split into volumes, each of which is presented in
a binder together with numbered 35mm slides of each
illustration. Each slide atlas volume also contains a list of
abbreviated slide captions for easy reference when using the
slides. Further information can be obtained from:

Gower Medical Publishing
Middlesex House
34—42 Cleveland Street
London W1P 5FB

Gower Medical Publishing 101 5th Avenue
New York, NY. 10003
USA

ILLUSTRATED TEXTBOOK OF

OBSTETRICS

GEOFFREY CHAMBERLAIN RD MD FRCS FRCOG

Professor of Obstetrics and Gynaecology
St George's Hospital Medical School
London, UK

CHARLOTTE R. GIBBINGS MB BS MRCOG DA

Formerly of Department of Obstetrics and
Gynaecology
St George's Hospital Medical School
London, UK

SIR JOHN DEWHURST MB ChB FRCSE FRCOG Hon.MD DSc FACOG
FRACOG FCOG(SA) FRCSI

Emeritus Professor of Obstetrics and Gynaecology
Queen Charlotte's Hospital
London, UK

Paediatrics contribution by:
DAVID HARVEY FRCP DCh

Consultant Paediatrician
Queen Charlotte's Maternity Hospital
London, UK

J. B. Lippincott Company PHILADELPHIA

Gower Medical Publishing LONDON • NEW YORK

Distributed in all countries except the USA, Canada and Japan by:
  Harper and Row International
  10 East 53rd Street
  New York, NY. 10022
  USA

Distributed in the USA and Canada by:
  J. B. Lippincott Company
  East Washington Square
  Philadelphia, PA. 19105
  USA

Distributed in Japan by:
  Igaku-Shoin Ltd.
  Foreign Book Department
  1-28-36 Hongo, Bunkyo-ku
  Tokyo 113
  Japan

Project editors: Michele Campbell
                        Catherine Moehrle

Design: Anne-Marie Shine

Illustration: Maurizia Merati

Line artists: Marion Tasker
                        Michael Rabess
                        Mark Willey

Series design: Michel Laake

Library of Congress Catalog Number: 88-80407
Library of Congress Cataloging in Publication Data are available
British Library Cataloguing in Publication Data:
  Chamberlain, Geoffrey, *1930–*
    Illustrated textbook of obstetrics.
    1. Obstetrics
    I. Title II. Gibbings, Charlotte R.
    III. Dewhurst, *Sir* C. John (Christopher John, *1920–*
    618.2
ISBN: 0-397-44580-6 (Lippincott/Gower)

Originated in Hong Kong by South Sea International Press Ltd.
Typesetting by IC Dawkins (typesetters) Ltd., London.
Text set in Sabon; captions and figures set in Univers.
Printed in Hong Kong by Imago Publishing Ltd.

Preface

There is no ideal book on obstetrics for the medical student. This may reflect the speed of change in the subject; the teaching of midwifery has mostly been replaced by that of reproductive medicine. Students no longer learn obstetrics as a first aid subject centred on the salvage of babies and mothers from difficult deliveries. Instead, they study the whole of pregnancy with its physiological changes as a part of normal life; the variations from normal are of course important, but in the developed world the extremes of these will always be dealt with by obstetricians who have been trained to deal with such emergencies. The emphasis for training all potential doctors has shifted rapidly towards the normal, for the abnormal is now taught after qualification to those doctors specializing in obstetrics.

Students vary in their methods of learning. Some like much detail, others general principles; all like relevant diagrams. With this in mind, we have written an account of the subject which covers more realistically what a student needs to know at qualifying level. To help learning, we have had excellent illustrations prepared by Maurizia Merati and Anne-Marie Shine. We are most grateful to them for the care with which they have reproduced our ideas. We have had very close cooperation with Gower Medical Publishing and happily acknowledge the help of several editors, the latest of whom, Michele Campbell, has put a great amount of effort into this book. Much of the good work in it is hers, any mistakes are ours.

We wish all students reading this book well for their final examinations. For the small proportion who wish to come into the specialty of obstetrics and gynaecology, we hope it will make a foundation for a lifetime of service in a very satisfying subject.

GEOFFREY CHAMBERLAIN
CHARLOTTE GIBBINGS
SIR JOHN DEWHURST

London 1988

Contents

1. Fetal Anatomy and Physiology

FETAL DEVELOPMENT AND ANATOMY

The growing fetus develops from a single fertilized cell to six billion cells in approximately thirty-eight weeks. The change in form of the blastocyst, embryo and fetus are considered in this section.

Fertilization

Before fertilization can occur, the ovum must mature. A period of growth is accompanied by meiosis in two stages: the first division is heterotypical, producing a large secondary oocyte and a polar body, both of which are haploid (that is, containing twenty-three chromosomes, which is half the number present in somatic cells). The second division does not occur until after fertilization.

After release from the ovary, the secondary oocyte is carried by ciliary action and peristalsis to the lateral end of the fallopian tube, where it is deposited. If intercourse occurs at this time in the menstrual cycle, the sperm which are deposited in the vagina travel up through the uterus to reach the ampullary section of the tube. Here, they encounter and surround the oocyte and penetrate the zona pellucida to enter the perivitelline space. One sperm then enters the oocyte itself (Fig.1.1 left). Once this has occurred, a rapid degranulation of surface vesicles inhibits penetration by more sperm. The tail of the sperm becomes separated from the head and is absorbed. The sperm's nucleus now represents the male pronucleus, which is haploid. The oocyte then completes the second stage of meiotic division, so producing the second polar body, and the mature oocyte containing the female pronucleus, which is haploid. The first polar body may also divide to produce a third polar body (Fig.1.1 centre). The diploid number of chromosomes (forty-six) is reconstituted by the fusion of the male and female pronuclei. The chromosomes arrange themselves on the spindle, and the cleavage furrow of future division is formed (Fig.1.1 right).

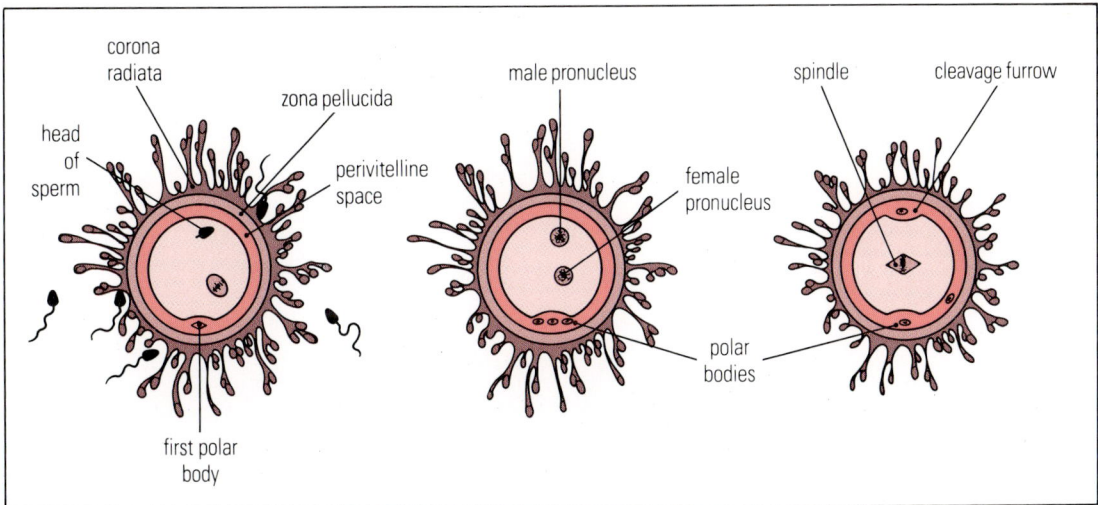

Fig.1.1 Fertilization of the ovum. Left: sperm surround the ovum but only one will penetrate the oocyte. Centre: the female pronucleus approaches the male pronucleus and they fuse. Right: the chromosomes arrange themselves on the spindle and a cleavage furrow circumscribes the ovum on the line of two of the polar bodies.

Cleavage

Cell cleavage commences a few hours later, and produces daughter cells, or blastomeres (Fig.1.2). The developing zygote takes approximately forty hours to reach an eight-cell stage. After further division, the sixteen-cell morula is formed. Fluid then accumulates inside the morula, which becomes a hollow blastocyst. Four or five days have now elapsed since fertilization, during which time the zygote has travelled down the fallopian tube, and arrived in the endometrial cavity at the blastocyst stage. An inner cell mass, the embryonic pole, develops in one region of the blastocyst (Fig.1.3).

Implantation

The blastocyst sinks into the endometrium with the embryonic pole pointing towards the endometrial epithelium (Fig.1.4 upper). After two days, it burrows through the layers of tissue.

The outer layer of the blastocyst is termed the trophoblast. The trophoblast cells penetrate the basement membrane of the endometrial epithelium and invade the stroma. Here, some of these cells fuse to form a syncytium, the syncytiotrophoblast. The remaining discrete cells constitute the cytotrophoblast (Fig.1.4 middle). The inner cell mass divides to form

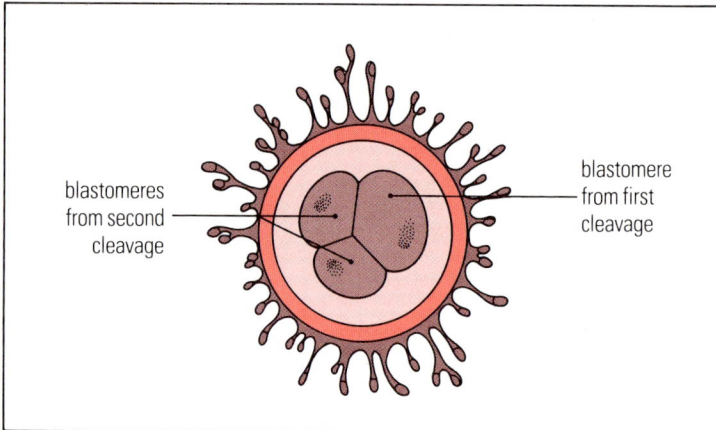

Fig.1.2 After division into two large cells (blastomeres), each with its full chromosome complement, one of the cells divides at right angles again. The other blastomere divides a short time later.

blastomeres from second cleavage

blastomere from first cleavage

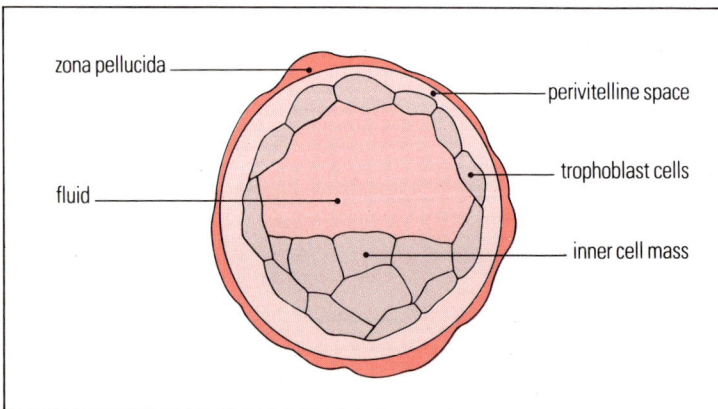

Fig.1.3 Development of the blastocyst. The zona pellucida starts to degenerate. Fluid is secreted by surface (trophoblast) cells and the centre becomes cystic. An inner cell mass forms at one pole; this will become the embryo.

zona pellucida

fluid

perivitelline space

trophoblast cells

inner cell mass

the embryonic disc, which consists of ectodermal and endodermal layers. Fluid soon accumulates between the trophoblast and ectoderm to form the amniotic cavity. Mesoderm is then formed between the amnion and trophoblast and on the inside of the blastocyst cavity, which is now called the yolk sac. This occurs by fourteen days after fertilization. The cytotrophoblast cells cover the surface of the growing blastocyst and the syncytiotrophoblast cells continue to invade the endometrium. The endometrial epithelium regenerates over the conceptus to bury it completely, leaving only a small operculum or fibrin

plug to show the site of implantation (Fig. 1.4 lower). The implantation process is completed by the fourteenth day after fertilization (Fig.1.5).

The endometrium is called the decidua once the pregnancy has started, that is, once implantation is complete. Implantation usually takes place in the upper part of the uterus, near the fundus. Rarely, the blastocyst travels down through the uterine cavity, rolling over on the endometrial wall to settle in the isthmus (the lower segment of the uterus); implantation at this site leads to a placenta praevia (see Chapter 5).

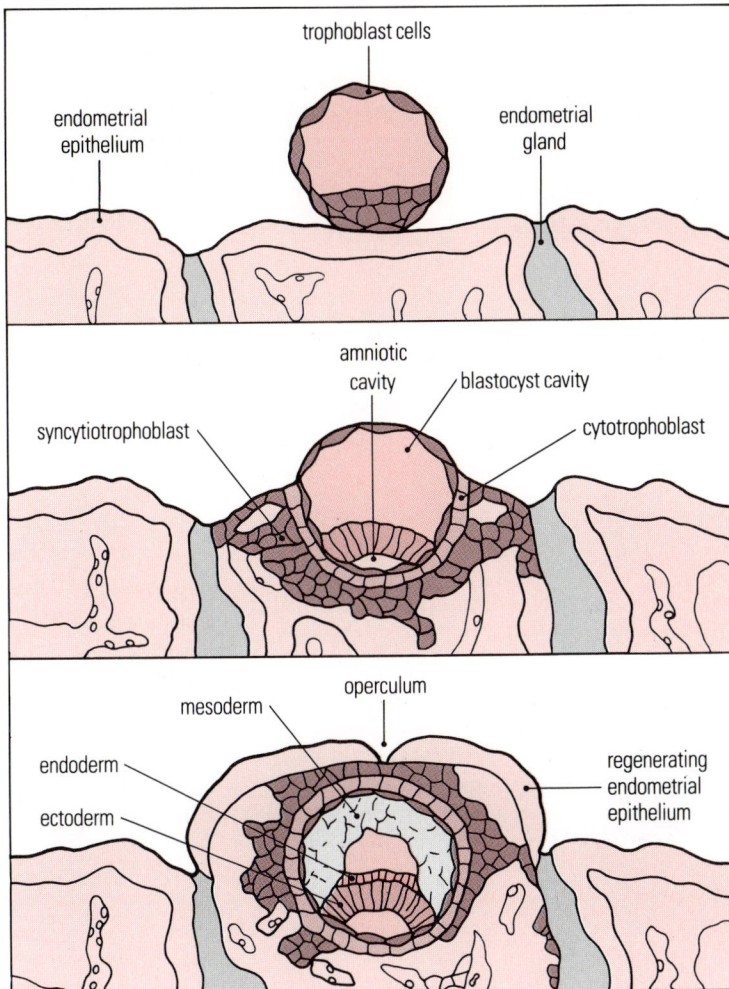

Fig.1.4 Implantation. Upper: the blastocyst usually settles between endometrial glands. The trophoblast cells closest to the endometrial cells begin to invade the uterine lining.
Middle: development of the amniotic cavity. Lower: the conceptus is now fully implanted.

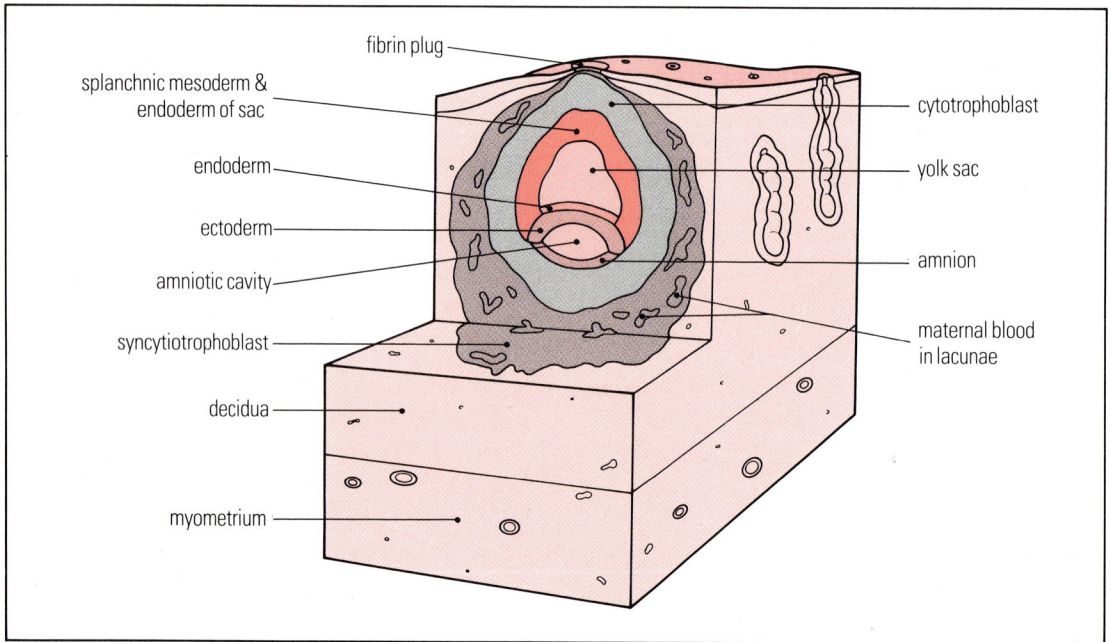

Fig.1.5 The conceptus is completely embedded in the decidua. The maternal blood vessels have been eroded so that maternal blood surrounds most of the conceptus.

Early development

At twelve to fourteen days after fertilization, a cavity forms in the extraembryonic mesoderm. This is the extraembryonic coelom, and it surrounds the yolk sac, bilaminar embryonic disc and amniotic cavity (Fig.1.6). The outer mesodermal layer and the trophoblast constitute the chorion.

At day fourteen, the bilaminar embryonic disc develops a groove, the primitive streak, at its caudal end. Cells spread out laterally from this to form a layer of somatic mesoderm separating the endoderm and ectoderm. The ectoderm will form the lining of the intestine, lungs and associated organs (liver, thyroid, pancreas). The dermis, skeleton, connective tissue, muscles, lymph, blood and kidney arise from the mesoderm.

At this time, lacunae form in the trophoblast and fuse with maternal capillaries. At fourteen days, the villous stems, with mesodermal cores, start to form. During the third week of embryonic life, the villous stems become vascularized and establish continuity with other vessels in the embryo.

After twenty-one days, the villi adjacent to the uterine cavity degenerate to form the chorion laeve, while those on the decidual side (the chorion frondosum), proliferate to form the placenta. The amnion grows rapidly to surround the embryo, which remains anchored to the yolk sac and chorion by the umbilical cord (Fig.1.7 left). The decidua overlying the implantation vesicle is called the decidua capsularis; the rest of the decidua, the decidua parietalis, lines the endometrial cavity; and the decidua underlying the chorion frondosum is called the decidua basalis.

By ten weeks post-fertilization, the extraembryonic coelom has been obliterated by fusion of the amnion and chorion. The uterine cavity is obliterated by fusion of the chorion and decidua basalis, and the decidual layers come into contact and begin to fuse (Fig.1.7 right). The yolk sac has gone but the communication from it to the fetus remains as the urachus, a fibrous cord found behind the anterior abdominal wall.

4

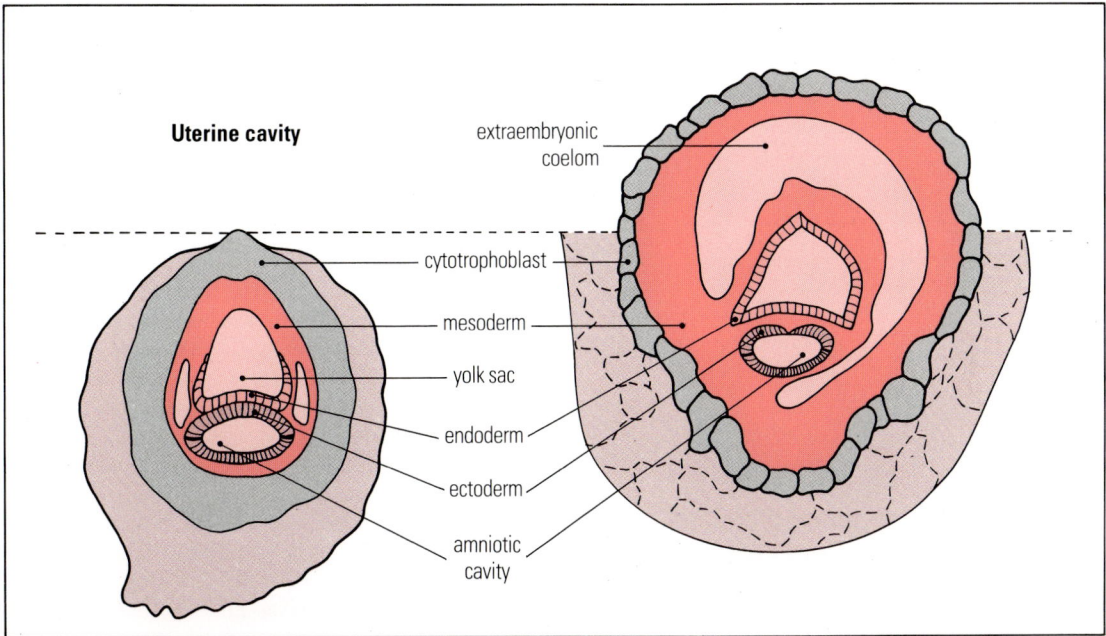

Fig. 1.6 Formation of the extraembryonic coelom. This cavity forms within the extraembryonic mesoderm and comes to surround the yolk sac, bilaminar embryonic disc and amniotic cavity.

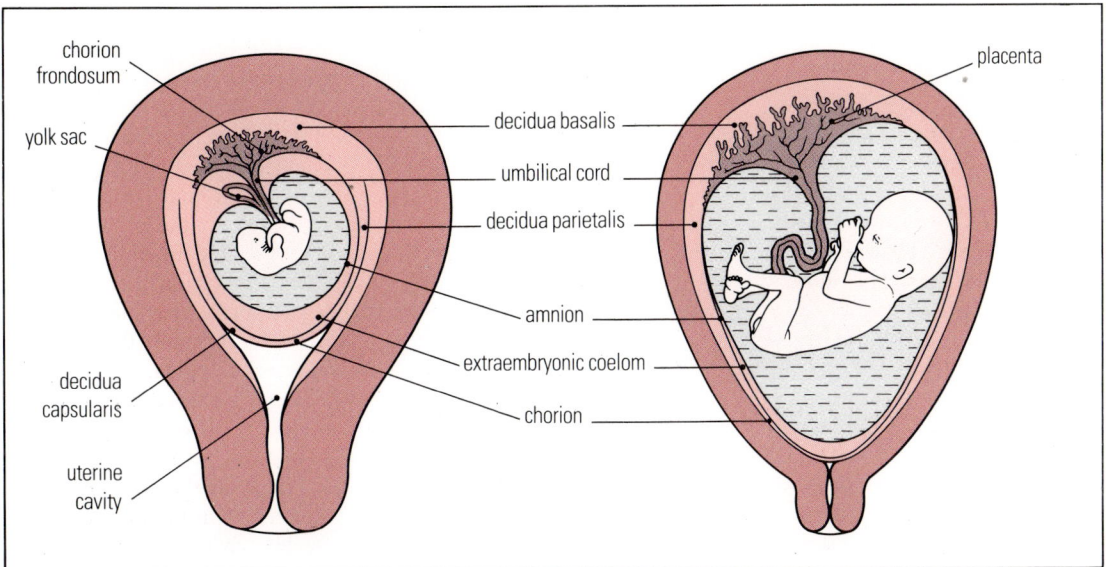

Fig. 1.7 Arrangement of fetal membranes at different stages of fetal development. Left: the yolk sac is still present alongside the umbilical cord in the extraembryonic coelom, between the amnion and the chorion. Right: at a later stage of development, there is no cavity in the uterus; the amnion and chorion are loosely bound together, the latter being attached to the decidua basalis.

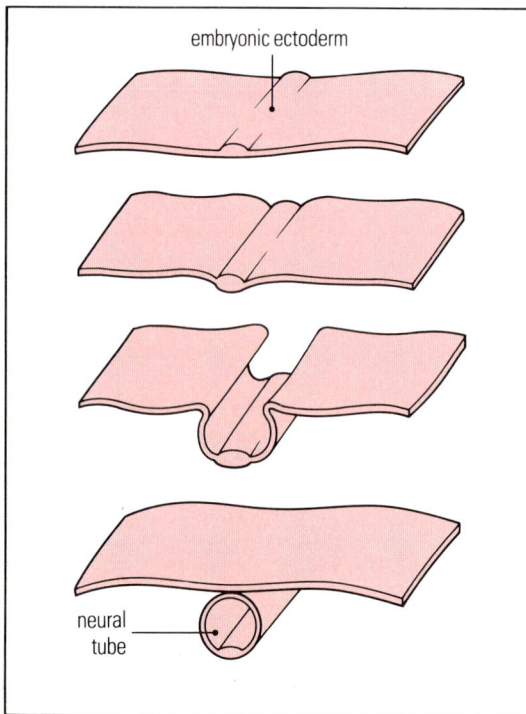

Fig.1.8 A ridge of ectoderm forms on the dorsum of the embryo and sinks below the surface. The two edges of the trough come together and fuse, producing the neural tube.

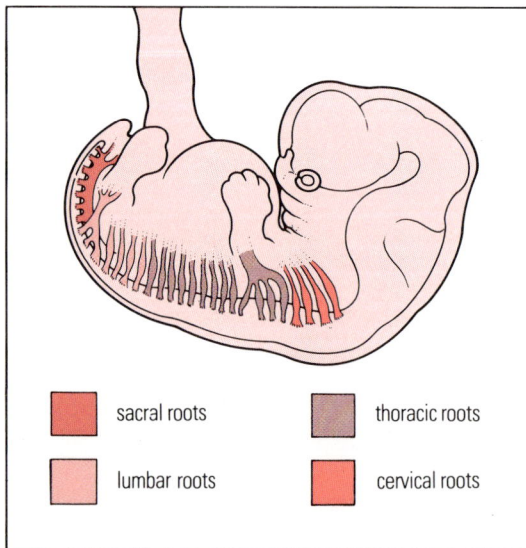

sacral roots

thoracic roots

lumbar roots

cervical roots

Fig.1.9 Development of the brain and nervous system.

Development of organs

Central nervous system

Nineteen days after conception, a ridge of ectodermal cells forms the neural groove. The cells sink beneath the surface of the embryonic disc along its length, thicken and form a trough (Fig.1.8). The edges of the trough come together, forming a tube under the skin. This is the basic central nervous system. The lower end becomes the spinal cord. The sealing-off process starts in the lower back region, moving upwards towards the head and downwards to the tail, starting at about twenty-eight days. Failure in the fusion process produces a number of congenital defects with relatively poor prognoses.

At the cephalic end of the neural tube, the nervous tissue expands in width and length, but growth is limited by the size of the embryo; therefore this region of the tube bends forward, kinks, convolutes and forms a complex pattern which becomes the brain (Fig.1.9). Two separate hollow processes of tissue grow sideways from the front end of the central nervous system; these form the specialized upper brain, or cortex. Growth continues and the surface becomes folded. The nerve roots, growing from the nervous tissue of the spinal cord, travel forwards and circumferentially in the body tissues. These develop into the peripheral nerves and their plexuses. There is a separate nerve root for each somite, or section, of the body. By fifty-five days post-fertilization, the central nervous system and peripheral nerves have been formed.

Eyes

Each eye is formed by the expansion of a hollow nerve process (extending from the central nervous system) which, as it approaches the skin of the face, becomes pushed inwards to form a cup (Fig.1.10). The epithelium over the surface of this cup sinks inwards to form a lens. A superficial ectodermal ingrowth forms the conjunctiva of the orbit and the eyelids.

Limbs

At approximately thirty days post-fertilization, limb buds develop just behind the head and half-way down the body of the embryo; the arms develop before the legs. These tubes of skin fill with mesodermal tissue, from which the bones and muscle of each limb will differentiate. At the end of each limb, the tissues flatten out into a fan, in which the small bones of the hand or foot develop. When the digits are first formed they are joined together. Later, they separate leaving only a small web of skin between them. Occasionally, however, this separation does not occur and fingers or toes remain fused into adult life. Horny plates, which become the nails, develop at the tip of each digit.

Within ten more days, the limbs, with their separate fingers and toes, are formed. Limb movements may start at about this time, but they usually cannot be felt by the mother until they are strong enough to

penetrate the myometrial barrier and impose upon her sensory nervous system. This occurs at about sixteen to twenty weeks in most women.

Cartilage forms within the undifferentiated mesoderm of the limb and the bones begin to ossify at approximately ten weeks, but this is not visible radiographically until sixteen weeks of gestation.

Alimentary system

The digestive system develops from a single tube which passes from the mouth to the anus (Fig.1.11). At the upper end, the tube fuses with a pit of epithelium, the stomatodaeum; the distal end joins with a similar pit, the proctodaeum. The tube grows rapidly and, being fixed at both ends, becomes convoluted. The alimentary tract is originally suspended from the back of the embryo by a mesentery but, as the convolutions loop around, it acquires secondary attachments, such as those between the stomach and transverse colon. Some parts of the tube dilate to form storage areas, for example the stomach and large intestine. The growth of the intestine is so rapid that it cannot be accommodated within the abdominal cavity and it is extruded into the amniotic cavity, whence it is withdrawn at ten weeks. If this fails to occur, exomphalos or gastroschisis result.

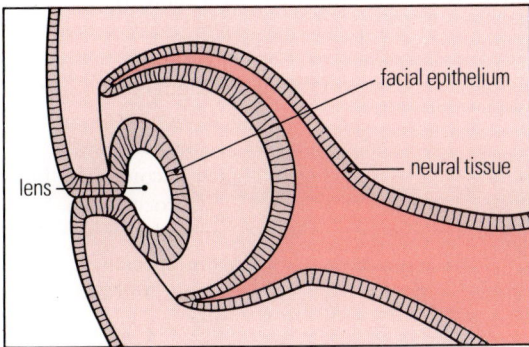

Fig.1.10 Formation of the eye. This stage of development is reached by 35 days of life.

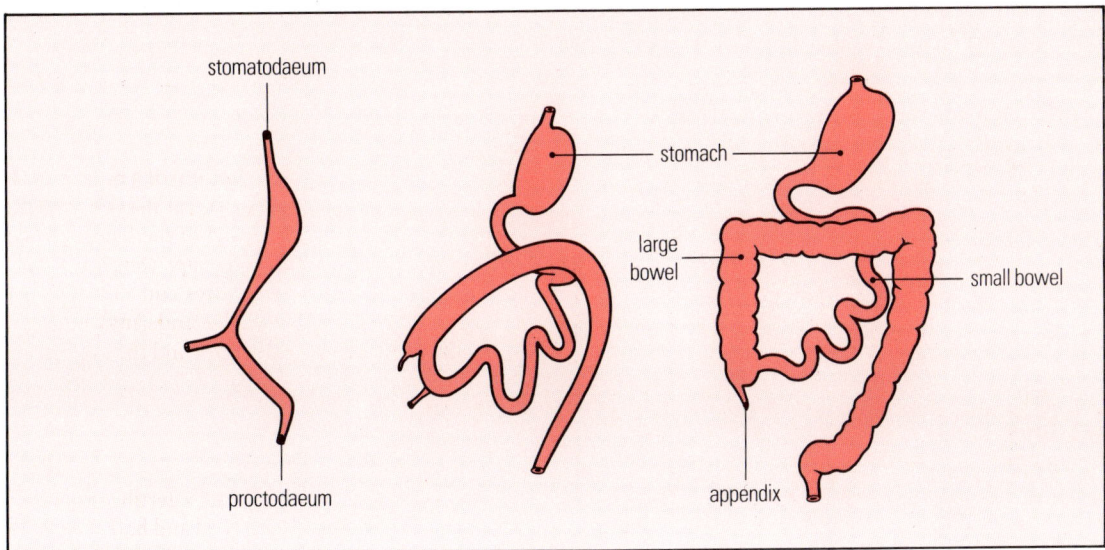

Fig.1.11 Formation of the alimentary tract.

Face

The face is formed by a series of buds growing in from the sides and down from the top of the head. The nose grows downwards as a central pillar. The eyes, initially lateral, move medially. The ears, initially low set, migrate cranially to their final position. Below the common nose and mouth, maxillary processes extend from the sides of the face towards the centre to form the floor of the nose and the roof of the mouth (Fig.1.12). The upper lip forms from two fused processes situated below the nose. Beneath this, harder tissue is laid down as cartilage, which later becomes the bones of the upper jaw. Small pits of skin sink into the jaw to form teeth, which are essentially hard pegs of bone covered with enamel. On the floor of the mouth, a bridge of muscle expands upwards to form the tongue, in which the taste buds develop.

Congenital malformations of the mouth occur when the fusion of the maxillary processes is incomplete or inadequate.

Cardiovascular system

Once an organism reaches a certain size, adequate oxygenation at its centre cannot be sustained by simple diffusion and a circulatory system is required. Approximately two weeks after conception, groups of blood-forming cells gather in various parts of the body. The channels between the clumps of cells become the future blood vessels. The central vessels run the length of the body, and in the pharyngeal area their mesenchymal layers enlarge to form the primitive heart (Fig.1.13).

The primitive circulation begins at around twenty-one days. Valves develop to ensure unidirectional flow, and a septum down the middle of the heart divides the organ into two sides. Many congenital heart defects result from lack of fusion of the septum.

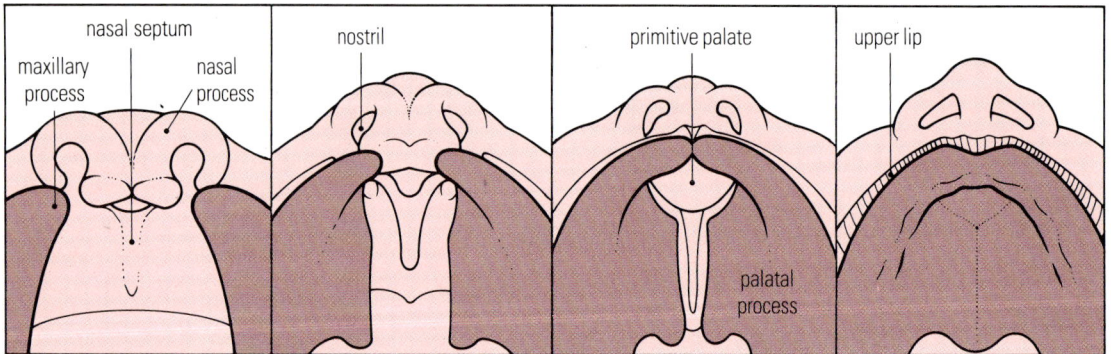

Fig.1.12 Formation of the hard palate occurs between the 6th-9th week. The maxillary processes grow from each side to join the nasal process; when they fuse the nostrils are formed.

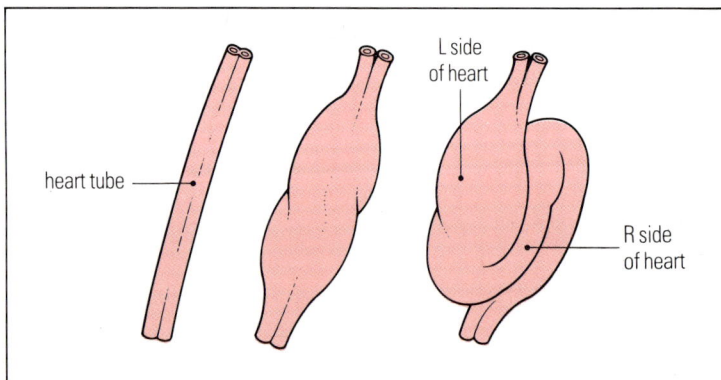

Fig.1.13 Development of the heart. The heart develops from a pair of blood vessels on the dorsal side of the embryo, initially in the pharyngeal region. The muscle layers of the tubes undergo hypertrophy to form the myocardium. Rapid growth forces the tubes into a convoluted shape, since they are fixed at both ends, and the left and right sides of the heart are produced.

Respiratory system

Although it is not needed in embryonic life, the respiratory system develops *in utero*. The trachea and major bronchi develop from pouches separated from the alimentary tract, forming a tubal system of lung buds in front of the gut (Fig.1.14).

Occasionally, the development of the trachea and oesophagus are not distinct and various abnormalities of conjunction can be found in the newborn. By twenty-two weeks of intrauterine life, the terminal bronchioles have developed. Alveoli are then formed, but the Type II respiratory cells, which produce surfactant, do not develop until much later.

The diaphragm grows inwards as a fibromuscular layer from the inner walls of the body cavity, starting high up in the cervical region and being pushed down as the lungs and heart develop. It eventually separates the thoracic and abdominal cavities.

Urinary system

This develops in the mesoderm on the posterior wall of the coelomic cavity. The three embryological stages are: the pronephros, the mesonephros and the metanephros (Fig.1.15).

The pronephros is a transient structure which exists for only a few weeks during development.

The mesonephros is comprised of a series of tubules which extend from the lower thoracic and upper lumbar region, and are joined to a longitudinal duct – the mesonephric, or Wolffian, duct. This develops a group of temporarily active tubular cells which act as an excretory organ for a few weeks. The definitive kidney develops from the metanephros system.

The metanephros, or permanent kidney, develops from two sources: the ureteric bud on the mesonephric duct, which forms the drainage system, and the metanephrogenic cap, which forms the

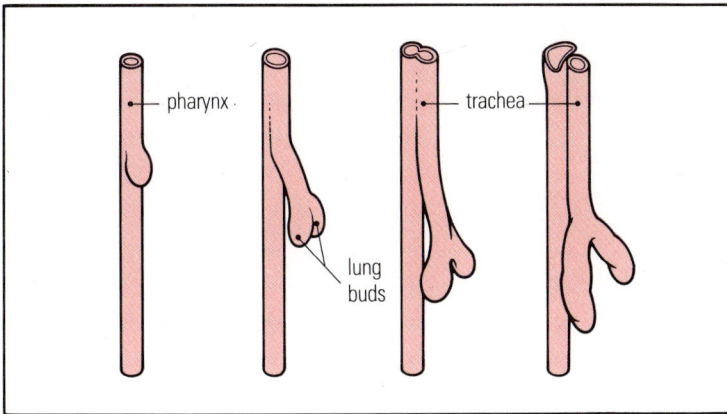

Fig.1.14 Development of the lungs. A diverticulum is formed at the front of the pharynx. This grows and divides, the bifurcations forming the beginning of the bronchi.

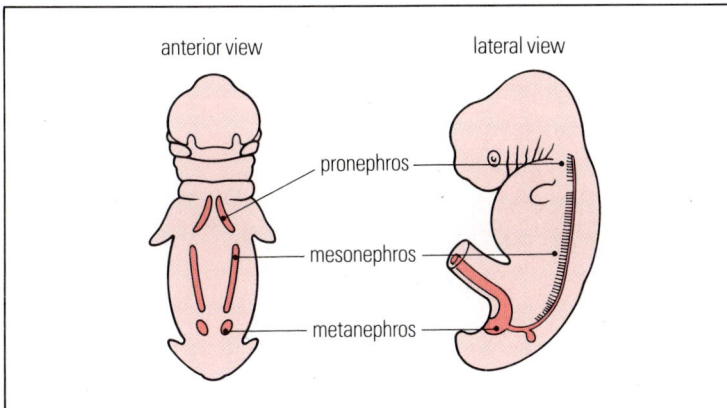

Fig.1.15 Sites of precursors of the urinary and renal systems, which develop from a series of primitive tubes.

9

substance of the adult kidney (Fig.1.16). The ureteric bud grows upwards to meet the metanephrogenic cap. The bud forms the ureter, renal pelvis and distal parts of the collecting tubules. The cap forms the glomerular capsules, convoluted tubules and loops of Henle.

Initially, the metanephros is entirely a pelvic organ, lying over the upper sacral segments and receiving its blood supply from the aorta. The apparent ascent of the kidneys in the abdomen is actually due to rapid caudal growth, drawing the kidneys upwards, so that in adult life they are at the level of the higher lumbar vertebrae. Congenital abnormalities of the urinary tract, such as renal fusion, hypoplasia and dysplasia, are not uncommon.

The trigone and posterior prostatic urethra develop from the mesonephric ducts. The remainder of the bladder and urethra develop from the urogenital sinus. From the upper end of the fundus of the bladder, the urachus, a remnant of the allantois, runs to the umbilicus. This is often hollow and accompanies the obliterated umbilical vessels. This,

in turn, represents the anterior portion of the early cloaca, a common ectodermal invagination into which the alimentary and urinary systems open.

Genital system

The sex of an embryo is established at fertilization, depending on the presence or absence of the Y chromosome in the fertilizing sperm. The gonads originate from germinal ridges located medially to the mesonephros on the posterior wall of the coelom (Fig.1.17). They are covered by a mesothelium, the coelomic epithelium, from which the sex cords arise; these sex cords develop into the gonads.

MALE
The sex cords develop in the medulla of the germinal ridge and form the seminiferous tubules. The testes then migrate down the path of the gubernaculum, gathering the duct systems in a secondary fashion

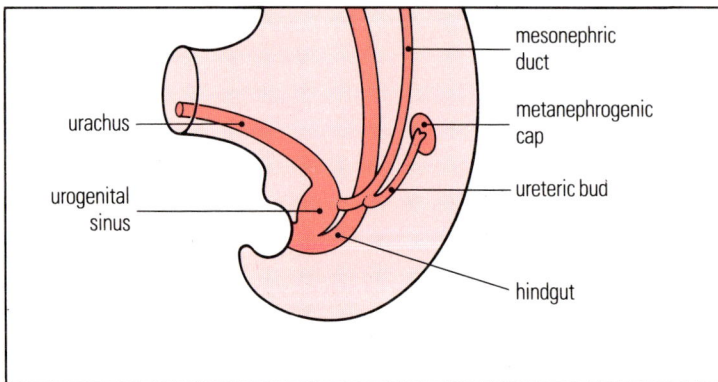

Fig.1.16 The urinary tract develops from the ureteric bud of the mesonephric duct. A metanephrogenic cap becomes the kidney, which then migrates upwards along the posterior abdominal wall. The bladder is formed from the anterior part of the urogenital sinus.

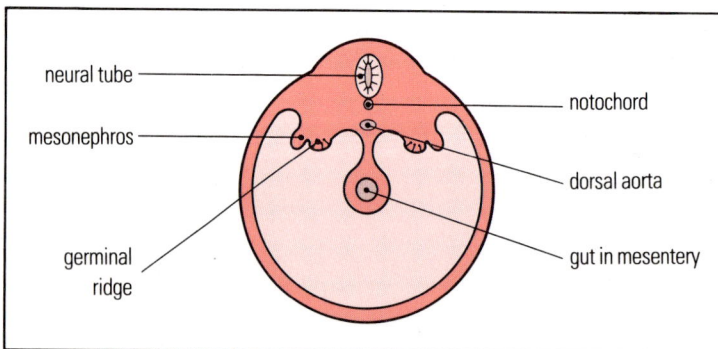

Fig.1.17 The gonads develop from the germinal ridges on the dorsal wall of the fetal coelomic cavity, medial to the mesonephros. They are covered with coelomic epithelium, from which the sex cords will develop and penetrate into the substance of the gonad.

from the mesonephric duct, and descend into the scrotum.

The seminiferous ducts become connected to the tubules of the mesonephros, which form the rete testis. These tubules, in turn, are connected to the mesonephric (Wolffian) ducts, which form the epididymis, vas deferens, seminal vesicles, ureters and trigone. The seminiferous tubules are solid until seven years of age. Spermatogonia in the testicular tubules will not enter the first meiotic division to form primary spermatocytes until puberty.

FEMALE

The ovaries differentiate later than the male gonads, usually between seven to eight weeks post-fertilization. In contrast to the testes, development takes place in the cortex of the gonadal ridge rather than the medulla, and a thinner tunica is formed on the surface of the gonad. The germ cells divide rapidly, by mitosis, to form oogonia.

Between eight and sixteen weeks, these oogonia enter the first stage of meiotic division and are then called primary oocytes. As soon as a primary oocyte is formed, it is surrounded by a single layer of cells from the ingrowing sex cords to form a primordial follicle.

The cells which surround the primary oocyte are granulosa cells and they secrete a substance which arrests the first meiotic division in prophase. The maximum number of primordial follicles is formed at sixteen to twenty weeks of gestation, after which their number gradually declines through atresia. By late fetal life, there are two million follicles in the ovaries. Many of these will degenerate before puberty, when only half a million remain.

The fallopian tubes and uterus develop from the paramesonephric, or Müllerian, ducts. The latter are formed by invagination of the mesothelium on the posterior abdominal wall, lateral to the mesonephric ducts. The paramesonephric ducts grow towards the pelvic region, cross in front of the metanephric duct and fuse in the midline during the ninth week of intrauterine life. Occasionally, a full fusion does not occur, so that either a double uterus or complete duplication of the female genital system may be found.

The vagina is formed in two parts (Fig.1.18). The upper end originates from the most caudal part of the paramesonephric ducts, and the lower part is an outpouching of the urogenital sinus. Fusion occurs just above the level of the hymen. A septum is present initially, but this breaks down before birth. The hymen itself is formed entirely from the urogenital sinus.

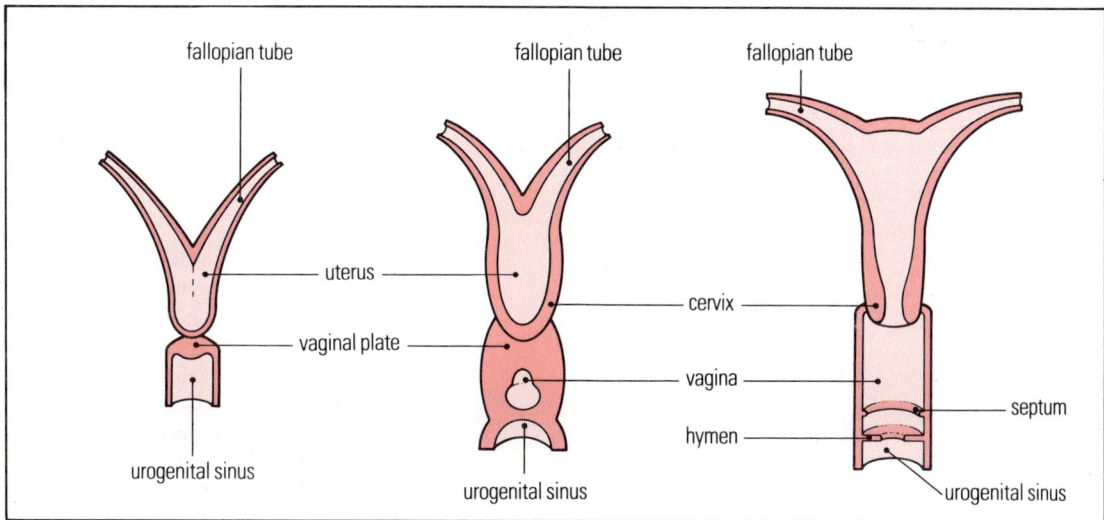

Fig.1.18 The vagina is formed from the vaginal plate of the urogenital sinus, which becomes canalized, and the lower end of the fused paramesonephric ducts. The fusion is at first partial, with a temporary septum between the two lumina.

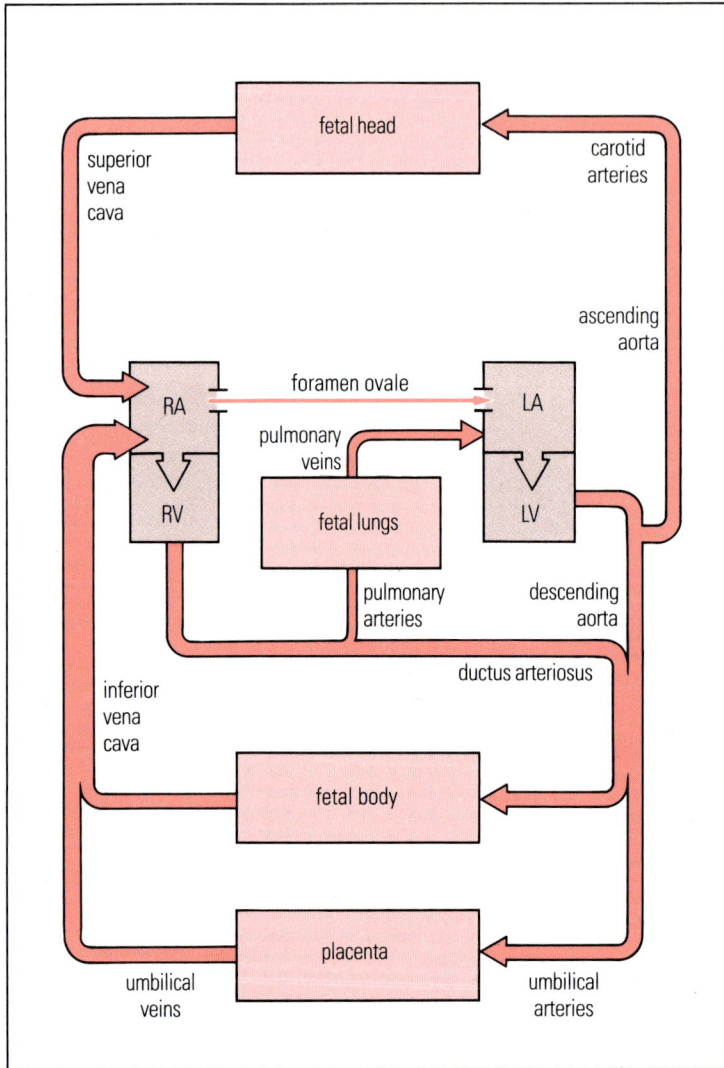

Fig.1.19 The fetal blood system. The right and left sides of the heart are separated by the pulmonary circulation.

NORMAL FETAL AND NEONATAL PHYSIOLOGY

After fertilization, the blastocyst grows rapidly in the uterus. It is conventionally called an embryo after organ formation starts (at two weeks), and a fetus after organogenesis is complete (at ten weeks). In combination with the placenta, the fetus crates a *milieu intérieur*, which permits its own survival and, in doing so, alters major maternal physiological processes.

One of the major differences between intra- and extrauterine life lies in the role of the placenta; this, rather than the lungs and alimentary tract, provides the fetus with oxygenation and nutrition.

Growth, particularly of the head, is the most notable feature of fetal physiology. The fetal head is larger in relation to its body and limbs than is that of an older child or adult.

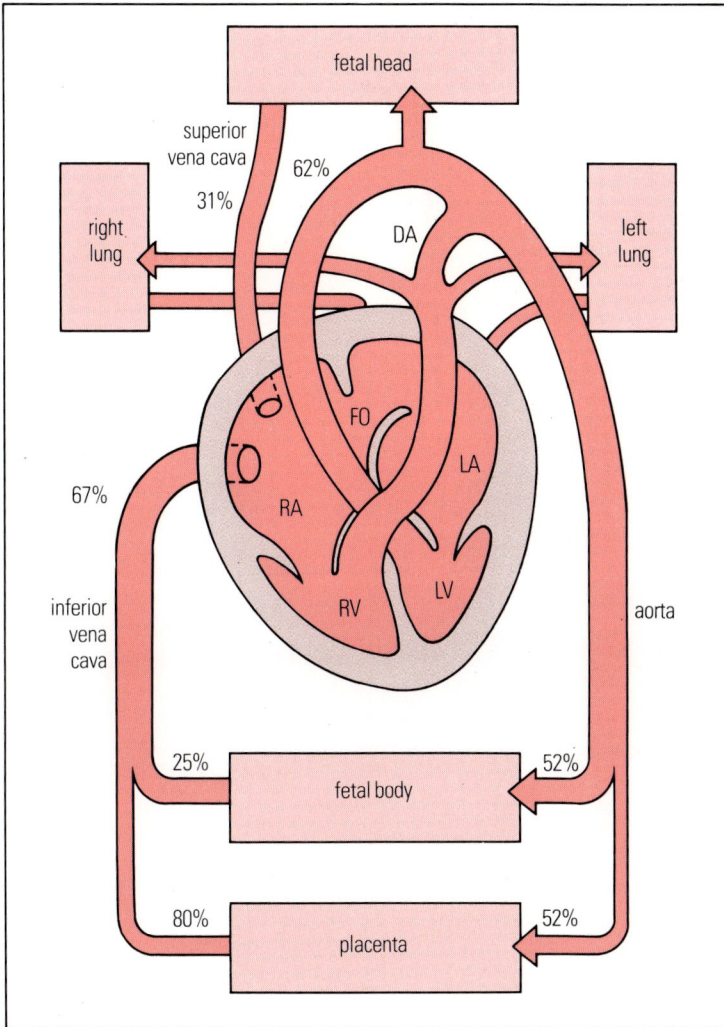

Fig.1.20 Fetal circulation showing the percentage oxygen saturation of the blood at various points.
RA = right atrium;
RV = right ventricle;
LA = left atrium;
LV = left ventricle;
FO = foramen ovale;
DA = ductus arteriosus.

Cardiovascular system

The fetal circulation serves the fetus *in utero*, but must be able to adapt rapidly to the adult pattern at birth.

The heart

Cardiac output in the fetus is high. Blood is pumped from the left ventricle into the aorta, whence it passes preferentially to the head (Fig.1.19). Blood returning to the heart from the inferior vena cava is more highly oxygenated, having come from the placenta. Blood briefly enters the right atrium. The majority of the

flow is then directed by a ridge of muscle, the crista galli, into the left atrium and so to the left ventricle and, thence, into the ascending aorta.

The less well oxygenated venous return from the superior vena cava passes, via the right atrium, to the right ventricle. It then flows into the pulmonary artery, where most of it passes into the ductus arteriosus and descending aorta. The remainer (about ten percent) flows through the lungs. Thus, the head of the fetus receives more highly oxygenated blood than the lower parts of the body (see Fig.1.20). There is little mixing of the oxygenated and deoxygenated blood; the bloodstreams pass each other in a swirling double spiral, with less than thirty percent intermixing.

13

In early pregnancy, the right and left sides of the fetal heart pump synchronously and the walls are of approximately equal thickness. In the second half of pregnancy, the right ventricular myocardium becomes thicker, providing the force required to pump blood around the lower part of the body. By term, however, the muscle walls of the ventricles are equally thick. The fetal heart rate is high in early pregnancy, and reduces slowly during gestation. At term, it is about 140 beats/minute.

At birth, cardiac output on a weight-for-weight basis is several times higher than in the adult. The systemic circulation now has to work harder to pump the blood around the body and the left ventricle becomes more muscular than the right by the end of the first year of life.

Fetal circulation

The blood passing to the fetus from the placenta has a high mean oxygen saturation (Fig.1.20). As this bypasses the liver, it mixes slightly with the blood coming from the inferior vena cava, causing a small decrease in oxygenation. Blood passes into the left side of the heart without a great decrease in oxygen content (sixty-two percent compared to sixty-seven percent).

Blood coming from the superior vena cava, however, has an oxygen saturation of only thirty-one percent, and this passes into the descending aorta for distribution to the lower part of the body. Its oxygen content is only slightly increased by mixing with blood from the placental circulation, the oxygen saturation rising to fifty-two percent. This is significantly less oxygenated than blood travelling in vessels to the upper part of the body (sixty-two percent).

Placental circulation

Approximately one-third of the combined left and right heart output passes through the placenta. A system of various bypass mechanisms allows some of the blood to flow to the villi for reoxygenation, while the remainder passes through the umbilical vein to the ductus venosus and into the general fetal circulation.

When the baby is born, the placenta separates from the maternal blood supply and up to one-third of the fetoplacental blood volume may remain in the placental circulation. No more oxygenation will take place once placental separation has occurred, at the end of the second stage of labour. In the minutes following separation, a proportion of the 100–150ml of blood in the placenta will return to the neonate, depending on the relative heights of the placenta and baby, and on when the cord is clamped and divided.

Pulmonary circulation

Pulmonary blood flow in the fetus is only about ten percent of that which circulates after delivery. The fetal lungs themselves are solid, and secrete lung fluid into the bronchi. The pulmonary arterioles have a high resistance, but these dilate with a rise in P_{CO_2} at birth.

Circulatory changes at birth

At birth, the fetal lungs very rapidly take over the function of oxygenation of the blood. After the placenta becomes detached from the placental bed, no further gaseous exchange can take place through it, since the fetal and maternal circulations are now separate. There is, therefore, little purpose in leaving the newborn attached to the placenta, and the cord is usually clamped within seconds of birth.

Several critical changes are necessary for oxygenation to occur in the fetal lungs (Fig.1.21). Pulmonary arterial pressure drops and the ductus arteriosus goes into spasm. Because of the low resistance in the pulmonary circulation, blood is pumped to the lungs and cannot bypass them by going into the aorta. The full decline in pulmonary arterial pressure takes place over several days after birth.

While the closure of the ductus arteriosus is initially by spasm, the raised P_{O_2} is followed by an increase in prostaglandin production in the smooth muscle, which perpetuates the constriction. In later weeks, the ductus is closed by fibrosis. If neonatal hypoxia follows, however, the functional spasm may be relaxed and the ductus become partly reopened.

The closure of the foramen ovale, between the left and right atria, follows the rise in left atrial pressure after blood returns from the lungs (Fig.1.22). The flap-like valve across the orifice is closed by the difference in pressure between the left and right atria.

14

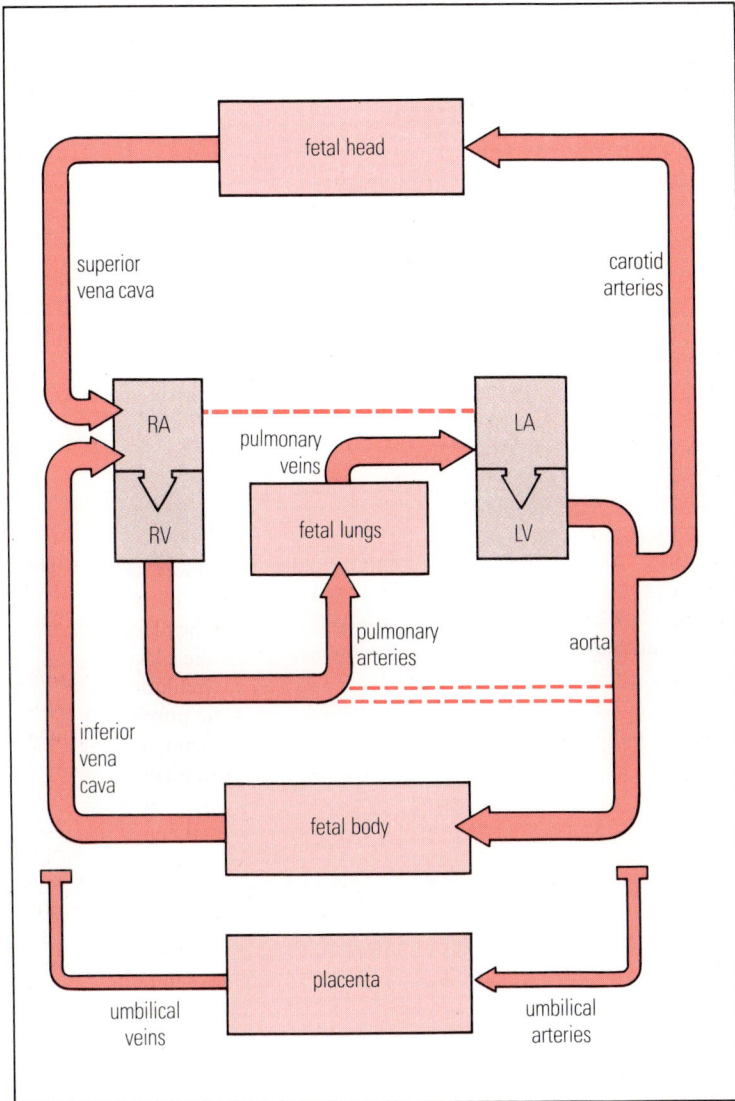

Fig.1.21 Changes in circulation at birth. The placental circulation is removed. The foramen ovale closes and the ductus arteriosus goes into spasm. Thus, all blood passes from the right side of the heart to the left side of the heart via the lungs, so that adult circulation is established.

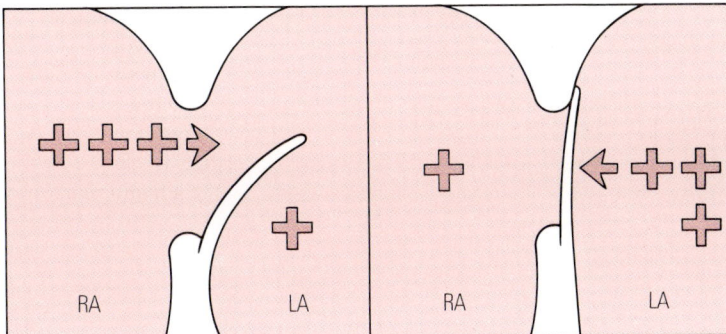

Fig.1.22 Closure of the foramen ovale. The foramen ovale remains open as long as the pressure on the right side of the heart is greater than that on the left. However, once the pulmonary circulation commences and the ductus arteriosus closes, pressure on the left side of the heart rises, closing the flap-like valve.

This closure converts the heart from being two pumps working on separate circulations to being a single pump working on one circulation in continuity. The functional closure by pressure of the foramen ovale is followed by a structural closure over the next few months, but it is not unusual for the foramen ovale to allow reversed flow in pathological circumstances.

Respiratory system

Alveoli begin to develop in the lungs at sixteen weeks of gestation, but they are too immature to support life until after the twentieth to twenty-second week. The surface tension of the lung fluids is responsible for keeping the alveoli and the air passages closed. Surfactant (composed of lecithin and sphingomyelin) helps to reduce this high surface tension. Lecithin and sphingomyelin are produced by the lungs, in increasing amounts, in the last weeks of pregnancy (Fig.1.23). Since lung fluid does not appear in appreciable amounts until after the thirtieth week of gestation, babies born prematurely have to overcome a deficiency of surfactant, to a greater or lesser degree.

In the intrauterine state, the alveoli are closed. They secrete lung fluid into the bonchi and trachea, which

are held open by cartilage rings. Lung fluid spills over from the larynx into the pharynx, and is usually excreted into the amniotic fluid or swallowed.

The fetus makes respiratory movements (detectable by ultrasound) in the uterus from about twenty-eight weeks. These movements shift a small amount of lung fluid (1–2ml) up and down the trachea. However, if there is hypoxia, the shift increases to 10ml and more amniotic fluid may be inhaled into the respiratory tract. Only in these circumstances does a large amount of amniotic fluid enter the respiratory tract, which is normally filled with lung fluid of a higher protein concentration.

The first breath taken by the baby has to overcome both the viscosity of the lung fluid in the airways and tissue resistance. The pressure on the chest wall during vaginal delivery pushes some lung fluid into the pharynx. Following delivery, there is elastic recoil of the thorax, which results in some air entering the lungs; increasing amounts follow with each breath. The lung fluid is not totally expelled through the larynx; some is absorbed through pores in the lungs and passes straight to the lymphatic system.

Respiration is induced by a series of stimuli. The removal of the fetus from suspension in amniotic fluid, combined with the mechanical chest squeeze

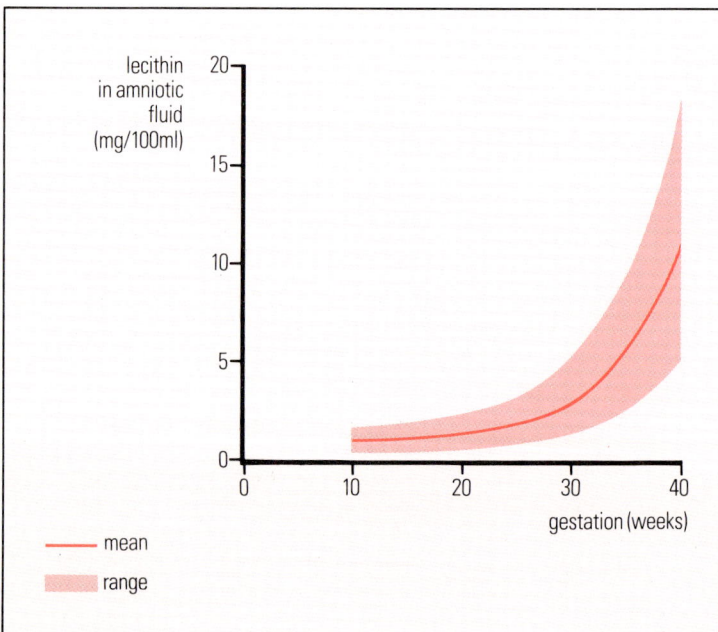

Fig.1.23 Lecithin concentration in the amniotic fluid. The concentration rises very sharply after 30 weeks gestation.

during vaginal delivery, may start respiration. The handling of the baby, temperature alterations on changing from an environment of 37°C to one of 20–25°C, and the accumulation of carbon dioxide, may also be important factors. The shut-down of the umbilical blood flow causes pressure changes, and these may also help stimulate respiration.

Spontaneous respiration will start even if the cord is not clamped and if there is no alteration in $P\text{co}_2$ or pH. Most babies probably start breathing due to a combination of the reduction in $P\text{co}_2$, detected by the carotid chemoreceptors, and a mixed group of sensations, for example touch and cooling of the skin, particularly in the nasopharyngeal area. The mechanisms are evidently efficient, as ninety-five percent of babies are breathing within thirty seconds of birth. Babies failing to breathe at birth should be managed by a competent paediatric and obstetrical team, with resuscitation offered as needed.

Alimentary tract

The gut develops from a hollow tube, as previously described. Once absorption begins, many low molecular weight substances pass across the surface, but the fetal gut is not as efficient as the neonatal bowel.

The liver produces bilirubin from the early weeks of gestation, and bile pigments are transferred across the placenta. Bilirubin moves easily across the placenta to the maternal circulation, where it presents a very small extra load because of the relatively large maternal plasma volume. After birth, the newborn loses this exchange route and depends on an immature liver for the excretion of bile. As the excess red cells break down and haemoglobin is denatured, the newborn baby often becomes jaundiced due to the increased amounts of bile breakdown products retained in the system.

Renal function

Although the kidneys form early in fetal development, they are immature. A smaller proportion of the total cardiac output passes through them than in the newborn baby, and the glomerular filtration rate is low. Much of the amniotic fluid in late pregnancy comes from the fetal kidney; this is a hypotonic solution compared with maternal plasma.

After birth, the kidneys have to take over excretory

functions. There is still a low glomerular filtration rate but this increases in the first week. The high urine flow of the newborn is reduced and tubular function improves in the first month of life. Sodium is absorbed into the bloodstream in the newborn, and the tubular concentration is low.

Fetal fluid balance

The fetus lives in its own private swimming pool – the amniotic cavity. In early pregnancy, most of the amniotic fluid is produced by the fetus and is secreted through the fetal skin. There is no organized keratinization of the epithelium and therefore water readily passes through this semipermeable membrane. Gradually, after twenty weeks of gestation, the fetal skin changes and lays down more keratin; the skin becomes organized, being formed from many layers of cells. Transudation is then sharply reduced and urine becomes the major fetal source of amniotic fluid. Dilute urine is excreted by the fetus in volumes of up to 0.5 litres/day at term; if the kidneys are missing (Potter's syndrome) or impaired, oligohydramnios can result.

A proportion of the amniotic fluid is produced by the amniotic membranes, which lie over the fetal surface of the placenta, over the umbilical cord and around the whole amniotic cavity. A much smaller contribution to the amniotic fluid (up to 30ml/day) is made by the fetal lung fluid.

Amniotic fluid has a rapid turnover, with a half-life of only two or three hours. Much is swallowed by the fetus; the rest passes straight to the maternal circulation, being absorbed through the amniotic membranes.

Fetal growth

An increase in size in the adult can be measured by many parameters, such as height, weight, and surface area of various dimensions, in unit time. The fetus *in utero*, however, can only be measured by non-invasive methods, such as ultrasound.

The weight/gestation charts in use are derived from measurements of fetuses that have left the uterus. It is important to note that these cannot be considered normal. Such fetuses would not have been expelled in the later weeks of pregnancy, nor would they have been removed at late terminations of pregnancy, if they had been normal. They may, for example, have been delivered after induction for severe pre-eclampsia at thirty-two weeks, or they may have followed a preterm labour after an abruptio placentae (premature detachment of a normally situated placenta) at twenty-eight weeks.

Consequently, the best measurements of growth are those made using longitudinal ultrasound, a technique which has only been available in the last two decades .

Fetal growth, expressed in weight gain per week, is slow and gradual until twenty weeks (Fig.1.24).

However, if examined incrementally, growth is at its greatest at this time. The rate of growth then becomes faster during the active phase, between twenty-four and thirty-four weeks of gestation. The growth rate of the head of the fetus is faster than that of the rest of the body, due to the preferential supply of blood to the cephalic end of the fetus. Using sequential ultrasound measurements, increases in size may be monitored throughout pregnancy. This provides the best prognostic indication of fetal wellbeing during pregnancy.

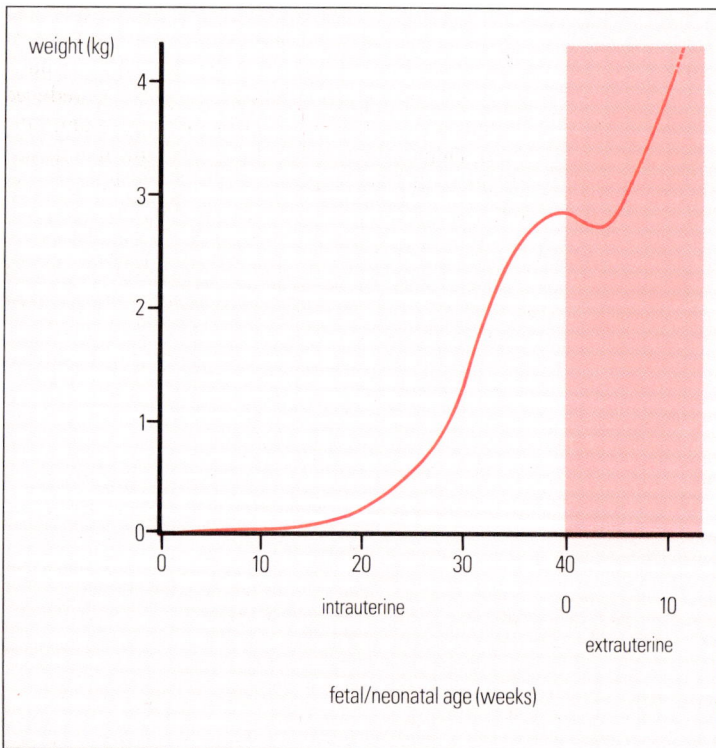

Fig.1.24 Mean rate of fetal and neonatal growth. After 34 weeks the growth rate is reduced until birth, when there is a minor decrease in weight due to fluid loss. During the first weeks of extrauterine life, growth proceeds at the same rate as the fast phase *in utero*.

2. Maternal Anatomy and Physiology

ANATOMY OF THE NORMAL FEMALE PELVIS

The bony pelvis

The general shape of the human bony pelvis can be compared to a saucer on top of a cup. The upper, or false, pelvis (represented by the saucer) is of little importance obstetrically. The true pelvis (represented by the cup) is, however, of great significance, the fetus passing through this during delivery. The true pelvis consists of a curved bony canal that is shorter anteriorly (behind the symphysis pubis) than posteriorly (in front of the sacrum).

The pelvic brim, where the upper and lower pelves meet, is approximately oval in shape with an anteroposterior diameter of 11cm and a transverse diameter of 13cm (Fig.2.1). The pelvic brim forms the inlet of the true pelvis, and the fetal head must pass through this when it engages in late pregnancy or labour. The transverse diameter is the maximum diameter of the pelvic brim and thus the largest diameter of the fetal head (the anteroposterior diameter) normally passes through this easily. When the fetal anteroposterior diameter engages with the face directed laterally, the fetus takes up a normal occipitolateral, or occipitotransverse, position.

Due to the curve of the sacrum, the midcavity of the pelvis is capacious and circular in outline, with a diameter of approximately 12cm.

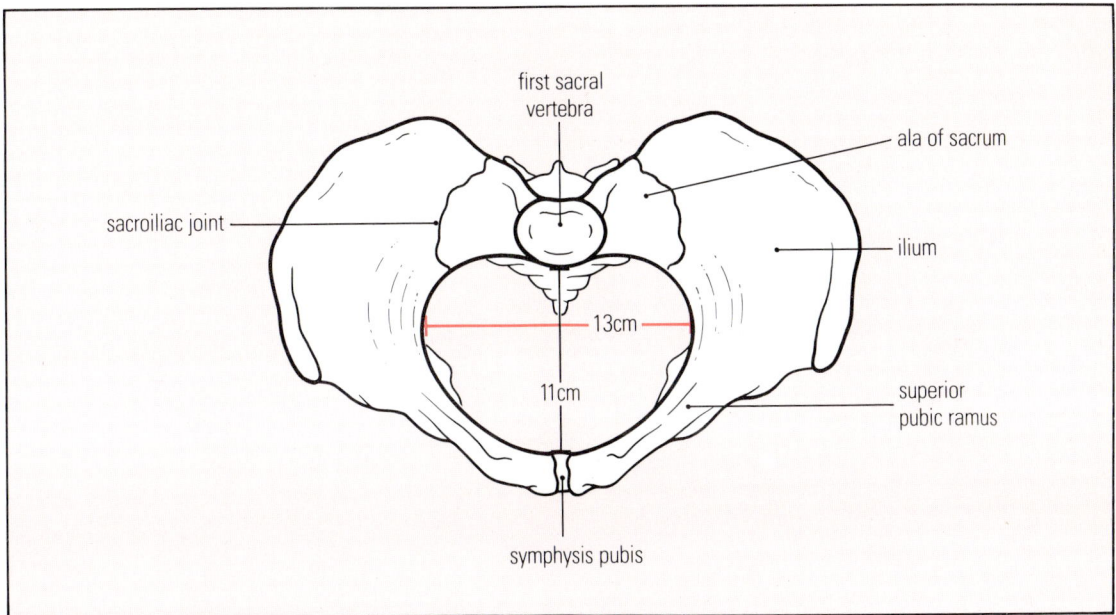

Fig.2.1 The pelvic brim. The outline of the brim follows the upper border of the first sacral vertebra, the alae, the sacroiliac joint, the ilium, the superior pubic ramus and the symphysis pubis.

The pelvic outlet is roughly diamond-shaped, and lies between several landmarks situated at different levels (Fig.2.2). The coccyx is usually pushed out of the way during delivery and is therefore not considered in making the posterior boundary. The anteroposterior diameter of the outlet, measured from the lower border of the symphysis pubis to the last fixed point of the sacrum, is 13cm, and the transverse diameter, measured between the ischial tuberosities, is 11cm.

The widest diameter of the pelvic canal, therefore, changes from the transverse diameter at the brim to the anteroposterior diameter at the outlet. Thus, cross-sections of the bony pelvis at different levels show a rotation of the maximum diameter (Fig.2.3).

To obtain the best fit of the fetal head, the anteroposterior diameter must pass through the maximum diameter of the outlet. The head must rotate from the lateral position through 90°, so that the anteroposterior diameter of the fetal head and the anteroposterior diameter of the outlet coincide. This accounts for the rotation of the fetal head during labour, the fetus presenting at delivery in either the occipitoanterior or direct occipitoposterior position.

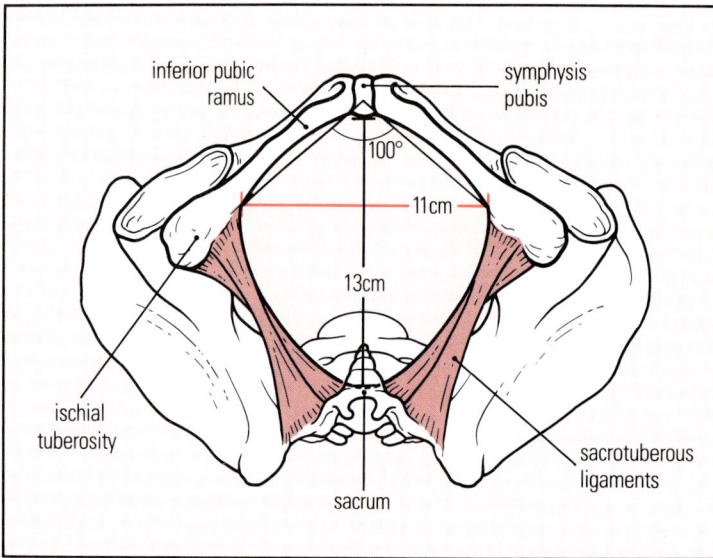

Fig.2.2 The pelvic outlet. The boundary of the outlet passes from the symphysis pubis, down the inferior rami of the pubic bones to the ischial tuberosities, and then obliquely upwards and posteriorly along the sacrotuberous ligaments to the tip fifth sacral vertebra.

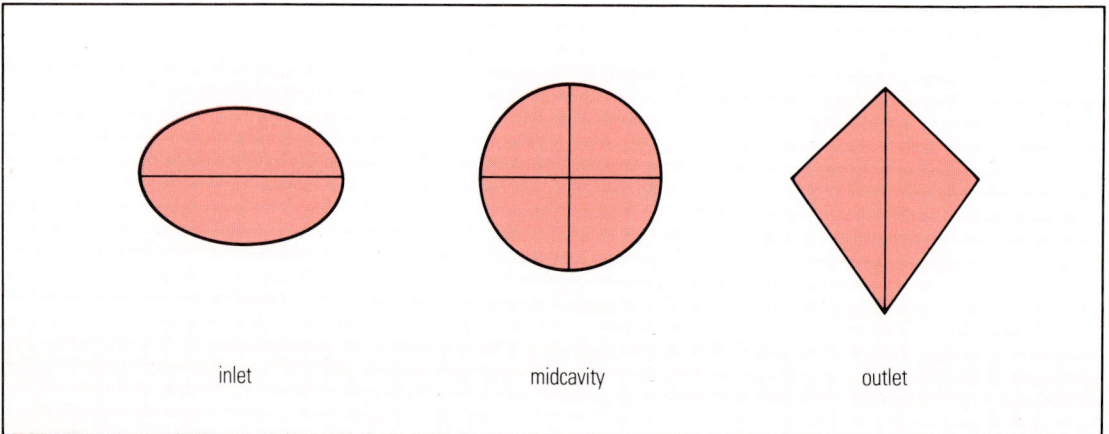

Fig.2.3 Diagrammatic representation of the pelvic canal showing the rotation of the maximum diameter from inlet to outlet.

The sub-pubic angle of the pelvis in the female is greater than in the male, being approximately 100° (see Fig.2.2). Any decrease in this angle diminishes the transverse diameters of the midcavity and outlet. In some women, the sub-pubic angle is reduced and the space between the pubic rami is lost to the descending fetal head, which is therefore forced posteriorly.

In the upright position, the plane of the pelvic brim is set at an angle of 55°–60° to the horizontal (Fig.2.4). A greater angle implies increased lumbar lordosis, which could lead to difficulties in engagement of the head in the inlet of the pelvis.

Soft tissues of the pelvis

In a lateral view of the pelvis and pelvic organs (Fig.2.5), the uterus usually lies in anteversion, so that the posterior fornix is deeper than the anterior fornix. The anterior wall of the vagina lies against the base of the bladder and urethra.

The ischiorectal fossae (Fig.2.6) lie lateral to the levator ani muscles, medial to the obturator internus muscles, and deep to the transverse perineal muscles. There is no barrier between this area and the retroperitoneal space higher up in the pelvis; thus,

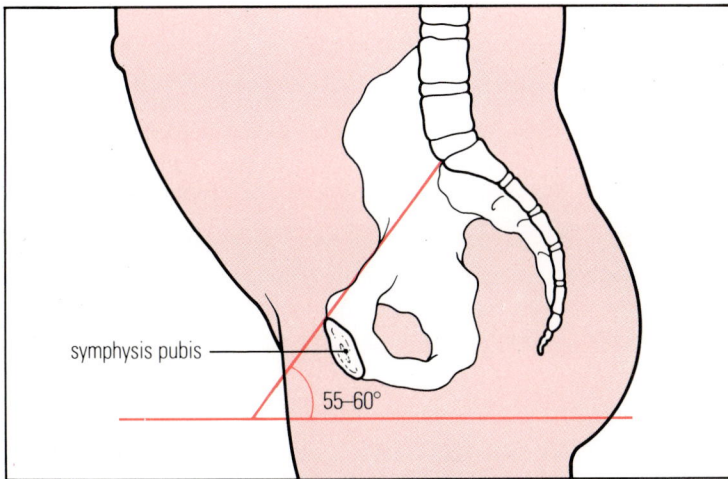

Fig.2.4 The angle of the pelvic inlet. When upright, the inlet usually subtends to the horizontal at an angle of 55–60°.

symphysis pubis

55–60°

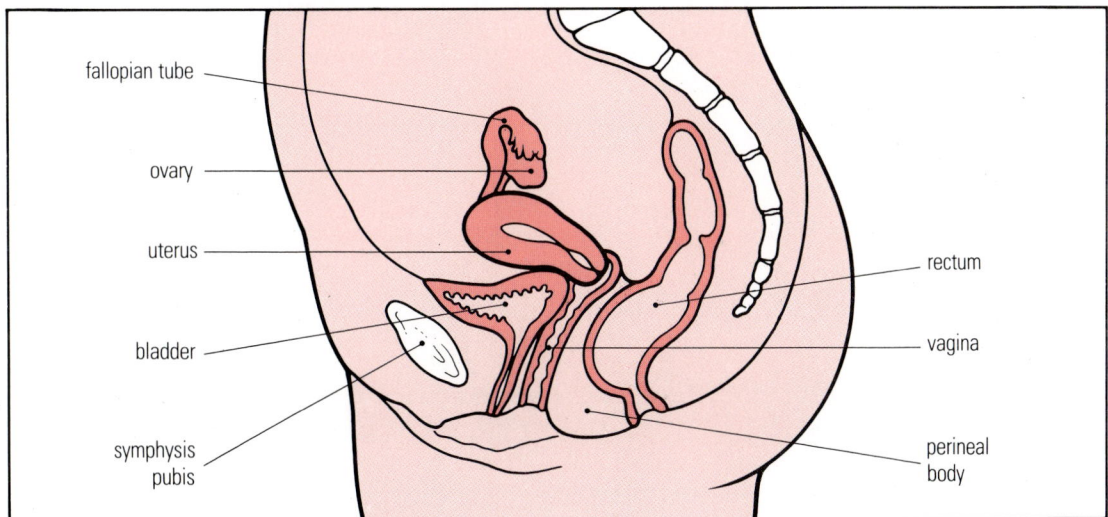

fallopian tube

ovary

uterus

bladder

symphysis pubis

rectum

vagina

perineal body

Fig.2.5 Lateral cross-sectioned view of the pelvic organs. The bladder and rectum lie anteriorly and posteriorly, respectively, to the reproductive organs.

21

infection or bleeding into the fossae can spread very rapidly into the pelvis.

The pudendal vessels and nerves pass along the floor of the ischiorectal fossae. On each side, the internal pudendal artery runs through the fossa and divides into the inferior haemorrhoidal, transverse perineal and perineal arteries, and also sends off small branches to the muscles. The internal pudendal nerve, arising from the second, third and fourth sacral nerves, also passes through this region, dividing into numerous branches to supply structures in the area.

Muscles, nerves and blood vessels

The muscles of the pelvic floor consist of the levator ani muscles, which lie at a deep level and other perineal muscles, which lie more superficially.

The levator ani muscles (Fig.2.7) arise on each side of the pelvis (from a line which passes backwards from the posterior surface of the superior pubic ramus) and pass over the internal surface of the obturator internus muscle to the ischial spine. From this origin, fibres from each side sweep downwards and backwards, interdigitating with each other in the midline around the upper portion of the vagina, bladder neck and rectum, and insert posteriorly into the lower portion

of the sacrum and coccyx. The levator ani muscles are bowl-shaped and form the pelvic diaphragm. Reflexes which raise the intra-abdominal pressure, such as coughing and sneezing, will relax these muscles.

External to the levator ani muscles are the deep and superficial perineal muscles, which provide support for structures in the lower pelvis (Fig.2.8). These consist of the bulbocavernosus muscle, the ischiocavernosus muscle, the superficial and deep transverse perineal muscles and the external anal sphincter.

The ischiocavernosus and bulbocavernosus muscles pass into the base of the clitoris. The superficial and deep perineal muscles extend from the sides of the pelvis and support the perineal body. They can be involved in tears and episiotomies at delivery.

The central point of the perineum is the perineal body. This is a musculofibrous structure, situated at a deep level between the vagina and the rectum. It acts as a keystone, with the transverse perineal muscles, bulbocavernosus muscle and the anal sphincter inserting into it. It is occasionally damaged during obstetrical tears. The anal sphincter is under voluntary control. Its contraction adds to the capacity to close the exit of the anus and prevent the passage of flatus or faeces.

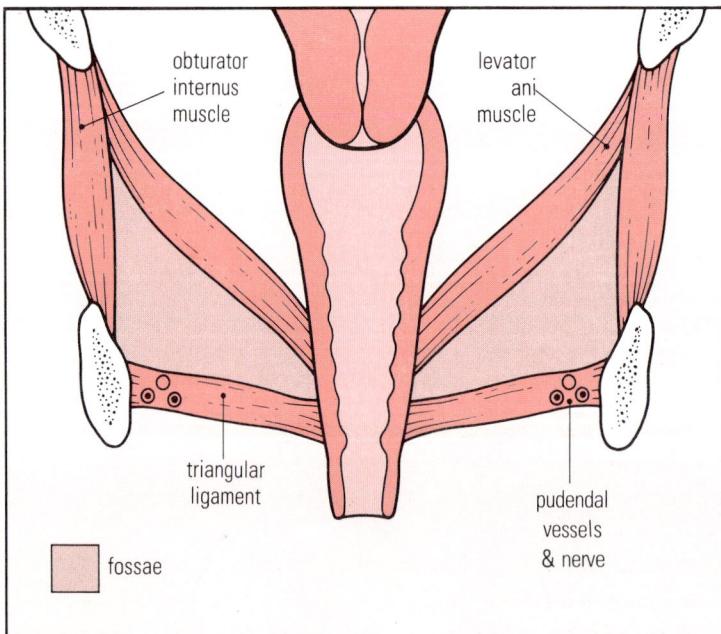

Fig.2.6 The ischiorectal fossae are triangular in section and lie on either side of the vagina, below the sloping levator ani muscles. They are filled with fat and loose areolar tissue.

obturator internus muscle

levator ani muscle

triangular ligament

pudendal vessels & nerve

fossae

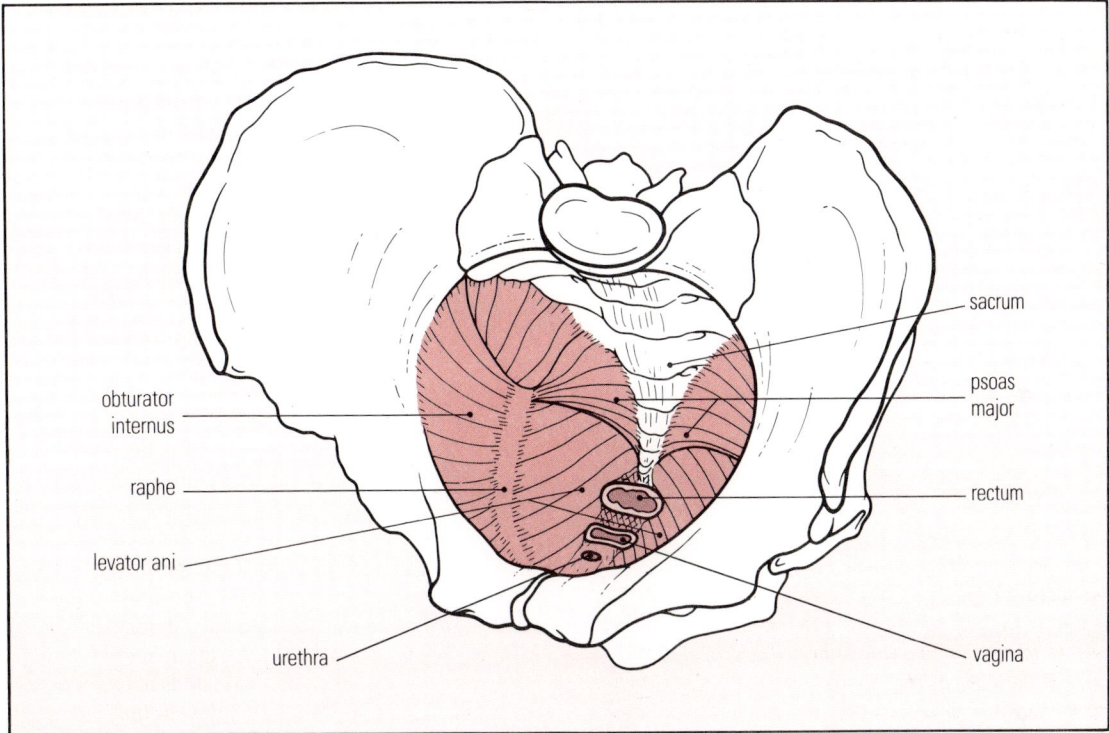

Fig.2.7 The pelvic diaphragm is predominantly composed of the levator ani muscles, which pass from the side walls of the pelvis down towards the midline.

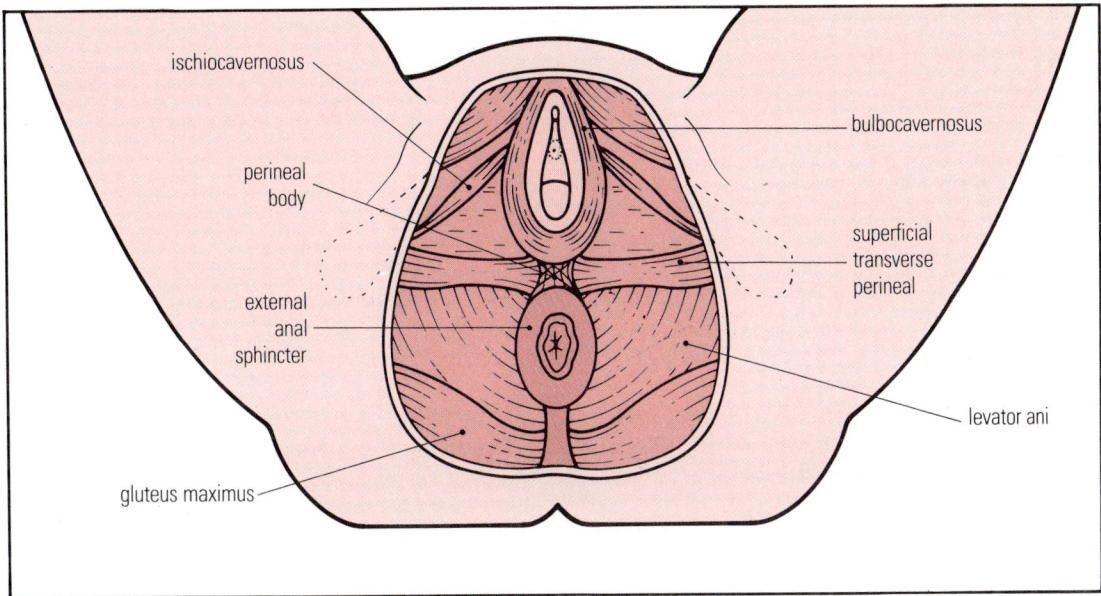

Fig.2.8 Deep and superficial perineal muscles of the pelvis.

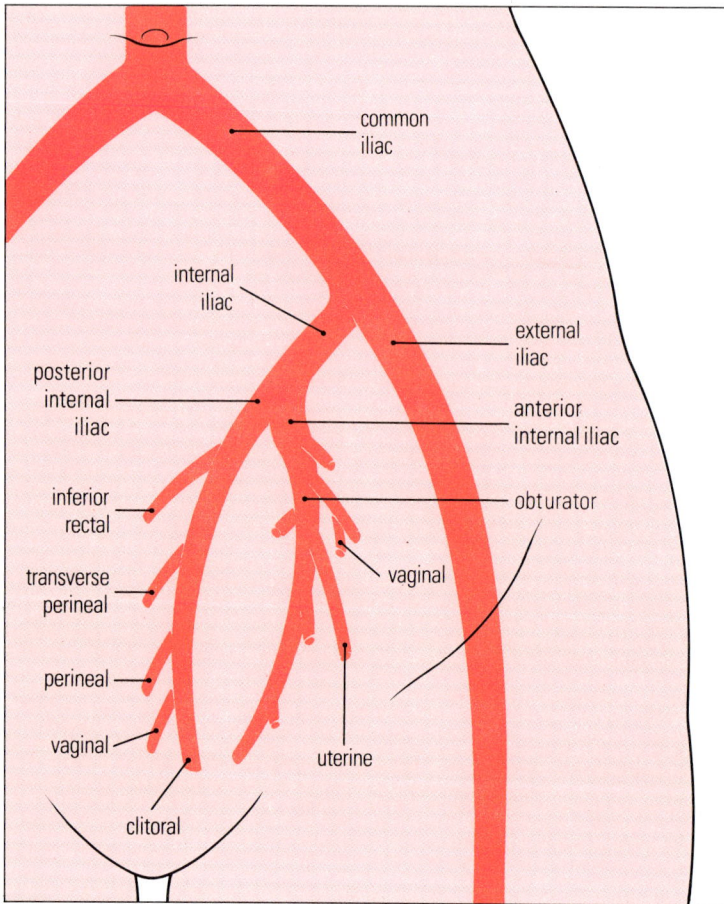

Fig.2.9 Arterial blood supply to the pelvic organs.

The blood supply to the uterus and vagina is provided mainly by the anterior branch of the internal iliac artery, which gives off the uterine, vaginal and obturator arteries (Fig.2.9). The uterus receives its blood supply from the uterine arteries, which extend from the side walls of the pelvis and divide at the upper part of the cervix (Fig.2.10). The upper branch passes upwards, often dividing into two branches, to supply the body of the uterus. The lower branch divides into a series of smaller vessels, which pass downwards alongside the vagina.

The ovaries obtain blood from the ovarian arteries. These arise from the dorsal aorta on the posterior abdominal wall and run down behind the peritoneum. They pass in a fold of peritoneum from the back wall of the pelvis, over the pelvic brim, towards each ovary; major terminal branches supply each fallopian tube and anastomose with the uterine arteries on the underside of the tube.

The pelvic organs are supplied by sympathetic and parasympathetic nerve plexuses (Fig.2.11). The sympathetic nerves arise from lumbar sympathetic ganglia one, two, three and four. They pass from the preaortic plexus down to the uterovaginal plexus and ovary. The uterovaginal plexus rests in loose areolar tissue at the side of the cervix, at the level of the uterosacral folds of peritoneum. Parasympathetic fibres come from the second, third and fourth sacral nerves, and supply the pelvis through the uterovaginal plexus.

Sympathetic nerve impulses relax the uterine muscle, especially during pregnancy. This effect is of pharmacological, rather than physiological, importance. Sensory impulses are also carried in the sympathetic nerves, and division of these nerves may relieve pain in the pelvis.

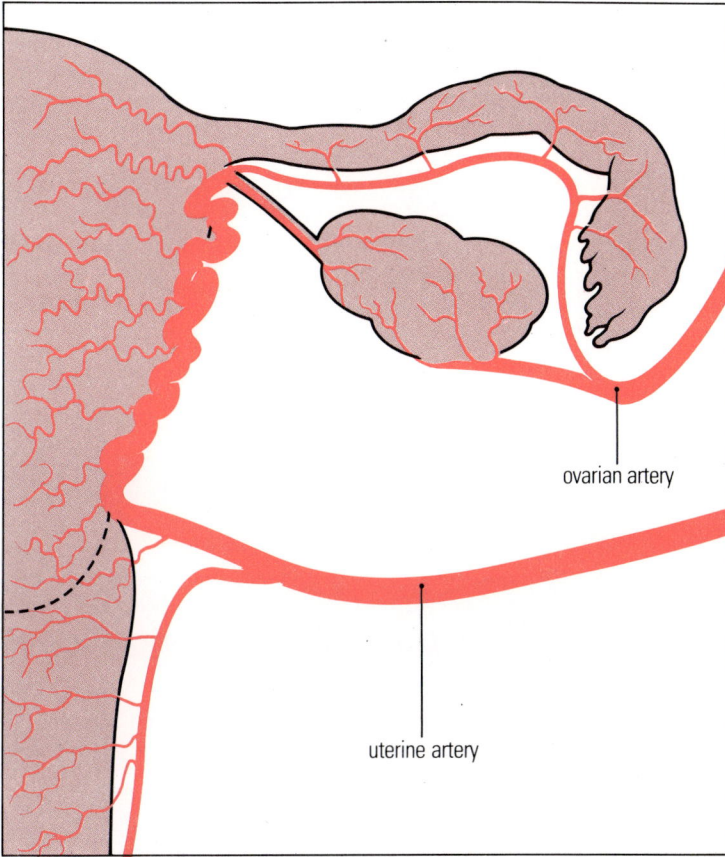

Fig.2.10 The uterine and ovarian arteries.

ovarian artery

uterine artery

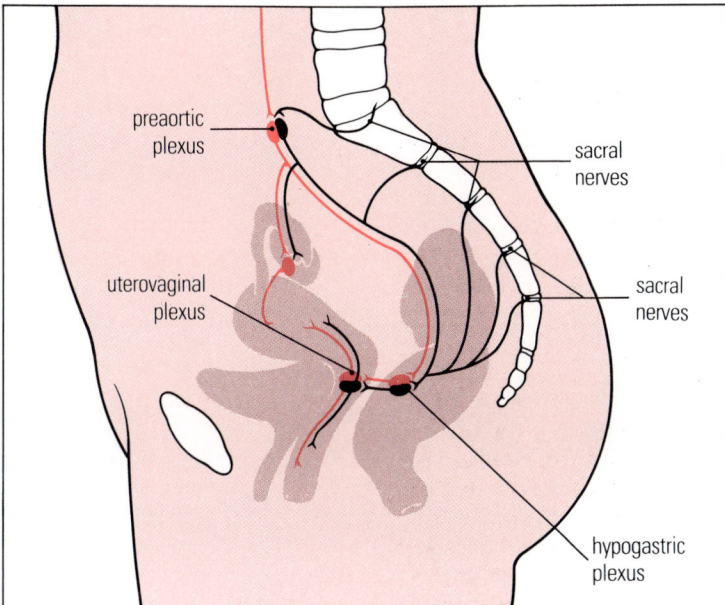

Fig.2.11 The sympathetic (red) and parasympathetic (black) nerve supplies of the pelvis. The sympathetic plexuses supplying the bladder and rectum are also shown.

preaortic plexus

sacral nerves

uterovaginal plexus

sacral nerves

hypogastric plexus

The uterus

The uterus is a pear-shaped organ, divided into the body and cervix; a thin segment, the isthmus, lies between them. During late pregnancy and labour, the isthmus is greatly expanded to form the lower uterine segment.

The uterine musculature is arranged in three ill-defined layers (Fig.2.12): a thin outer layer of longitudinal muscle, which passes anteriorly from the front of the isthmus, over the fundus of the uterus and down to the cervix; a thick layer of spiral myometrial fibres which encircles the cavity; and an inner layer of poorly defined circular muscle surrounding the ostia of the fallopian tubes and the internal and external ora of the cervix. Synchronous contractions of the spiral myometrial fibres make the uterus shorten in length and cause compression of the uterine vessel.

The uterus normally lies in anteversion and anteflexion and is held in place by muscular and fibrous supports. The important muscular supports are the levator ani muscles and, to a lesser extent, the perineal muscles superficial to them. On the deep surface of the levator ani muscles, and wrapped

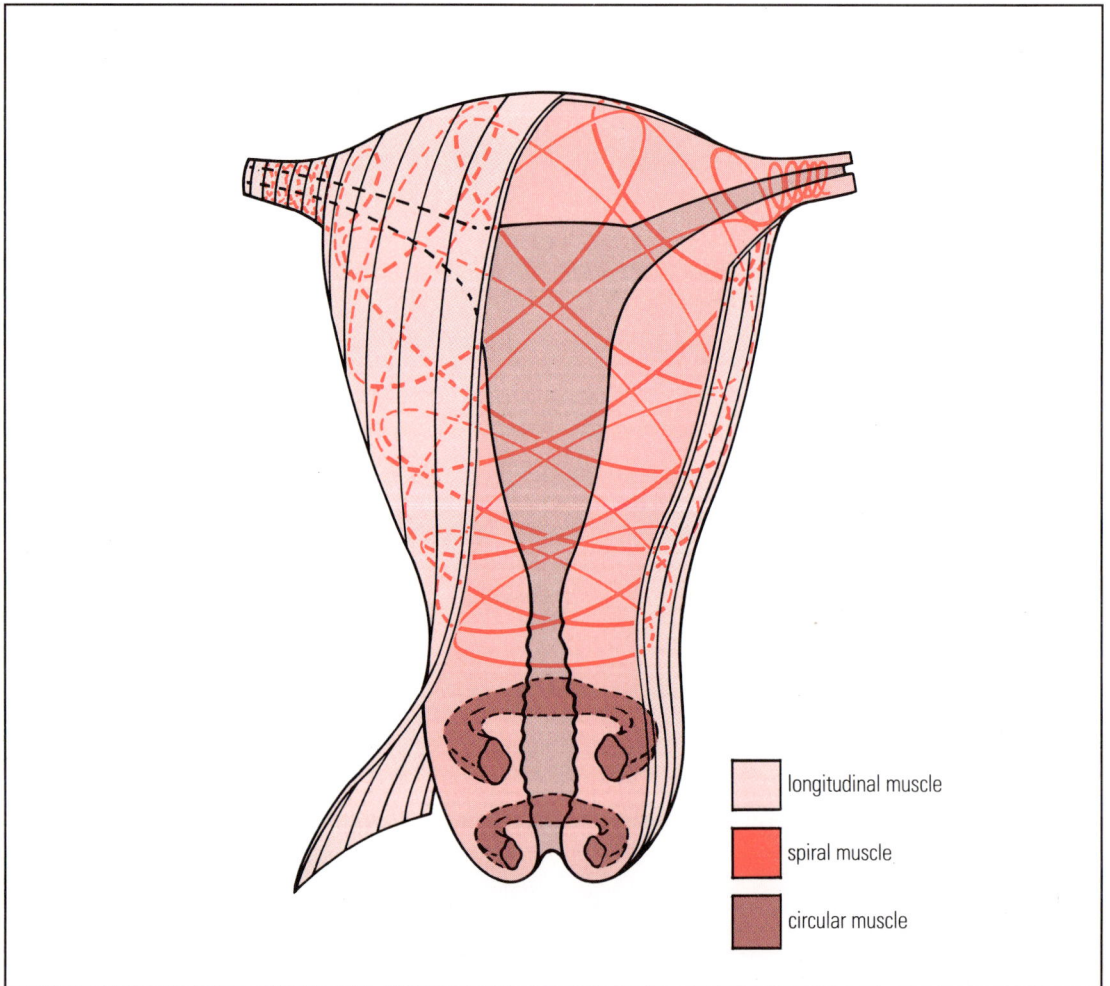

longitudinal muscle

spiral muscle

circular muscle

Fig.2.12 Uterine musculature.

around the pelvic organs, is the pelvic fascia, which is firmly condensed in certain areas to produce the fascial supports (Fig.2.13). The areas of special condensation are:

• Anteriorly, the round ligaments, which stretch from the top of the uterus just in front of the cornu, along the path of the gubernaculum, around the side of the pelvis, under the peritoneum, enter the inguinal canal and terminate by fusing with the pubic orifice; they offer no major support.

• Laterally, the transverse cervical ligaments, which pass from the lateral pelvic wall to the cervix near the internal os and which contain, in addition to compressed fibrous tissue, the uterine vessels. In the upright position, the ligaments suspend the uterus in a sling.

• Posteriorly, the uterosacral ligaments, which are thinner and less effective as a support; they pass from the back of the cervix and fornices of the vagina to the anterior surface of the sacrum.

The broad ligament, although referred to as a ligament, merely helps to hold the uterine fundus in anteversion and has no major support function.

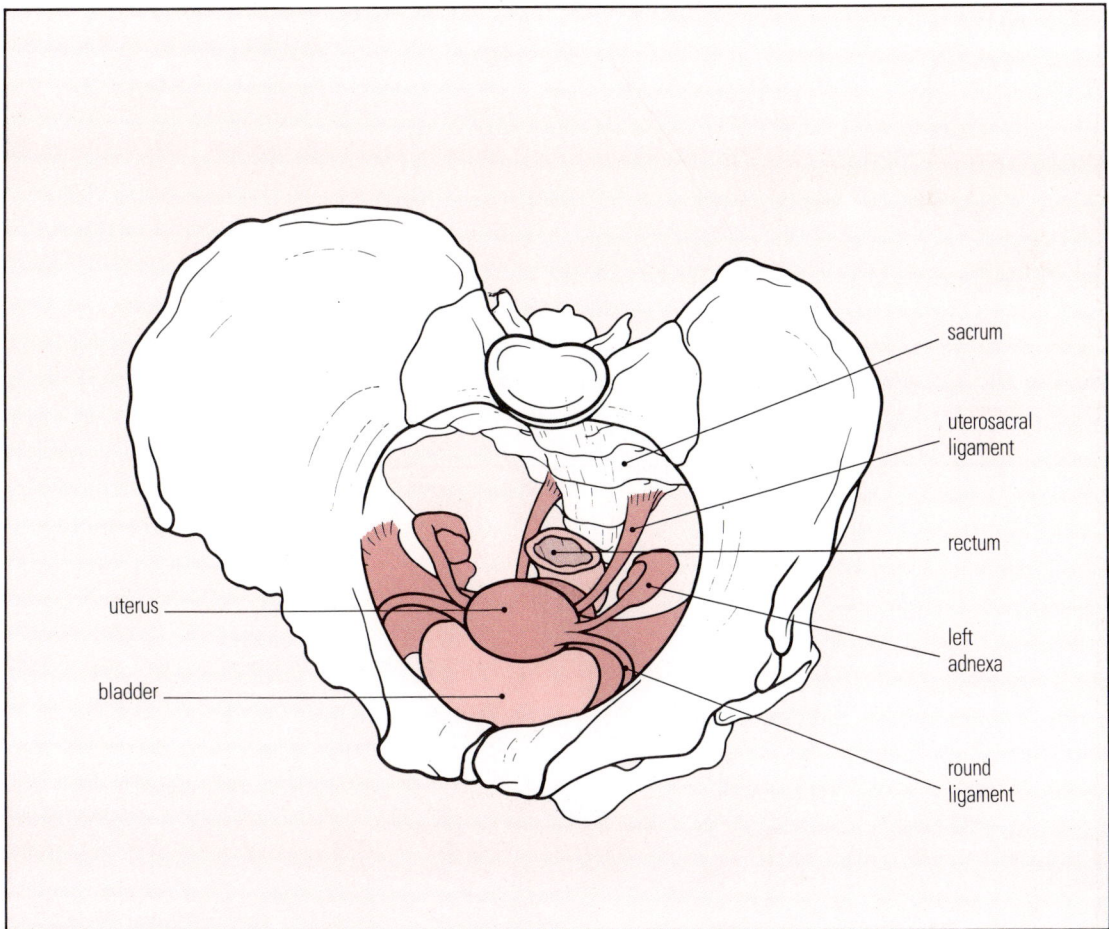

Fig.2.13 Uterine ligaments. These are: anteriorly, the round ligaments; laterally, the transverse cervical ligaments; and posteriorly, the uterosacral ligaments.

The size of the uterine body in relation to the cervix changes at different times during a woman's life (Fig.2.14). At birth, the uterine body is comparatively large, due to stimulation by oestrogens from the placenta, and is equal in length to the cervix, the ratio of body to cervix being one to one. After birth, the placental source of oestrogen is no longer available and the uterine body shrinks, the cervix remaining relatively longer, with a body to cervix ratio of one to two. At puberty, the uterine body is stimulated to grow, reversing this ratio.

The bladder

The bladder is a hollow muscular organ, lying extraperitoneally in the anterior part of the pelvis (Fig.2.15). The size and shape of the bladder vary with the amount of urine contained, but usually it takes the form of an inverted pyramid, with the apex behind the pubic symphysis and the base against the wall of the peritoneal cavity.

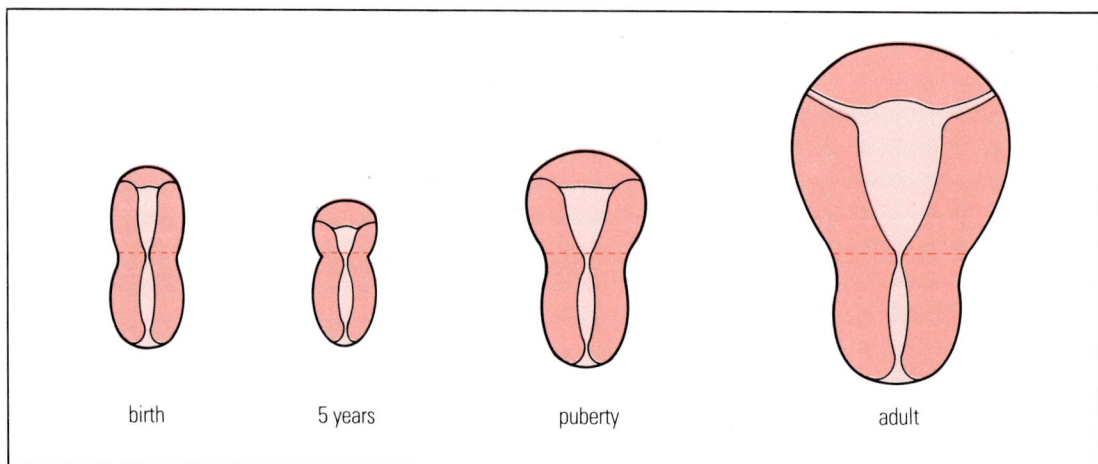

Fig.2.14 The length of the cervix in relation to the length of the uterine body. The ratio changes as the genital tract matures.

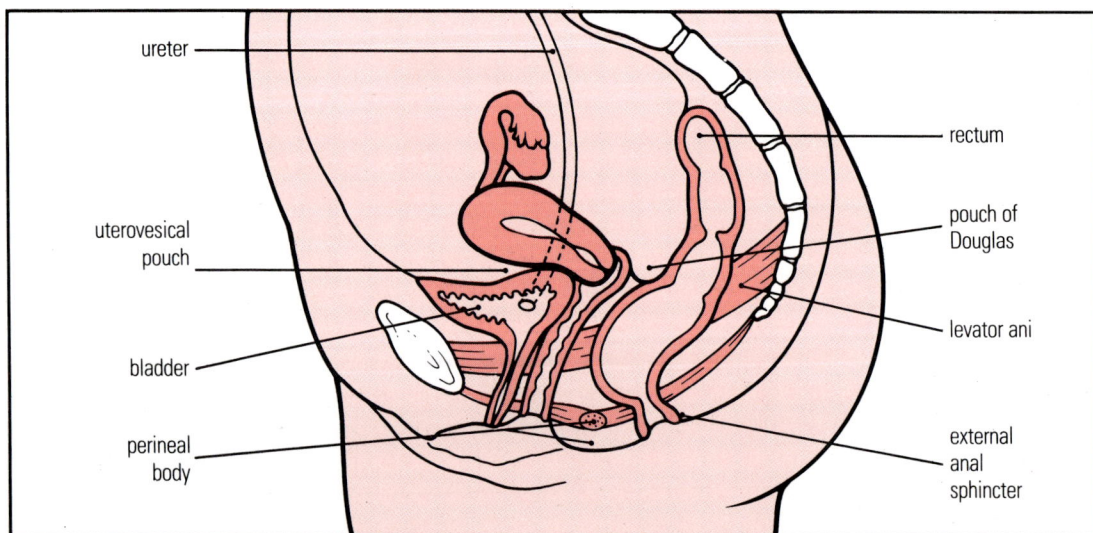

Fig.2.15 The bladder and rectum in relation to other pelvic organs and muscles.

The ureters enter the bladder at the posterolateral angles of the base, and the urethra leaves it inferiorly. The uterovesical pouch is formed by a reflection of the peritoneum covering the uterus and the superior surface of the bladder. The arterial blood supply is provided by the inferior and superior vesical branches of the internal iliac artery. The sympathetic nerve supply arises from the first and second lumbar segments, and the parasympathetic fibres from sacral segments two, three and four.

The rectum

The rectum is a hollow tube, approximately 12cm long, which joins the sigmoid colon to the anal canal. The lower third is embedded in pelvic fascia, the middle third is covered anteriorly by peritoneum, and the upper third is covered anteriorly and laterally by peritoneum. There is no mesentery, the posterior border being retroperitoneal at all levels.

Posterior to the rectum lie the superior rectal artery, the third, fourth and fifth sacral nerves, the sympathetic trunk, and the sacral artery (the terminal branch of the aorta). Blood is supplied from the rectal arteries (branches of the internal iliac artery) which anastomose with branches of the inferior mesenteric artery superiorly, and the pudendal artery inferiorly.

Lymphatic drainage of the pelvic organs

The lymph nodes are located around the external and internal iliac arteries and the aorta. The lower abdominal wall and the bladder drain into the external iliac nodes. The cervix drains into the internal iliac and obturator nodes, as does the body of the uterus; the uterine fundus may drain with the ovary into the para-aortic nodes. The perineum drains into the inguinal and femoral nodes. The external and internal iliac lymphatic vessels pass to the common iliac nodes and thence to those adjacent to the aorta.

NORMAL MATERNAL PHYSIOLOGY IN PREGNANCY

The physiological changes in the mother's body during pregnancy occur in response to hormonal variations and to the growth of the fetus.

Weight

Hormonal changes are responsible for a considerable increase in weight during pregnancy (Fig.2.16); women gain an average of approximately 18kg (39.69lb). The weight gain is partly due to the increase in size of the uterus and to its growing contents, and partly to fat laid down in the mother's body. The weight gain of a woman in pregnancy may be apportioned as follows:

Fetus	3.5kg
Placenta	0.5kg
Amniotic fluid	1.5kg
Uterus	1.0kg
Increase in blood volume	1.5kg
Breasts	1.0kg
Extracellular fluid	3.0kg
Fat and protein storage	6.0kg
Total	18.0kg

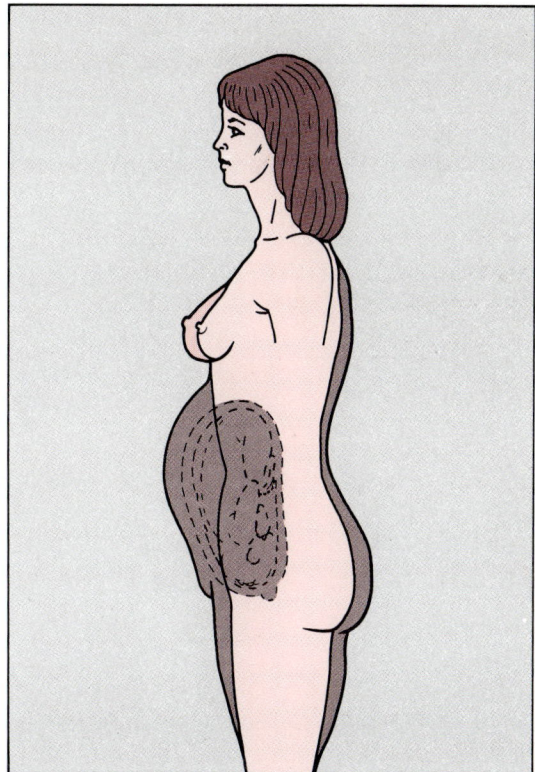

Fig.2.16 Distribution of weight gained in pregnancy due to fluid retention, and increases in body fat on the shoulders, buttocks and thighs. Half the weight gain is due to the increase in reproductive tissues, i.e. the uterus and its contents and the breasts.

Metabolism

During pregnancy there is an increase in all basic physiological processes, such as respiratory rate and cardiac output, to accommodate the metabolic demands of the fetus and placenta. A normal woman requires approximately 2500cal/day to cope with these changed circumstances.

Carbohydrate metabolism alters to provide the fetus with a readily available energy source; maternal tissues involved with lactation and rapid growth during pregnancy also require an immediate carbohydrate supply. Blood glucose levels are sustained during fasting by hormone-induced gluconeogenesis, but normal glucose homeostasis after a meal requires increased post-prandial insulin secretion. If the pancreas cannot meet this demand, gestational diabetes will develop. Some sugar may be lost in the urine, since the renal threshold for glucose is reduced during pregnancy.

Gastrointestinal system

A number of characteristic changes occur in the gastrointestinal system during pregnancy. Nausea and vomiting are present in approximately two-thirds of women during early pregnancy. These symptoms are most pronounced in the fourth to twelfth weeks of pregnancy, when gonadotrophin concentrations are at their highest level. Thereafter, nausea and vomiting become less troublesome. Thus, prolonged or excessive symptoms should be considered pathological.

Constipation is common in pregnancy and is probably due to progesterone relaxing the smooth muscle. The motility of the intestinal tract is reduced and the passage of food slowed. One beneficial effect is that the absorption of nutrients is improved.

Gastric acidity is usually reduced during pregnancy and a relative achlorhydria frequently occurs. This, together with reduced gastric motility, often has a beneficial effect in women with a history of peptic ulcer. Nevertheless, relaxation of smooth muscle involves the cardiac sphincter, and reflux heartburn is a common complaint.

Cardiovascular system

There is an increase in blood volume of thirty to forty percent during pregnancy (Fig.2.17). The increase in

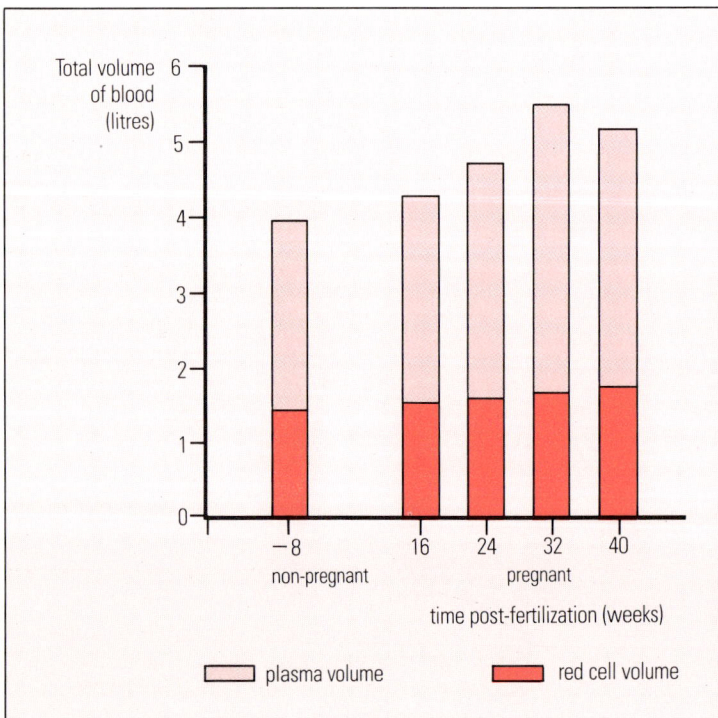

Fig.2.17 Increase in blood volume during pregnancy. The increase in plasma volume is greater than that of the red cell mass.

plasma volume is greater than the expansion in red cell mass, so a relative dilution of blood takes place, leading to a lower haemoglobin concentration. This is sometimes incorrectly termed the physiological anaemia of pregnancy. Cardiac output also increases by around forty percent, and this is accomplished mainly as the result of an increase in stroke volume from 70ml to 90ml.

Blood pressure is little affected in normal pregnancy; occasionally, a small reduction characterizes the second trimester, with a rise to prepregnancy levels in the third trimester. Pre-eclamptic toxaemia may affect pregnancy in the late second and early third trimesters, with a consequent rise in blood pressure.

As the pregnant uterus increases in size, it exerts greater pressure on the blood vessels lying over the lumbar vertabrae in the lower abdomen (Fig.2.18). The aorta is relatively thick-walled and is more resistant than the inferior vena cava. Thus, a damming of blood occurs in the lower limbs and pelvis, particularly when the woman is supine and the uterus lies across the great vessels. This may lead to a diminution in blood return to the heart, and so to a relative hypotension, which leads to faintness – the supine hypotension syndrome.

Respiratory system

True respiratory difficulties are seldom encountered during pregnancy. However, some women may become conscious of difficulty in breathing in the last weeks of pregnancy, when the enlarging uterus pushes the lower ribs upwards and outwards and presses on the diaphragm. This displacement of the ribs alters the stresses placed on them and occasionally, if a pregnant woman develops a severe cough, a fracture may occur.

Alterations in lung volume become more marked as the pregnancy advances (Fig.2.19). As the growing uterus presses against the underside of the diaphragm, there is a diminution in total lung capacity. The vital capacity remains unchanged, but the inspiratory capacity is increased by approximately 300ml and the functional residual capacity is decreased by the same amount. The respiratory rate does not alter during pregnancy. There is, however, an increased tidal volume and this enhances gaseous exchange, with an increase in P_{O_2} and a decrease in P_{CO_2}.

Urinary system

Renal function in normal patients is not impaired by pregnancy. The renal blood flow increases, starting from the first missed period. The glomerular filtration rate increases in a similar fashion. Despite these changes, pregnant women with a normal fluid intake have a urinary output comparable to, or even slightly less than, non-pregnant women. This is due to an increase in tubular reabsorption of water and electrolytes.

Dilatation of the renal pelves and ureters occurs from the twelfth week of pregnancy onwards, due to the relaxing effect of progesterone on smooth muscle. This may lead to urinary stasis and may consequently give rise to renal infection. To some extent, there is also pressure from the enlarging uterus on the lower ends of the ureters.

An increased frequency of micturition is a

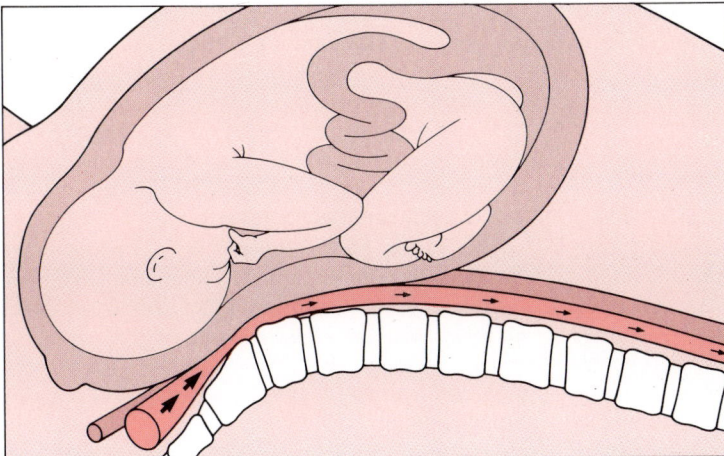

Fig.2.18 The growing uterus and its contents press on the major blood vessels over the lumbar vertebrae. This may lead to supine hypertension syndrome.

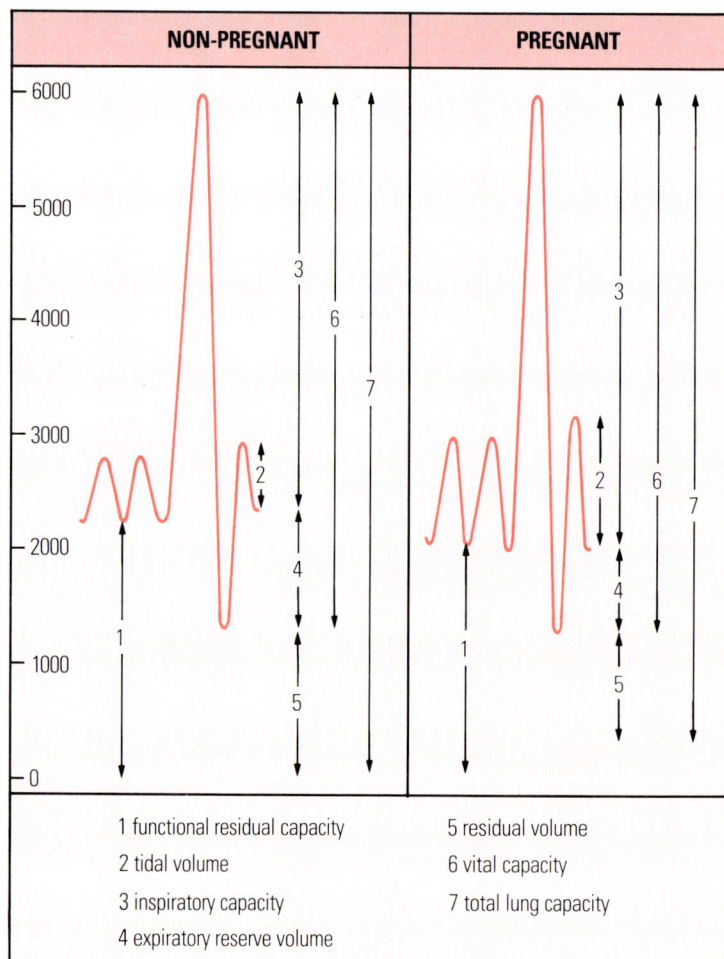

NON-PREGNANT	PREGNANT

1 functional residual capacity
2 tidal volume
3 inspiratory capacity
4 expiratory reserve volume
5 residual volume
6 vital capacity
7 total lung capacity

Fig.2.19 Changes in respiratory excursion during pregnancy. The scale represents volume in ml. Modified from Chamberlain, G. (1980) *Lecture Notes on Obstetrics (4th edition).* Oxford: Blackwell Scientific Publications.

commonly quoted symptom of early pregnancy. It is probably caused by the enlarging uterus, still in the pelvic cavity in early pregnancy, exerting pressure on the bladder.

Other changes

The breasts increase in size considerably during pregnancy, in response to altered levels of progesterone and oestrogen. This is notable even in the comparatively early stages, and the patient may be aware of a tingling sensation and increased tenderness if the breast is touched. Hyperaemia later becomes pronounced, and dilated veins can be seen in the subcutaneous tissues. The areola darkens and a secondary, ill defined but pigmented areola is usually evident, especially in dark-haired women. The sebaceous glands of the areola become enlarged and protrude as Montgomery's tubercles. It is possible to express colostrum from the breast from the end of the first trimester of pregnancy onwards.

The skin sometimes develops a coarse appearance during pregnancy, and it may become more greasy than usual. Hair tends to thicken, although there is considerable variation in this effect.

The pelvic joints loosen in all pregnancies. Normally this is asymptomatic but occasionally, when considerable separation of the symphysis pubis occurs, a looseness of this region is noticed, especially when walking. If the condition deteriorates, permanent damage may follow in the form of pelvic arthropathy.

3. Antenatal Care

PRINCIPLES AND ORGANIZATION OF ANTENATAL CARE

Introduction

Antenatal care is the systematic examination of the mother and growing fetus throughout pregnancy. It aims to ensure that the mother and her unborn child come to delivery in the best possible condition. The problems of pregnancy, as they present clinically, are managed at antenatal clinics. More recently, however, antenatal care has expanded to include the detection of potential problems before they appear clinically. This aspect of antenatal care is provided as a screening service for presymptomatic disease. For such screening to be effective, the total population must be examined and certain members designated as being at higher risk for various disorders.

Antenatal visits are usually monthly at first, fortnightly later, and then weekly in the last month of pregnancy. Obviously, the frequency of visits will vary with individual patients, depending on their particular risks and problems.

Diagnosis of pregnancy

Pregnancy is diagnosed from the patient's history, clinical examination and investigations.

History

A history of amenorrhoea is found in most pregnant women and can be used to estimate the expected date of delivery (Fig.3.1). There is a ninety percent chance that delivery will occur within ten days on either side of this date. Estimation is most accurate under the following conditions:
- precise date of last menstrual period
- previously regular cycle (25–35 days)
- no bleeding
- not a post-pill conception

Among women in the reproductive age group who have had unprotected intercourse, a persistent lack of periods is usually considered to be an indication of pregnancy. However, in some pregnant women, a

ESTIMATION OF DELIVERY DATE	
First day of last menstrual period	15 • 10 • 88
Add one year	+ _____1
	15 • 10 • 89
Add seven days	+ 7 _____
	21 • 10 • 89
Subtract three months	− 3 _____
Estimated delivery date	= 21 • 7 • 89

Fig.3.1 Estimation of delivery date. This is only an approximate estimate and depends on the features mentioned in the text.

little bleeding may occur at monthly intervals after the last normal menstrual period.

About sixty percent of women complain of nausea or vomiting (see Chapter 5). Some have tenderness and tingling of the breasts, particularly around the areolae; breasts may start to enlarge very early in pregnancy (five to six weeks gestation).

Many patients, particularly parous women, feel different in pregnancy in a way which they find difficult to describe. Pregnancy may be diagnosed by the woman herself, even before she has missed a period, from this non-specific sensation of well-being.

Examination

The signs of pregnancy often present later than the symptoms. Breasts become enlarged, veins may appear on their surface and the sebaceous glands around the edge of the areolae may enlarge, producing Montgomery's tubercles.

The uterus enlarges but usually this cannot be felt by abdominal examination until after twenty weeks gestation (Fig.3.2). The first pelvic signs are detected by bimanual examination; the uterus becomes cystic, soft and rounded by about five to six weeks gestation. Later, after about eight weeks, some enlargement may be detected, but softness is the primary feature.

Investigations

Biological animal tests on rabbits and frogs have now been outdated by immunological tests. These depend upon the presence of human chorionic gonadotrophin (hCG) in the urine, detected usually by the agglutination test (Fig.3.3).

It is conventional to use early morning urine for the pregnancy test, since this contains the highest concentration of the hormone. The β subunit of hCG can be detected by a radioimmunoassay (RIA) from as early as eight or nine days after fertilization, that is, four or five days before the woman has missed her period. This particularly sensitive test need only be performed if there is an unusual or urgent reason to know if the woman is pregnant.

Conventional pregnancy tests become positive about ten days after the missed period (that is, two or three weeks after fertilization). False positive results occasionally occur, particularly in the later years of reproductive life when a high concentration of pituitary gonadotrophins, instead of hCG, causes the test to become positive. These hormones are produced by the pituitary to stimulate the older, more resistant ovary. False negative results usually occur due to a low concentration of hCG in the urine; a repeat test carried out one week later is often positive.

The level of hCG continues to rise until about sixteen weeks gestation and then falls slowly after that. If, for some reason, the embryo has perished, as in an incomplete abortion, some trophoblast tissue may remain viable in the decidua. This small nidus of tissue can produce enough hCG to keep the pregnancy test positive; thus a pregnancy test is of no use in assessing the prognosis of spontaneous abortion.

Pregnancy can also be diagnosed by an ultrasound scan (Fig.3.4). The fetal sac can be detected at about five weeks gestation, and embryonic tissue by about

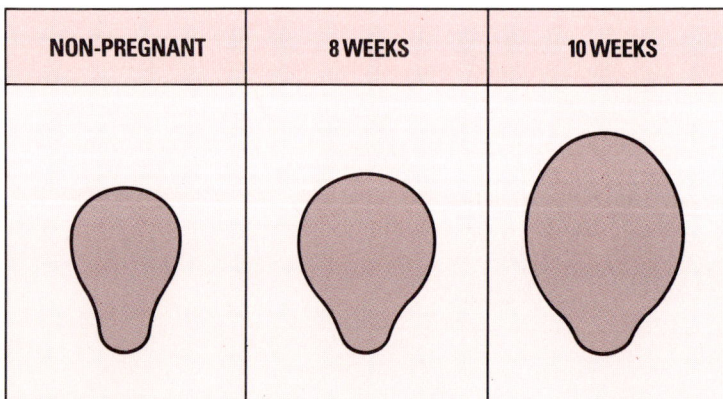

Fig.3.2 Growth of the uterus. In early pregnancy, this is usually in width rather than length, so that the uterus appears fuller and softer.

NON-PREGNANT	8 WEEKS	10 WEEKS

AGGLUTINATION PREGNANCY TEST

Pregnant urine	Non-pregnant urine
No agglutination	Agglutination

anti-hCG   ▲ hCG   ✦ hCG–coated RBC

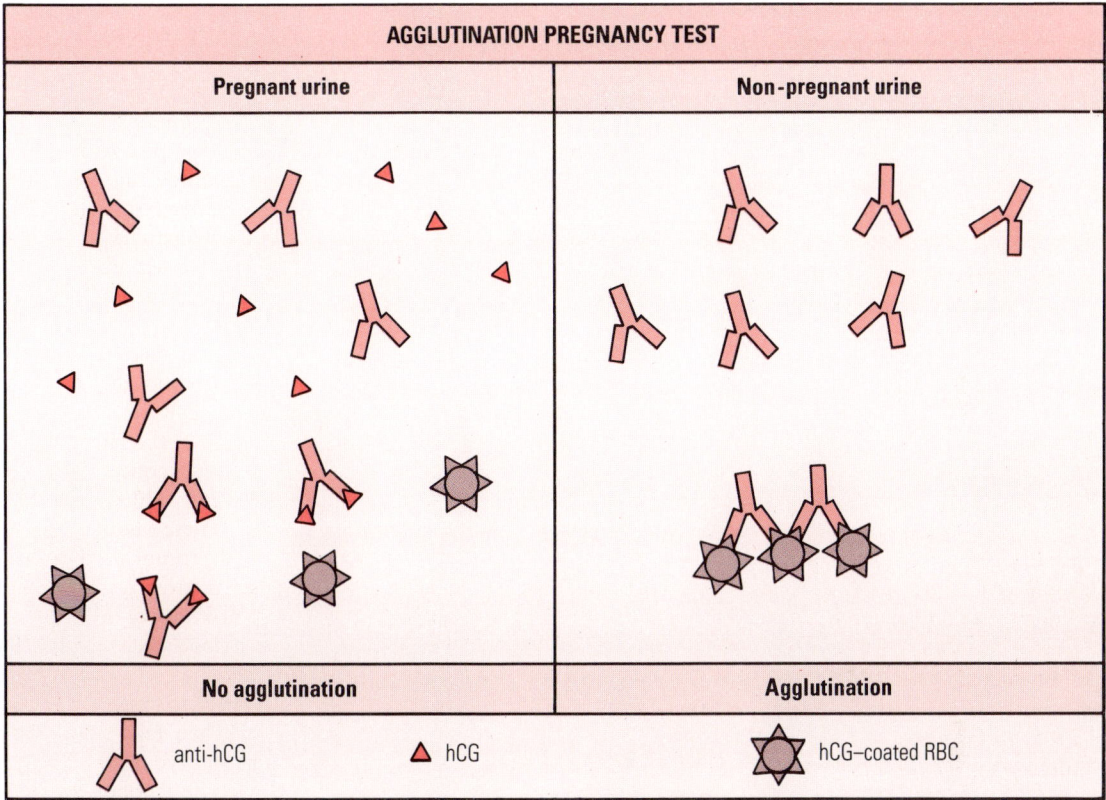

Fig.3.3 Agglutination pregnancy test. Anti-hCG is added to the urine to be tested. Red blood cells coated with hCG are then added. The red blood cells will agglutinate if no hCG is present in the urine (i.e. if the woman is not pregnant). If hCG is present, it will bind to the anti-hCG molecules and the red blood cells will not agglutinate, indicating a positive test.

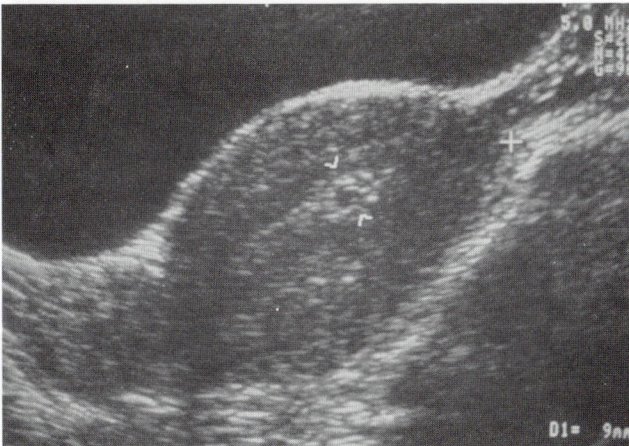

Fig.3.4 Ultrasound appearance of gestational sac in early pregnancy. This scan was taken at 5 weeks after the last menstrual period, the lower limit of when one would expect to detect a sac in pregnancy. Courtesy of Dr. R. Patel.

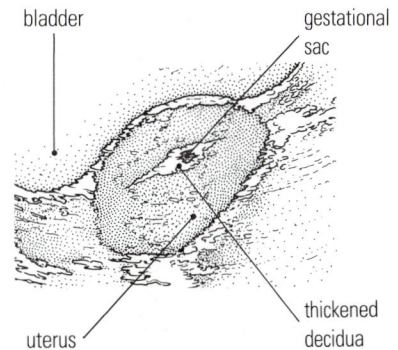

six weeks. The sac can sometimes be present without embryonic tissue, for example in a missed abortion or blighted ovum.

X-rays are not usually used as a pregnancy test for a number of reasons. Firstly, they may be dangerous in the early weeks of gestation and secondly, they will not show a fetus until calcification of the fetal bones has taken place; this usually occurs after sixteen to eighteen weeks, by which time pregnancy has nearly always been diagnosed by other methods.

Very occasionally pregnancy is diagnosed incidentally, for instance in an X-ray of a girl who has not reported her missed periods but is having an abdominal X-ray for some other reason.

The booking visit

The woman should book at a hospital in early pregnancy. The first visit to the antenatal clinic is the longest and yields predictive information about the likelihood of problems.

History

A history is taken of:
- Menstrual cycle, in particular the date of the last normal menstruation, some idea of regularity of cycle length and any history of recent use of oral contraception.
- Past obstetric history, if multiparous.
- Past illnesses, such as tuberculosis or renal disease.
- Family history, particularly of twins or diabetes.

Examination

The patient's general health must first be assessed, paying particular attention to any evidence of anaemia. The cardiovascular system (including blood pressure) is thoroughly checked. The spine and legs are examined for skeletal abnormalities, which may be associated with pelvic variations. The abdomen is examined for scars and masses. If the pregnancy is sufficiently advanced, the uterus can be felt arising from the pelvis but this rarely occurs before twelve weeks gestation.

A vaginal examination is usually performed at the first visit to confirm that the woman is pregnant and to check the uterine size against the date of gestation (see Fig.3.2); uterine or ovarian masses can be

excluded at the same time. The bony pelvis is usually assessed not at this visit, but later in the pregnancy when the fetal head is used as a check of pelvic size.

Investigations

An early morning specimen of urine should be analysed for protein and glucose levels. If protein is present, a second midstream specimen should be checked to exclude contamination. If protein is still present, the specimen should be examined for the presence of white cells, which indicate urinary infection. If there is no infection, the presence of protein in the urine implies glomerular damage. If glucose is present, the test should be repeated, and if glycosuria is found again, a glucose tolerance test should be performed using a 75g oral load.

Blood is checked for:
- α-fetoprotein, indicating open abnormalities of the fetal CNS (usually performed at 16 weeks).
- Sickle cell trait or disease.
- Wassermann reaction.
- Australia antigen.
- Rubella antibodies.
- Haemoglobin and red cell size on a blood film.
- Blood groups (ABO and rhesus). If the patient is rhesus negative, the presence or absence of antibodies should be checked.
- HIV.

Other tests include a cervical smear and ultrasound investigation (best done at sixteen to eighteen weeks).

Management

Ideally, all patients attending antenatal clinics should feel that the staff have adequate time to be asked any questions and to give factual and reassuring answers. This is particularly important at the booking visit. If there are relevant problems the woman should see a medical social worker. She should also be informed about any welfare benefits which she is entitled to receive, usually outlined in government pamphlets.

The patient must be advised on her dietary requirements, as these change in pregnancy; the phrase 'eating for two' is both inaccurate and misleading. A pregnant woman should not eat extra food, but rather food that provides specific nutrients in sufficient quantity. Ideal daily requirements vary, but the generally accepted values are:

- 2500–3500kcal
- 60–80g protein (particularly plant protein)
- 1g calcium
- 500µg folate

Most antenatal clinics have a book or pamphlet providing dietary advice and culinary suggestions.

A normal mixed diet contains adequate supplies of all the required vitamins, with the exception of folate, which is necessary for fetal and increased maternal tissue growth. In view of this, folate (300 – 500µg/day) is offered routinely. Similarly, many women live on diets with borderline iron deficiency. If they cannot obtain their iron from an improved diet, such women should be advised to take iron tablets in the second half of their pregnancy to maintain the maternal circulating haemoglobin and to help build up fetal iron stores. Iron is absorbed from the intestine only in the ferrous state and a high concentration is necessary in the lumen before uptake will take place. Consequently, prophylactic iron should provide at least 100mg of elemental iron per day. The tablets commonly used have an elemental iron content greater than this.

In summary, information given at the booking visit should include general advice on diet, welfare benefits, antenatal and parentcraft classes, and details of future visits.

Subsequent antenatal visits

Patients are seen at regular intervals throughout their pregnancy. A plan of visits is discussed with the GP and hospital if wished. At all visits, the woman is asked about symptoms that concern her or problems arising in relation to the pregnancy. She is weighed, and the change in weight from the previous visit is noted. Blood pressure is checked and urine is examined. After mid-pregnancy, the actual growth of the uterus and its contents is compared with the expected growth for that stage of pregnancy.

Specific aspects are assessed at different stages in the pregnancy.

SIXTEEN TO EIGHTEEN WEEKS

A routine ultrasound scan is performed to measure the biparietal diameter of the fetal head (Fig.3.5). Growth of the fetal head proceeds at a rate of 3mm/week between sixteen and twenty-nine weeks, slowing to less than 2mm/week between thirty and forty weeks. Determination of gestational age by this method is most accurate in early pregnancy (twenty-six weeks or less), when the range is narrow. The ultrasound scan also enables the examiner to check for obvious abnormalities such as anencephaly.

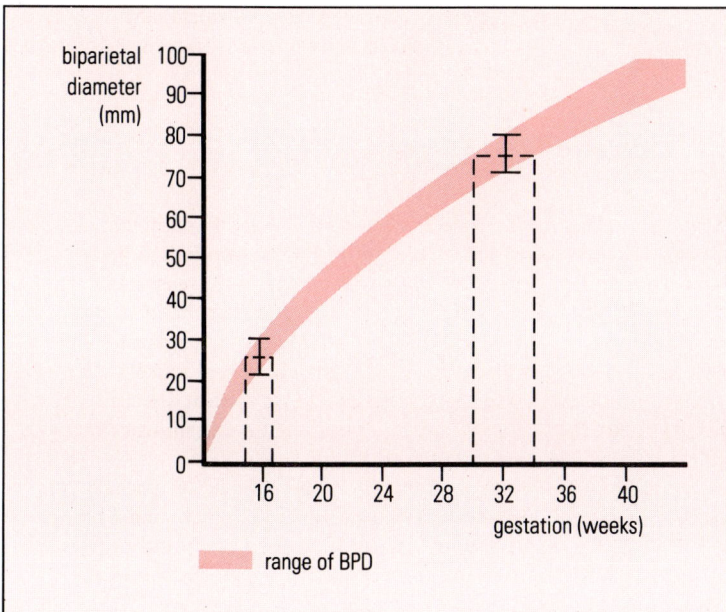

Fig.3.5 Biparietal diameter (BPD) of the fetal head throughout pregnancy. The range (the mean ± 2SD) of values from a large population of normal babies is shown. Determination of gestational age is more accurate in early pregnancy, when the range is small.

TWENTY-SIX TO THIRTY-THREE WEEKS

At this stage the examiner should be able to confirm clinically the number of fetuses, in most cases only one. The haemoglobin level should be rechecked and if the woman is rhesus negative, her antibodies should also be rechecked.

A second ultrasound scan may be needed to exclude intrauterine growth retardation.

THIRTY-FOUR TO THIRTY-SIX WEEKS

The lie of the fetus can be confirmed at this stage. By this time it should have settled into a longitudinal lie and, commonly, a cephalic presentation. The bony pelvis may also be assessed on this occasion (Fig.3.6). The examining fingers should seek the promontory of the sacrum, although this usually cannot be felt. If, however, it can, the pelvis is probably small, particularly in the anteroposterior diameter of the brim.

THIRTY-SEVEN TO FORTY WEEKS

The lie of the fetus should remain longitudinal and, if a cephalic presentation, the engagement of the head should be assessed. The maximum diameter of the fetal head enters the brim of the pelvis at engagement (Fig.3.7). In a primiparous woman this usually occurs in the last weeks of pregnancy, although it may not occur until the onset of labour. Furthermore, women of Negro origin often have delayed engagement of the fetal head owing to the different angle of inclination of their pelvic inlet.

If the head has not engaged by this stage, the woman should be propped up on her elbows (Fig.3.8). Should the head not engage by this manoeuvre, cephalopelvic disproportion may be suspected and a series of investigations should be performed.

OVER FORTY WEEKS

If gestation continues to this stage, the imminence of labour should be checked. Softening and ripening of the cervix occurs in late pregnancy and early labour. The cervical canal is effaced from above as the lower uterine segment pulls on the top of the internal os. It becomes conical in section and as further traction pulls from the sides, it is flattened out completely. The cervical os then starts to dilate. These changes

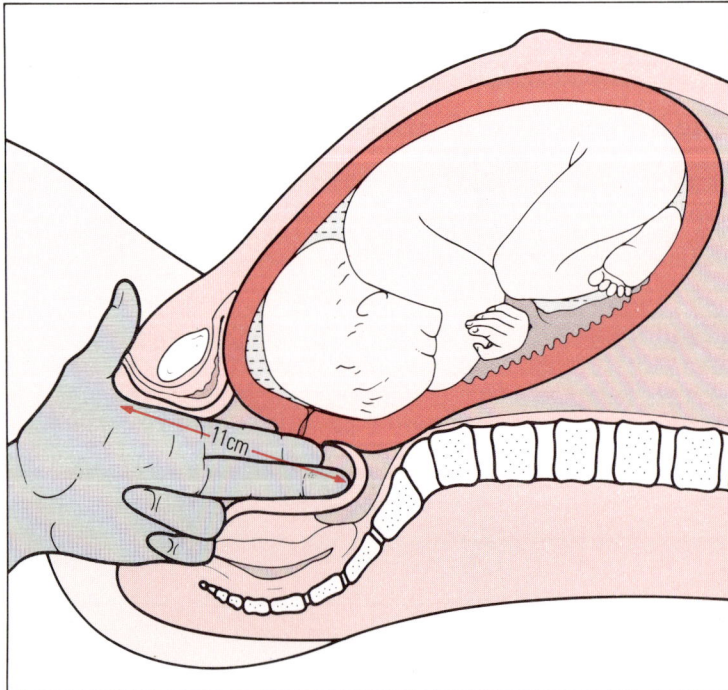

Fig.3.6 Assessment of bony pelvis by vaginal examination in late pregnancy. If the examiner's fingers cannot reach the sacral promontory, the anteroposterior diameter of the inlet is greater than 11cm.

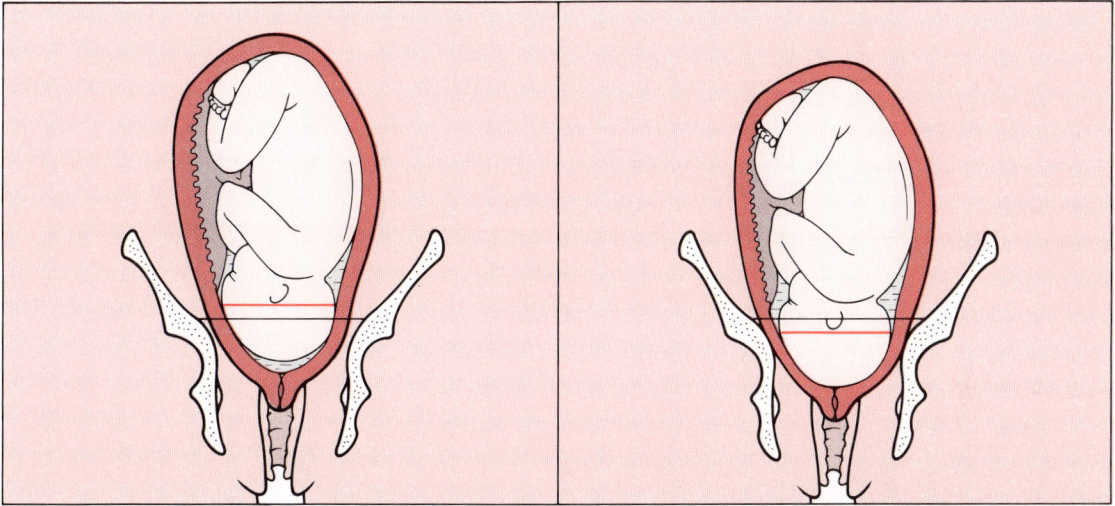

Fig.3.7 Engagement of the normal, well flexed fetal head in late pregnancy. The maximum diameter of the head (red line) descends below the maximum diameter of the pelvic brim (black line).

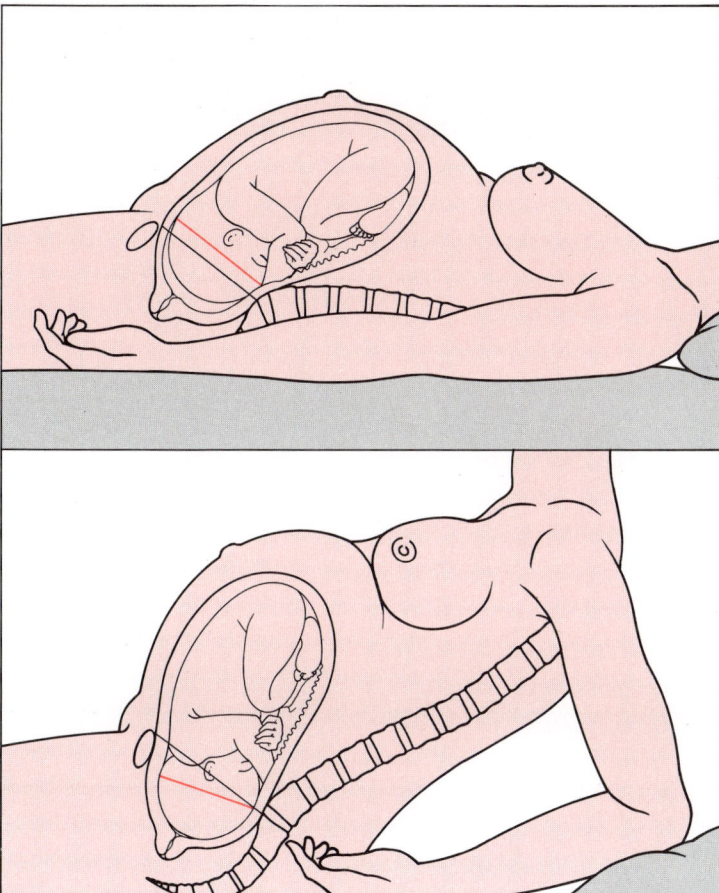

Fig.3.8 If the fetal head has not engaged in the last weeks of pregnancy a simple test is to prop the patient on her elbows. In this position (lower), the elevation of the uterus causes the head to sink down into the pelvis and become engaged.

BISHOP'S SCORE					
	Criteria	Score			
		0	1	2	3
A	dilatation of cervix	closed	1–2cm	3–4cm	≥5cm
B	effacement of cervix	0–30%	40–50%	60–80%	fully effaced
C	consistency of cervix	firm	medium	soft	———
D	position of cervix	posterior	central	anterior	———
E	level of fetal head in relation to ischial spines	3cm above	2cm above	1–0cm above	1–2cm below

	RIPENING OF THE CERVIX		
A	0	1	3
B	0	1	3
C	0	1	2
D	0	1	2
E	0	0	1
Total score	0	4	11

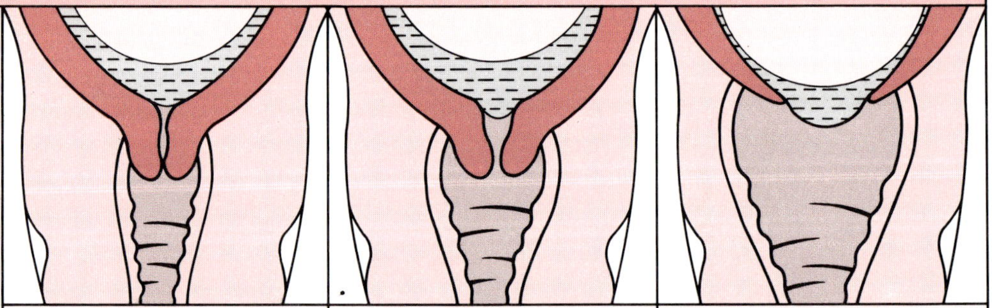

Fig.3.9 Bishop's score (upper) and ripening of the cervix (lower), with scores for each stage. Criteria C and D are topographical factors for which there are only 3 points. A, B and E are expressed as measurements, each having four scores.

occur simultaneously and are know as ripening of the cervix; they can be assessed and recorded using Bishop's score (Fig.3.9), which gives an indication of the likely success of an induced labour. The system has five criteria for assessment, each of which has a number of possible scores. Induction is likely to be successful when the total score is greater than nine; a score of five indicates a less favourable outcome. Careful fetal monitoring, often with a cardiotocograph, should also be undertaken.

Many obstetricians believe that pregnancy should not continue past forty-two weeks, as postmaturity places the fetus at higher risk (Fig.3.10). However, if pregnancy is allowed to continue, the woman should be seen at half-weekly intervals until she goes into labour, checking the fetus carefully at all visits.

Antenatal education

All antenatal clinics should now have antenatal instruction classes to which the woman and her partner are welcome. A typical programme should include a visit to the delivery area and demonstration of any equipment which may be used, such as the machines for the self-administration of analgesia and cardiotocograph machines.

The women attending antenatal classes generally do so from twenty-four weeks gestation onwards. The classes consist usually of six to twenty women, and involve discussion of a relevant topic and the practice of relaxation techniques. Plenty of time and encouragement must be given to questions which people are often very hesitant to ask in a group. Antenatal classes should endeavour to remove the natural fear of the unknown element of pregnancy; for example, the problem of the abnormal or dead baby should not be ignored. With a perinatal mortality rate of ten per thousand in the United Kingdom, mothers can be assured that ninety-nine out of one hundred babies are born alive. Similarly, with a major abnormality rate of 1.7 percent, they can be informed that ninety-eight percent of babies are born normal.

Antenatal classes and clinics help pregnant women to meet each other. It can be reassuring to know that others have similar feelings about seemingly trivial matters. Some of the best antenatal instruction is given individually by the doctor or midwife while the woman is at the ordinary clinic.

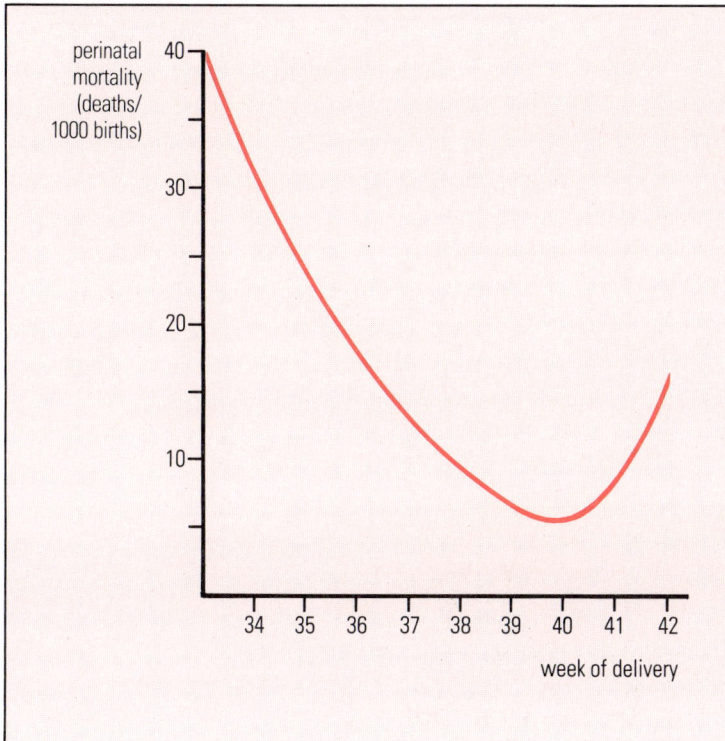

Fig.3.10 Perinatal mortality rate. The rate is lowest at around 40 weeks but increases steeply thereafter.

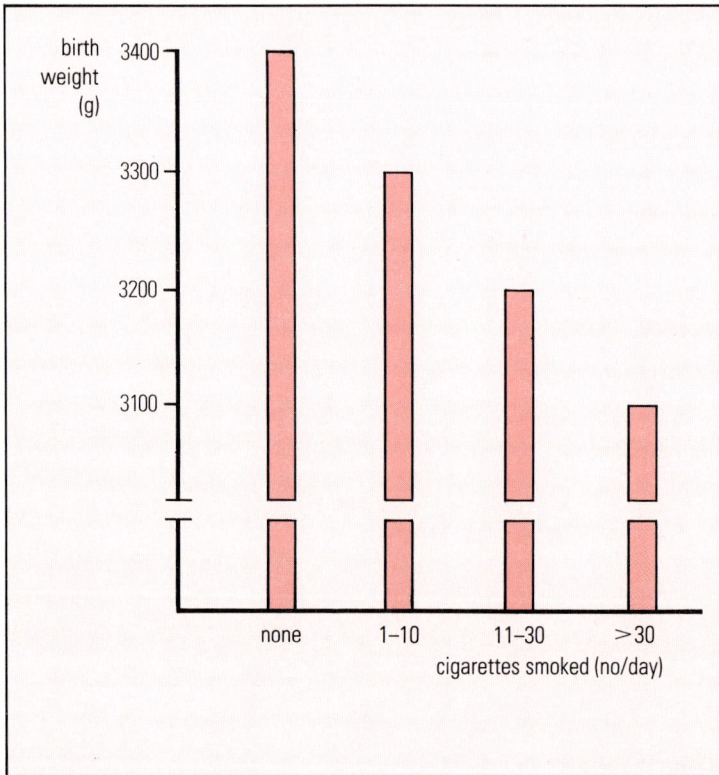

Fig.3.11 The effect of maternal smoking habits on birth weight of the baby.

Smoking

Habitual cigarette smoking is associated with smaller babies and some degree of diminished development (Fig.3.11); the effect is related to the number of cigarettes smoked. Women can often be persuaded to stop smoking voluntarily; if they do so by sixteen weeks gestation, the fetal effects are usually greatly reduced.

Alcohol

Occasional alcohol may cause no harm, however, heavy alcohol drinking affects the growth and development of the fetus. This applies to both chronic heavy drinking and occasional binges.

Sexual intercourse

Sexual intercourse may continue throughout a normal pregnancy unless there has been recent vaginal bleeding. Women can be reassured that labour and fetal infection are not caused by intercourse.

Rest, work and exercise

Questions related to rest, work and exercise are often asked. The best answer is to tell the woman to be guided by how she feels. She is likely to need more rest, particularly in late pregnancy, and may wish to stop work. Similarly with exercise, she should not exert herself but should allow her level of fatigue to guide her level of activity.

Travel during a normal pregnancy is not contra-indicated. Although air travel is safe, airlines can stop a pregnant woman flying after thirty-four weeks gestation. In cars, safety belts should be worn at all stages of gestation.

Clothes

The woman can be informed of specialist maternity clothing stores which provide excellent ranges of attractive clothes. Special brassieres will be required later in pregnancy; some women may have enlarged breasts at an early stage and they should be prepared to change into a good supporting brassiere as soon as the breasts feel heavy.

Onset of labour

Many women, even those who have had a baby before, are unaware of the variations in the onset of labour. Expectant mothers should be warned that the onset of painful, regular contractions coming from the small of the back to the lower abdomen is the commonest sign of the onset of labour. Rupture of the membranes with expulsion of warm liquor, or a mucoid or bloody discharge are less common signs.

The patient must be assured that it is best to present at the hospital if she thinks she is in labour, rather than waiting at home. Although it is easy to be sure about uterine contractions in established labour, it is often more difficult at the onset; hence, the woman must be encouraged to develop a low threshhold of suspicion and come into the hospital in good time.

ASSESSMENT OF FETAL WELLBEING

Clinical monitoring

In order to assess fetal wellbeing, a full and detailed clinical history of the mother must be taken. Information obtained from the history in conjunction with that gained from a thorough examination should be used to evaluate any potential risks to the unborn child (Fig.3.12).

The history

Factors that should be noted when taking the mother's history are:
- Maternal age. Risk to the fetus increases at the extremes of reproductive age (Fig.3.13).
- Social circumstances. Perinatal mortality is increased in the underprivileged classes and the unemployed (Fig.3.13).
- Domestic circumstances, for example whether the father of the child is supporting the mother.
- Current and past medical health.
- Current or long-term drug therapy. Special note

should be made of any drugs taken in early pregnancy.
- Smoking habits and alcohol consumption.
- Gynaecological history. Details of the menstrual cycle before pregnancy, of contraception close to the start of pregnancy and of any treatment for infertility (for example induction of ovulation) should be noted.
- Past obstetric history. The parity and gravidity of the mother can be graded using the system outlined in Fig.3.14. After the second pregnancy the risk of perinatal mortality rises with each subsequent pregnancy (see Fig.3.13).

The history is assessed with particular reference to dating the pregnancy and the health of the woman since conception; any current medication should be detailed. The obstetrician should enquire about the occurrence of episodes of vaginal bleeding, lower abdominal pain, vomiting and urinary symptoms. Throughout the visit the woman should be guided to answer relevant questions to help assess the potential risks to the fetus.

The examination

The woman should be fully examined in comfortable surroundings, with attention to privacy. An examination to assess her general health is made.

Of particular importance in the clinical assessment of fetal risk is abdominal palpation of the uterus and fetus. The growing uterus normally enters the abdomen at twelve weeks gestation. It reaches the umbilicus at twenty-two weeks gestation and is just under the costal margin by thirty-six weeks. This does not give a precise indication of fetal age because the amount of amniotic fluid can add to the uterine bulk. A series of estimates from successive antenatal visits gives a measure of uterine growth. Bimanual palpation of the uterus is often useful up to about twenty weeks gestation, allowing the observer a more precise palpation of the lower pole so that the uterine size is estimated more accurately. Fetal parts are usually palpated from about twenty-six to twenty-eight weeks gestation. Later on the lie, presentation and size of the fetus are assessed at each visit.

Once the fetus can be palpated, its lie in relation to the mother can be determined. In a longitudinal lie, the fetus presents with its long axis parallel to that of the mother (Fig.3.15). Thus, the fetus will be able to

MATERNAL FACTORS AFFECTING PREGNANCY		
Score	1 2 3 4	
Maternal age		
20–29		
<20 & 30–34	▭ (score ~1)	
≥35	▭ (score ~1.5)	
Parity		
1 & 2		
0 & 3	▭ (score ~1)	
≥4	▭ (score ~1.5)	
Social class		
I & II		
III	▭ (score ~1)	
IV, V & unemployed	▭ (score ~2)	
unsupported mothers	▭ (score ~2)	
Previous obstetric performance		
abortion	▭ (score ~4)	
antepartum haemorrhage	▭ (score ~2)	
postpartum haemorrhage	▭ (score ~4)	
immature delivery (≤36 weeks)	▭ (score ~2)	
low birthweight (≤2500g)	▭ (score ~2)	
caesarean section	▭ (score ~4)	
stillbirth	▭ (score ~4)	
neonatal death	▭ (score ~4)	
Medical history		
hypertension	▭ (score ~4)	
diabetes	▭ (score ~4)	
cardiac disease	▭ (score ~4)	
chronic respiratory disease	▭ (score ~4)	
chronic renal disease	▭ (score ~4)	
endocrine disease	▭ (score ~4)	
Sociobiological		
height ≤ 62″	▭ (score ~1)	
≥5 cigarettes/day	▭ (score ~1)	

Fig.3.12 Maternal factors affecting pregnancy. The degree of risk associated with each factor is indicated on a scale of 1 to 4. Hypertension is defined as a BP of 140/90 or more before 20 weeks of gestation.

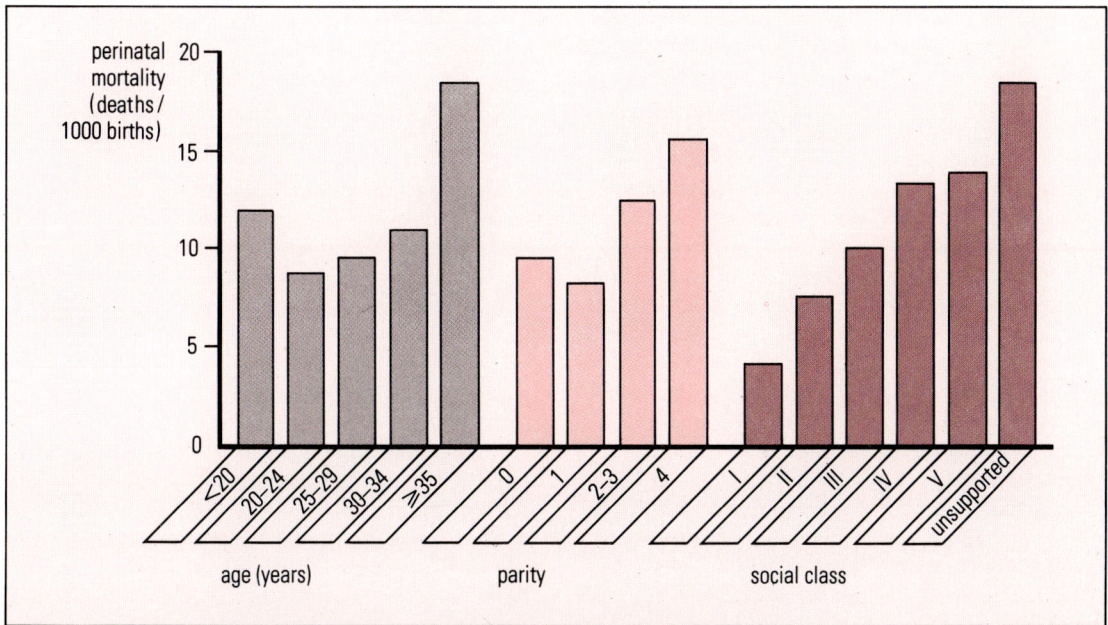

Fig.3.13 Perinatal mortality associated with age, parity and social class of the mother.

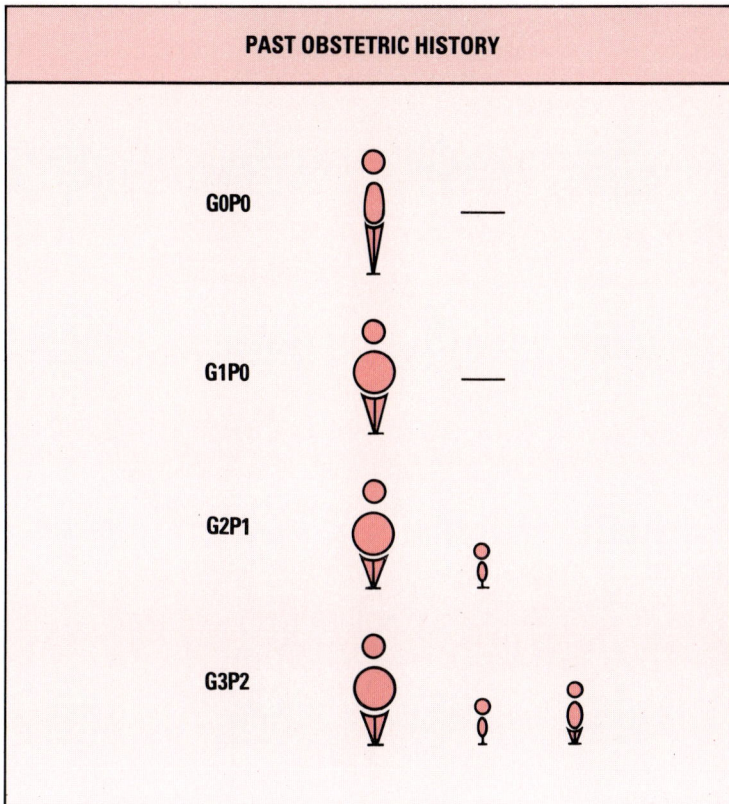

PAST OBSTETRIC HISTORY

G0P0

G1P0

G2P1

G3P2

Fig.3.14 Grading of gravidity and parity. Gravity (G) refers to number of pregnancies and parity (P) refers to number of children. A woman who has never been pregnant is G0P0. In her first pregnancy, she is gravid but has not had any children and so is G1P0. After birth of the child, she would be G1P1, and in the next pregnancy G2P1. After birth of the second child, if she becomes pregnant again, the woman would be G3P2. If, however, the second pregnancy is aborted, the next pregnancy would be her third but she has only one child, and is therefore G3P1.

be delivered vaginally. The presenting part of the fetus in a longitudinal lie is either the head (cephalic) or the buttocks (breech). These can be determined by abdominal palpation and confirmed, if necessary, by vaginal assessment. Oblique or transverse lies, where the fetal long axis is at an angle to that of the mother (Fig.3.15 right), are incapable of vaginal delivery and, if neglected, may lead to obstructed labour and a ruptured uterus.

Fetal size can be estimated by gently grasping each pole and trying to visualize the fetus out of the uterus (Fig.3.16). It is important to master this technique so that fetal weight can be guessed to within 500g. The accuracy of this method of estimation improves with practice. It is far more precise than judging the fundal height from external landmarks in the maternal abdominal wall.

In the later weeks of pregnancy, an estimate of the ability of the fetal head to pass through the mother's pelvis should be made. When the maximum cephalic diameter has passed below the pelvic brim, the head is engaged. It usually does this in the last three to four weeks of pregnancy (that is, after thirty-six weeks). If the head has not engaged by thirty-eight weeks, one should check that it can be engaged (see Fig.3.8).

The fetal heart

The fetal heart may be heard using a Doppler ultrasound machine from the twelfth week of gestation, and a Pinard stethoscope from the twenty-sixth week of gestation.

The presence of fetal heart sounds are reassuring to the mother and one should attempt to allow her to hear them at the antenatal visits. Little qualitative assessment can be made from the fetal heart rate, which usually becomes slower as gestation advances.

Amniotic fluid

In the later weeks of pregnancy, a clinical estimate should be made of the volume of amniotic fluid, paying particular attention to the exclusion of extreme conditions, that is, an excess of fluid (polyhydramnios) or a deficiency (oligohydramnios). Both conditions may be associated with fetal compromise.

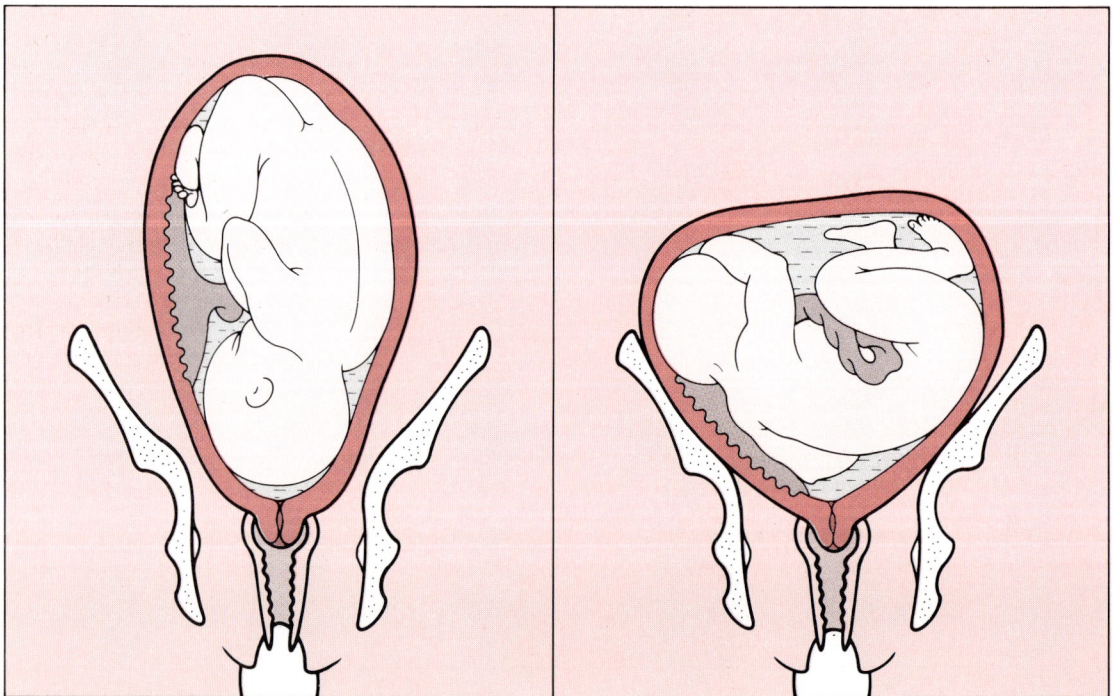

Fig.3.15 Lie of the fetus. Left: longitudinal lie; Right: transverse lie.

Biochemical monitoring

Several biochemical tests are used to assess fetal wellbeing. Individual results are of limited use and, in general, it is the pattern of results over several readings that provides useful information. The measurements made reflect placental metabolism. Although metabolism and transfer are loosely associated, specific tests of placental transfer are badly needed.

Alpha-fetoprotein

Alpha-fetoprotein (AFP) is a single-chain glycoprotein (molecular weight 69,000), produced initially by the yolk sac and subseqently by the fetal liver. It may be detected in the maternal serum and in the amniotic fluid (Fig.3.17). The maximum maternal serum level of AFP occurs at about thirty-two weeks gestation.

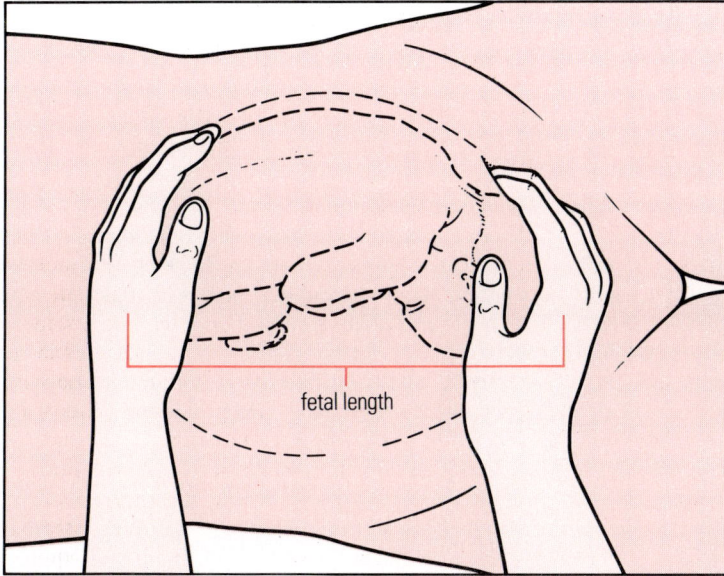

Fig.3.16 Estimation of fetal size.

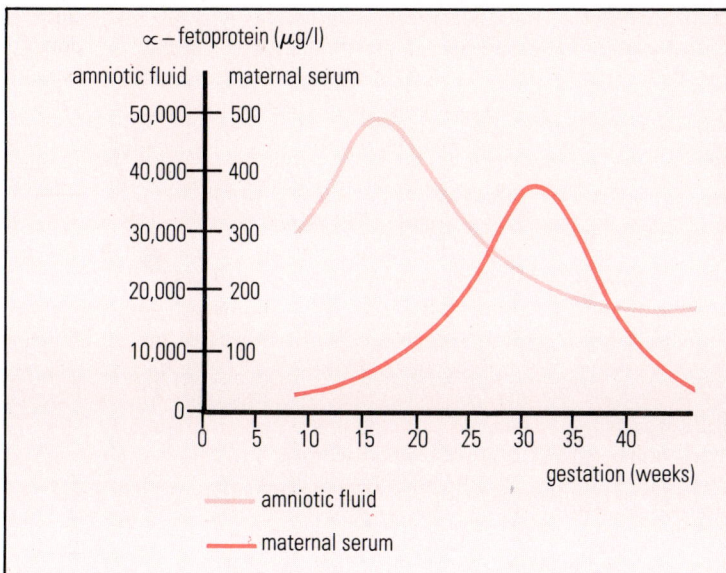

Fig.3.17 α–fetoprotein concentrations. The peak in concentration in the amniotic fluid occurs at about 16 weeks, while that in the maternal blood occurs much later. Note the significant difference in concentration between the two peaks.

In the presence of open central nervous system abnormalities in the fetus, increased amounts of AFP are secreted into the amniotic fluid. Amniotic absorption leads to raised levels in the maternal serum. There may also be an increased concentration of AFP in the presence of exomphalos, multiple pregnancy and after a threatened abortion.

The level of AFP taken to be the upper limit of normal is in debate; in most laboratories, two and a half times the median is used. The exact week of gestation is critical as AFP levels alter markedly from one week to the next and false positives may be obtained if the dating of a woman's pregnancy is inaccurate.

In practice, serum AFP levels are measured in the woman's blood at sixteen weeks; ultrasound dating of the pregnancy is usually carried out at the same time to obtain the accurate gestational age of the fetus. If the AFP is elevated, a repeat test is carried out. If the increased concentration is confirmed, an amniocentesis is recommended to check the AFP level in the amniotic fluid. Fewer false positive results occur in measurement of the amniotic fluid levels. If AFP concentrations are still elevated (and other causes for this are excluded) the parents should be advised about the probability of having a baby with a central nervous system abnormality and a termination of pregnancy may be recommended. Since this is the only treatment that can be offered, the full position should be explained to the mother before she starts the first AFP test.

Recent research shows that the measurement of other chemicals may assist in the diagnosis of fetal disorders. Acetylcholinesterase levels in the amniotic fluid are also elevated in association with open neural tube defects.

Placental protein hormones

HUMAN CHORIONIC GONADOTROPHIN

Human chorionic gonadotrophin (hCG) is a glyco-protein (molecular weight 47,000) consisting of an α and a β subunit joined by a disulphide bond. The α subunit is very similar to that of the other gonadotrophins from the pituitary gland (for example LH, TSH and FSH) and therefore cannot be differentiated from them. The β subunit, however, can be detected by radioimmunoassay nine days after conception, that is, before the date of the missed period. Production of hCG increases rapidly until about the sixteenth week of gestation (Fig.3.18) and then levels off in the latter weeks of pregnancy.

The urine pregnancy test depends on the presence of hCG. It is usually performed on an early morning specimen of urine (the most concentrated) and detects the hormone by immunological means (see Fig.3.3).

Estimations of hCG are not usually used to assess fetal wellbeing; they are useful in indicating the presence of trophoblastic tissue and thus that the woman is pregnant. Unfortunately, hCG estimation gives no indication of whether the fetus is alive. After early embryo death or in a blighted ovum, for example, small fragments of trophoblast tissue can survive and are enough to maintain an elevated hCG level in the blood and urine for several days.

HUMAN PLACENTAL LACTOGEN

Human placental lactogen (hPL) is a single-chain polypeptide (molecular weight 22,000). It is secreted by the trophoblast and is similar in biological activity to human pituitary growth hormone, but is initially much weaker. Levels of hPL can be measured in the maternal serum initially by radioimmunoassay and later, when there are larger amounts circulating (Fig.3.19), by enzyme immunoassay.

Levels of hPL in maternal serum decrease after a reduction in placental metabolic function; thus, a fall may be seen in the weekly readings from a woman who is at higher risk, for example due to pre-eclampsia or hypertension. Single low readings are not necessarily indicative of fetal hazard. It must be remembered that this is a retrospective investigation and, as such, measures past events rather than giving an indication of fetal prognosis.

OTHER PLACENTAL PROTEIN HORMONES

The placenta synthesizes several other proteins in increasing amounts during pregnancy, all of which are secreted into the maternal blood.

Pregnancy-associated plasma protein A (PAPP-A) is a glycoprotein which increases in concentration until the onset of labour. It can inhibit glycolysis and may be associated with disseminated intravascular coagulopathy. Altered concentrations may be found in pre-eclamptic women. PAPP-B is a larger glyco-protein, and the concentration in maternal blood follows similar patterns to those of hPL. Pregnancy-associated plasma protein 5 (PAPP-5) is a small

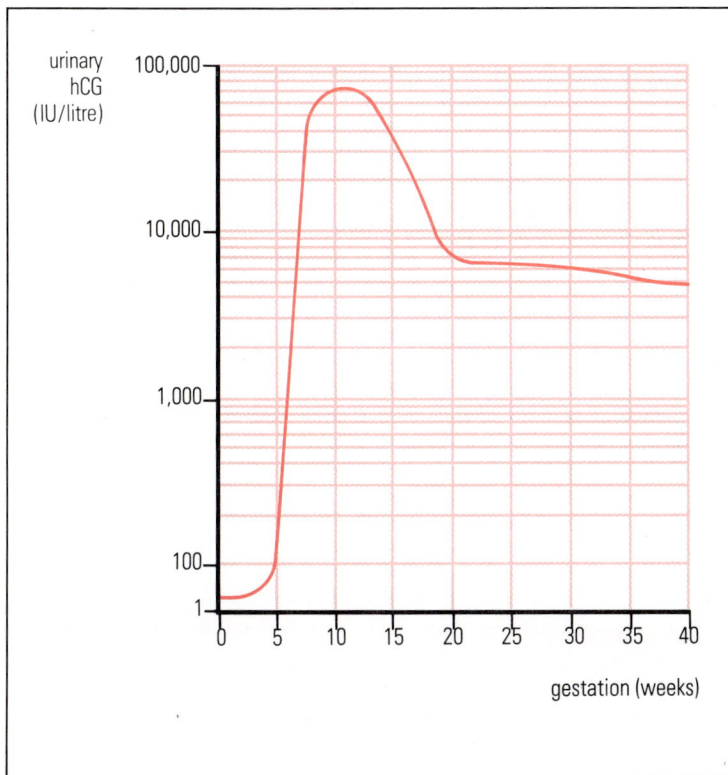

Fig.3.18 hCG concentrations in the urine throughout pregnancy. Note that this is a log scale and therefore some hCG can be detected even in the first days of pregnancy.

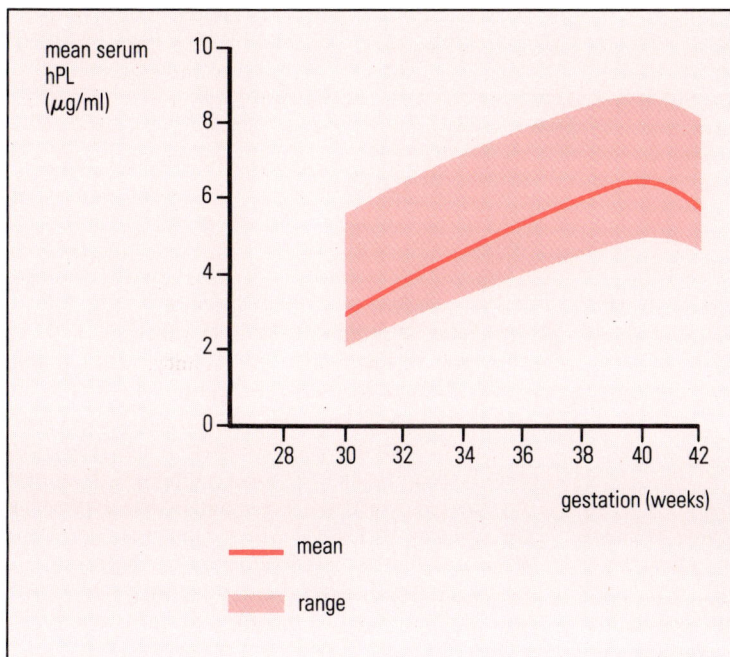

Fig.3.19 Serum hPL levels in late pregnancy. The mean ± 2 SD is shown; note that the range is wide.

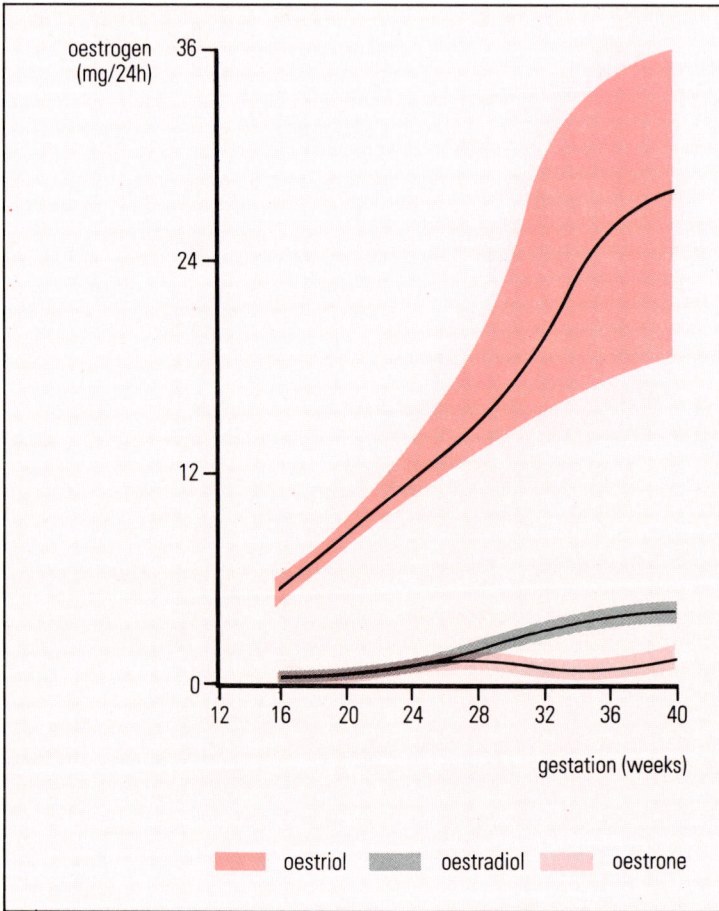

Fig.3.20 Concentrations of oestrogens throughout pregnancy. Oestrone and oestradiol levels increase only slightly but the production of oestriol increases greatly as the pregnancy progresses. For each hormone, the mean ± 2 SD is shown.

glycoprotein which may inhibit protease activity in the placenta.

Schwangerschaftsprotein (SP1) is a glycoprotein, the concentration of which increases in pregnancy. It provides a measure of placental activity, particularly in suspected placental dysfunction. It can be measured by radioimmunoassay and by immuno-assay in late pregnancy.

Placental enzymes

Cystine aminopeptidase and heat-stable alkaline phosphatase are produced by the placenta. Their levels have been reported as reduced with poor placental function and raised in severe toxaemia, although their measurement is not considered a standard test.

Fetoplacental steroids

OESTROGENS

Three main oestrogens are found in the maternal serum: oestrone, oestradiol and oestriol, the ratio of their concentrations being one to two to thirty. Oestrone is very active but is not found in high concentrations in young women. Oestradiol is the major oestrogen in the human; it has a weak hormonal action. In pregnancy, the fetal liver metabolizes increased concentrations of oestriol precursors, which are subsequently metabolized in the placenta to form the fully functional steroid. In the last weeks of gestation, eighty-five percent of the oestrogen produced is oestriol. Although it is a weaker hormone, its presence swamps that of the others (Fig.3.20).

The concentrations of plasma oestrogens generally

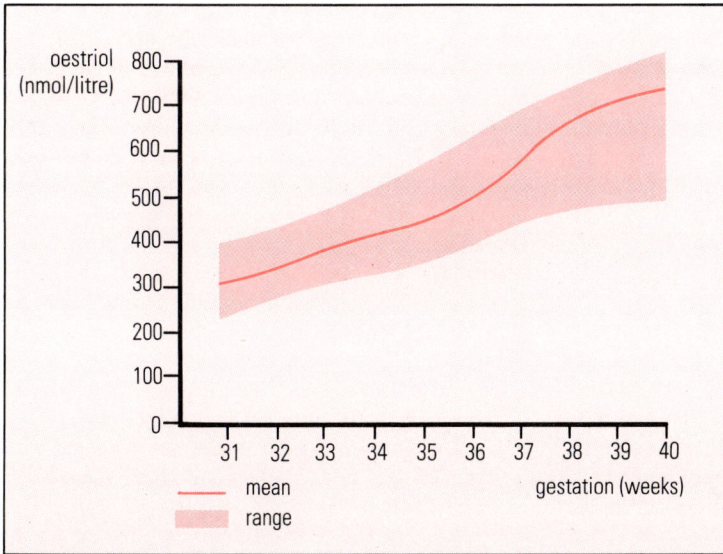

Fig.3.21 Concentration of plasma oestriol in late pregnancy. The mean ± 2 SD is shown.

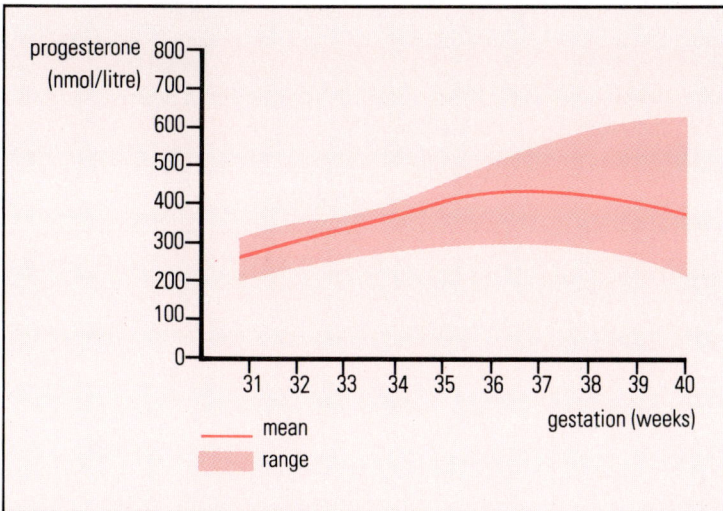

Fig.3.22 Progesterone concentration in the maternal blood in late pregnancy. The range is wide and reflects mostly variation in placental bulk rather than in placental function.

rise during pregnancy but there are diurnal variations and other fluctuations. Consequently, twenty-four hour urine specimens, rather than single samples of plasma, are used for the determination of hormone levels, thus eliminating the short-term variations. A decline in fetoplacental growth and metabolic activity may be associated with a reduction in the level of oestriol.

Oestrogen measurements are most useful when carried out as serial assays in a woman at high risk. It is important to note that the range of variation is large and action should not be taken on a single reading (Fig.3.21). However, after several readings, trends may appear which can alert the obstetrician to chronic ill health of the fetus.

PROGESTERONE
During pregnancy, progesterone is produced in large quantities by the syncytiotrophoblast, being secreted into both the maternal and fetal circulations (Fig.3.22). It can be easily measured by simple biochemical methods but is not useful in assessing the fetal state. It reflects the bulk of the placenta and thus may be raised in conditions associated with placental hypertrophy.

Biophysical monitoring

Biophysical tests measure the physical changes of the fetal body and are an increasingly popular method of monitoring fetal wellbeing. They are non-invasive, harmless to the mother and fetus, and can be repeated, hence a series of tests can be used to build up a dynamic picture of fetal development.

Ultrasound

The reflection of ultrasound waves by tissues of differing acoustic density can be used to measure distances very precisely. At the interface of fluids and solids, and differentially between certain solids, sound waves are reflected with different intensity. Ultrasound waves are transmitted in a narrow beam. Those which strike the reflecting surface at right angles are reflected back along the same course to a receiver. Those which strike at other angles are deflected and so are lost to measurement. When the source of the ultrasound waves and the receiver of the reflected waves are aligned, the distance from the source to the reflecting surface can be measured

accurately, knowing the speed of sound. If a second reflecting surface is also aligned with the source, then the distance between the two surfaces of the object can be measured. Thus, diameters of bony objects like the fetal skull can be measured with great precision (Fig.3.23) and a series of such measurements taken through the stages of gestation will reflect the growth of the biparietal diameter of the fetal head.

The modes of ultrasound are:

- A-scan. The reflected wave height varies with the acoustical density of the reflecting tissue. The biparietal eminences, being bone, stand out, so that two dense points may be identified and the distance between them measured (Fig.3.24).
- B-scan. The ultrasound waves are reflected as a series of dots and, as the transducer is moved, a picture can be built up on a retard VDU. This presents problems if the fetus is moving, as the image becomes blurred.
- Real time scanning. A pulsatile picture of the intrauterine contents is obtained by moving a transducer which contains a crystal rotating every 0.025 seconds. This represents a moving picture of the area under the transducer.

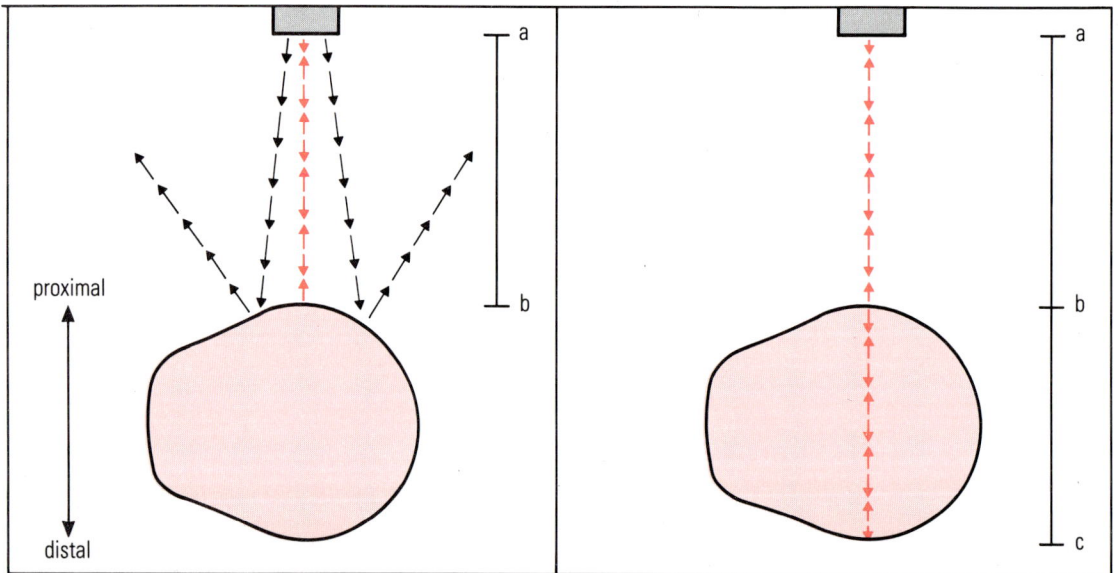

Fig.3.23 The use of ultrasound to measure biparietal diameter. Left: measurement of the distance (ab) from the machine to the proximal biparietal eminence. Reflected waves are shown in red and deflected waves in black. Right: measurement of the distance(ac) from the machine to the distal biparietal eminence. The biparietal diameter (bc) is easily calculated by subtracting ab from ac.

ULTRASOUND IN EARLY PREGNANCY

The amniotic sac can be identified from five to six weeks of gestation; the embryo can just be seen at about this time. A missed abortion can thus be diagnosed and confirmed. The fetal heartbeat may be detected from about seven weeks, and fetal movements at nine weeks. The presence of two sacs can be shown, indicating a multiple pregnancy. However, very often one of the sacs is anembryonic, and only later in gestation is it apparent that just one fetus is present. Hydatidiform mole, which has a characteristic appearance on the ultrasound (see Chapter 5), can also be diagnosed at this stage.

The estimation of fetal gestational age can be made in early pregnancy by measurement of the crown to rump length. However, the variable degree of flexion of the fetus renders this an imprecise measure of fetal size after about twelve weeks of gestation. At an early stage, the parietal eminences of the fetal skull have not formed and therefore the biparietal diameter cannot be determined.

ULTRASOUND IN MID-PREGNANCY

In the second trimester, ultrasound scanning of the fetal head can measure the biparietal diameter very precisely (Fig.3.25). A series of readings between fourteen and twenty-four weeks provides an accurate assessment of gestational age (Fig.3.26). Growth of the biparietal diameter is approximately 3mm/ week

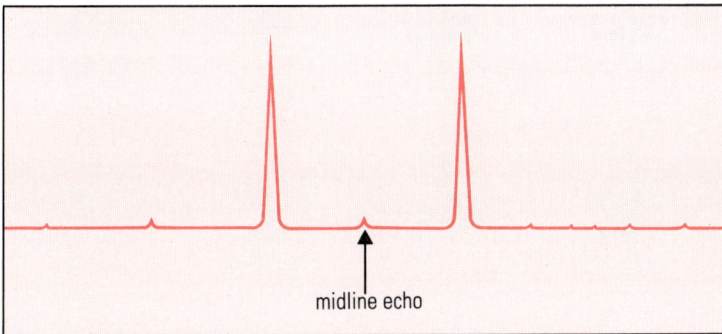

Fig.3.24 A-scan mode ultrasound. Between the waves produced by the biparietal eminences is a smaller midline echo, produced by reflection of waves from the double fold of dura mater lying between the cervical hemispheres.

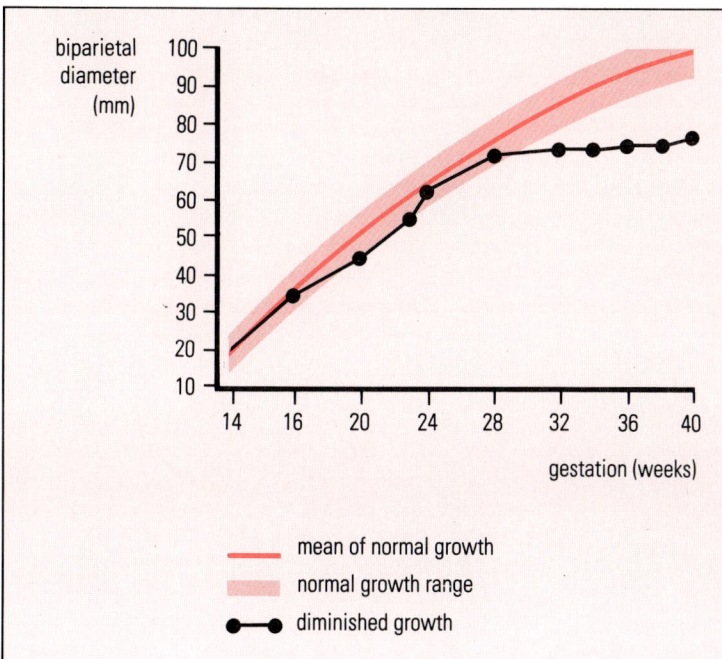

Fig.3.25 The mean ± 2 SD of the biparietal diameter throughout pregnancy. Note the narrowness of the range at any given week, and therefore the great precision of the test. Normal growth of the fetal head is compared with an abnormal pattern of diminished growth.

53

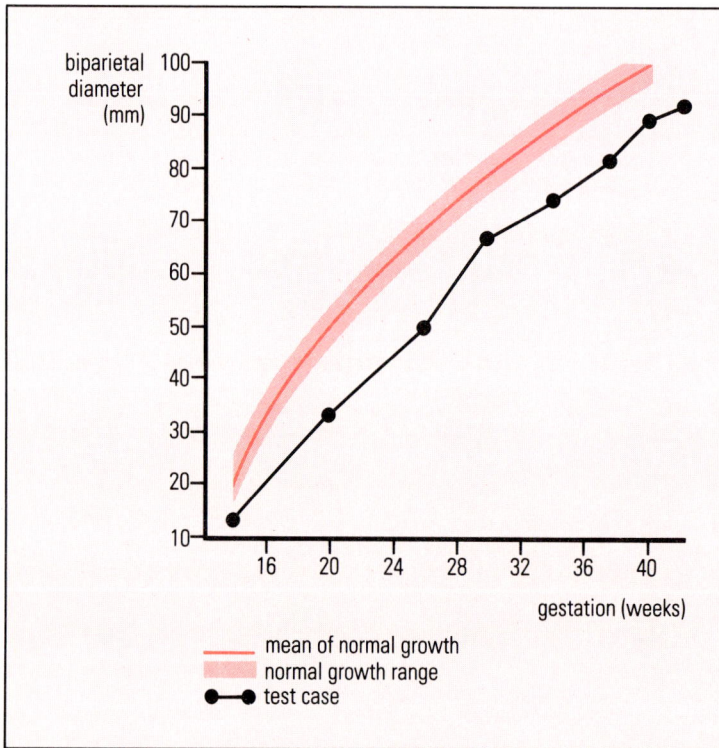

Fig.3.26 Biparietal diameter used to determine gestational age. The baby's growth is normal, but the mother was wrong in her dates. If the growth line is put back by 4 weeks, it fits the normal range.

and the range of variation is narrow. A standard scanning programme at an antenatal clinic will include one reading of the biparietal diameter at fourteen to eighteen weeks and a second at about thirty weeks. Any variation from normal growth patterns can be seen by comparison of these readings with normal growth curves, and intrauterine growth retardation can be detected.

When used skilfully, ultrasound can detect congenital abnormalities in mid-pregnancy. Anencephaly, hydrocephaly and spina bifida can be visualized, and appropriate counselling given. The kidneys and bladder can be examined and any distension can be diagnosed. The heart may be scanned and all the chambers, septa and major vessels identified. Limbs can be measured and shortening detected. The amount of amniotic fluid can be estimated and this guides the obstetrician to look for other abnormalities, such as oesophageal atresia, immediately after birth.

ULTRASOUND IN LATE PREGNANCY

Measurement of the biparietal diameter in the third trimester is not as predictive as measurements taken earlier in pregnancy. The rate of growth slows and the range of variation is wider (Fig.3.27). However, the abdominal circumference can be readily measured. This gives an estimate of fetal liver size. Since the head of the fetus is relatively spared during placental malperfusion, measurements of the abdomen can provide an earlier indication of the intrauterine state of the fetus than measurements of the head alone. Serial plots of the cephalic circumference to abdominal circumference ratio can detect babies who are suffering from intrauterine malnutrition (Fig.3.28). This ratio is of little use when the fetus is symmetrically growth retarded, as the abdominal and cephalic circumferences are similarly affected.

Amniocentesis is used in the early stages of pregnancy to check for fetal abnormalities. It can also be useful later on for assessing the degree of rhesus effect in the fetus and fetal lung maturity (by measuring lecithin to sphingomyelin ratios). Such penetration of the amniotic sac should always be done under ultrasound control. The placenta and fetus should be localized and the pool of liquor which is most easily available should be pierced.

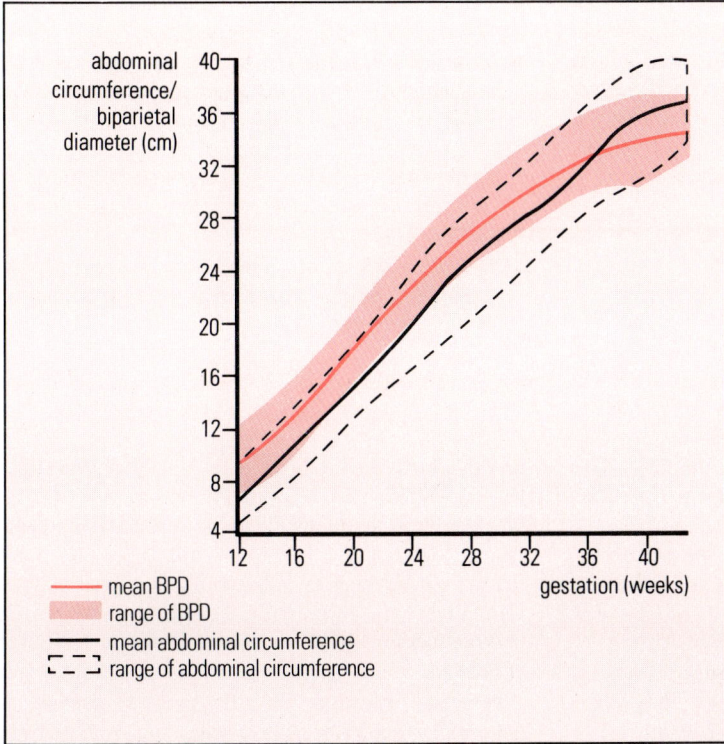

Fig.3.27 Ultrasound measurement of biparietal diameter and abdominal circumference in late pregnancy. There is a diminution of cephalic, but not of abdominal growth in the last weeks of pregnancy.

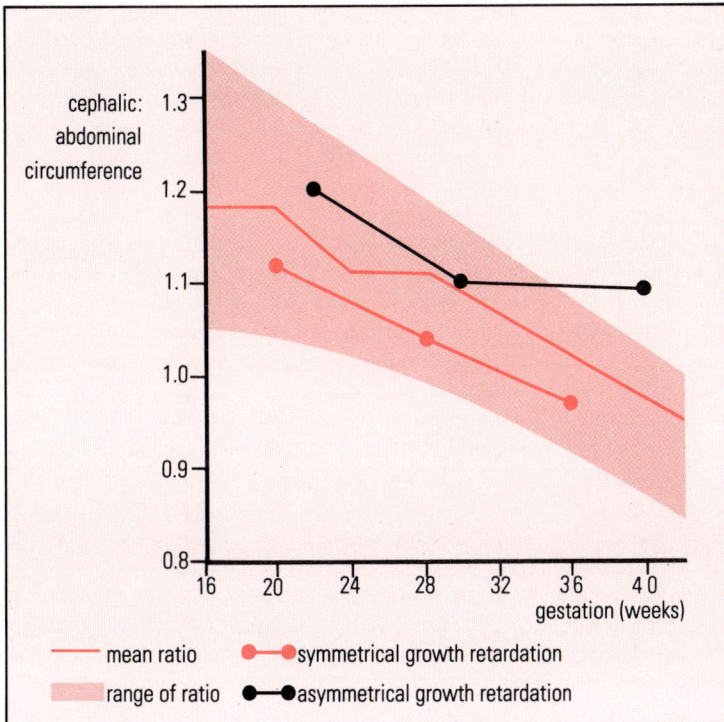

Fig.3.28 Cephalic to abdominal circumference ratio. The mean ± 2 SD is shown. Since the rate of growth of head circumference decreases as pregnancy advances, the ratio diminishes. If there is symmetrical growth retardation, the ratio will decrease at the normal rate. In asymmetrical growth retardation, the ratio in the last weeks of pregnancy is high and lies outside the normal range.

A rough dynamic assessment of fetal wellbeing in late pregnancy can be made using ultrasound to estimate the amount of time the fetus spends in rotation and performing limb movements. Fetal chest wall movements (fetal breathing) have been measured and their associations investigated. Correlations with alterations in fetal wellbeing are not strong.

Cardiotocography

Monitoring of both the fetal heart rate and the uterine pressure allows the heart pattern to be assessed in response to external constraints. This has the advantage over biochemical tests of giving an immediate result, monitoring what is actually happening to the fetus at any precise moment. The following signals from the fetal heart are used to monitor its rate:

- Sound. This can be picked up by a carbon microphone placed on the mother's abdomen. This is less efficient with an obese patient or a very active fetus.
- Electrical output. This can be picked up by external electrodes on the mother's abdominal wall or, once the membranes have ruptured in labour, by internal electrodes applied to the presenting part of the fetus.
- Reflection of ultrasound. The Doppler effect from the moving column of blood in major vessels can be detected with ultrasound waves. This is the commonest method now used antenatally.

Uterine pressures are usually monitored simultaneously with the fetal heart rate, so that the effect of uterine muscle activity on the fetus may be assessed. Externally, this is done with a displacement transducer, placed on the mother's abdomen, which measures the frequency and duration of contractions but not their intensity.

Internal pressure monitoring can be carried out only after rupture of the membranes. A fluid-filled catheter allows measurement of the displacement of the fluid, or a catheter with a pressure transducer at its distal end may be used. Using either method, the intensity of contractions and their frequency and duration may be assessed.

Cardiotocography can be undertaken from about twenty-six weeks gestation, becoming more precise as pregnancy advances and the fetus becomes larger. Assessment of the cardiotocograph trace is based on the interpretation of four criteria:

- The baseline heart rate. This should lie between 120 and 160 beats/min (Fig.3.29).
- A variability in the baseline heart rate of at least 5 beats/min. This is expected on a normal trace. Single or multiple receivers may be used during cardiotocography, making it an easy method of monitoring. Since the signal is averaged, variability cannot be accurately assessed, but a general idea of variance can be gained.
- Periodic accelerations. These occur when the heart responds to stimuli, for example uterine activity or fetal movement. This is expected on a normal trace.
- Periodic decelerations. External stimuli should not provoke a deceleration in fetal heart rate.

Baseline tachycardia in the fetus before labour might be associated with chronic hypoxia, but this is unusual. It is more likely to be due to a maternal factor; for instance, the mother might be receiving a tocolytic drug such as salbutamol. The fetus may be immature with an underdeveloped parasympathetic nervous system or it may be anaemic, as in rhesus effect.

Maternal infection may be present, leading to maternal pyrexia and tachycardia, and consequently a fetal tachycardia. A compensatory burst of speeded fetal heart rate may occur after a period of bradycardia; this is physiological and usually settles.

A bradycardia is commonly associated with fetal acidosis. It might also be associated with high uterine tone, maternal hypotension, or a defect in the fetal cardiovascular system, all of which reduce fetoplacental exchange.

Reduced variability (Fig.3.30) may be due to fetal acidosis following chronic hypoxia, or drugs given to the mother. In the latter case, the variability improves as the effect of the drug wears off. The fetus sleeps in the uterus, and during these times the trace is often flat (Fig.3.31), but variability improves on waking.

Accelerations are the normal physiological response to any stress. A tracing with no accelerations may indicate a fetus, for example one which is growth retarded, that is not able to respond as efficiently as normal, but is not actually in any distress.

If decelerations occur, it is important to determine when they occur in relation to the uterine contractions. Decelerations occurring coincidentally with a contraction, and recovering immediately after the contraction wears off, are called synchronous,

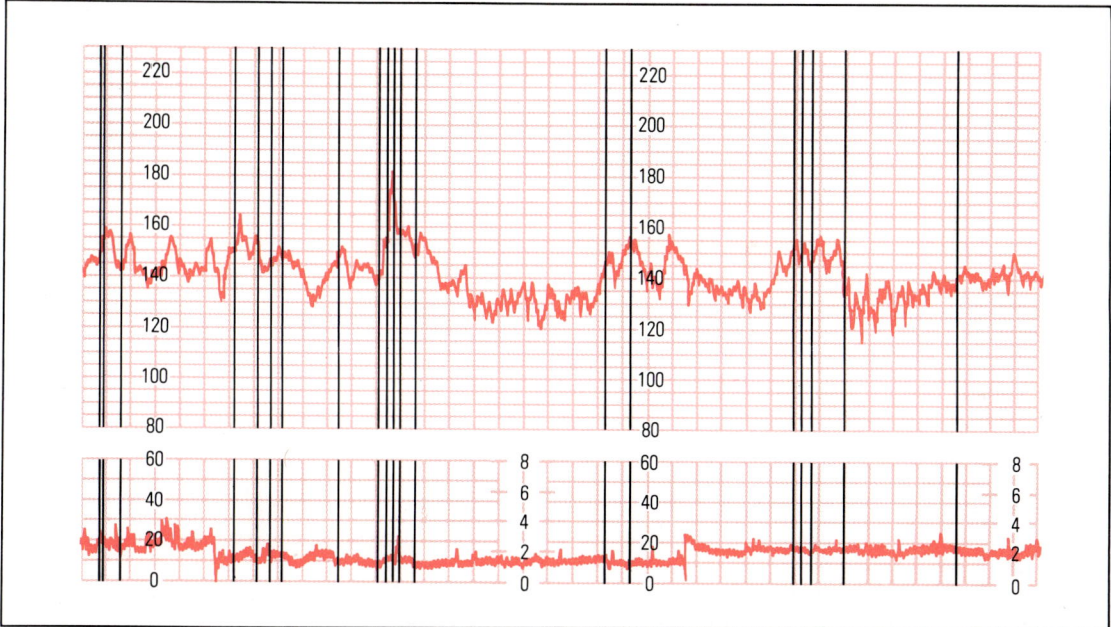

Fig.3.29 A normal antenatal cardiotocograph trace which shows a normal fetal heart rate above and uterine muscle tone below. The heart rate is 120–140 beats/min ; there is good baseline variability. Accelerations of the heart rate are seen, particularly in association with fetal movements (indicated by vertical bars).

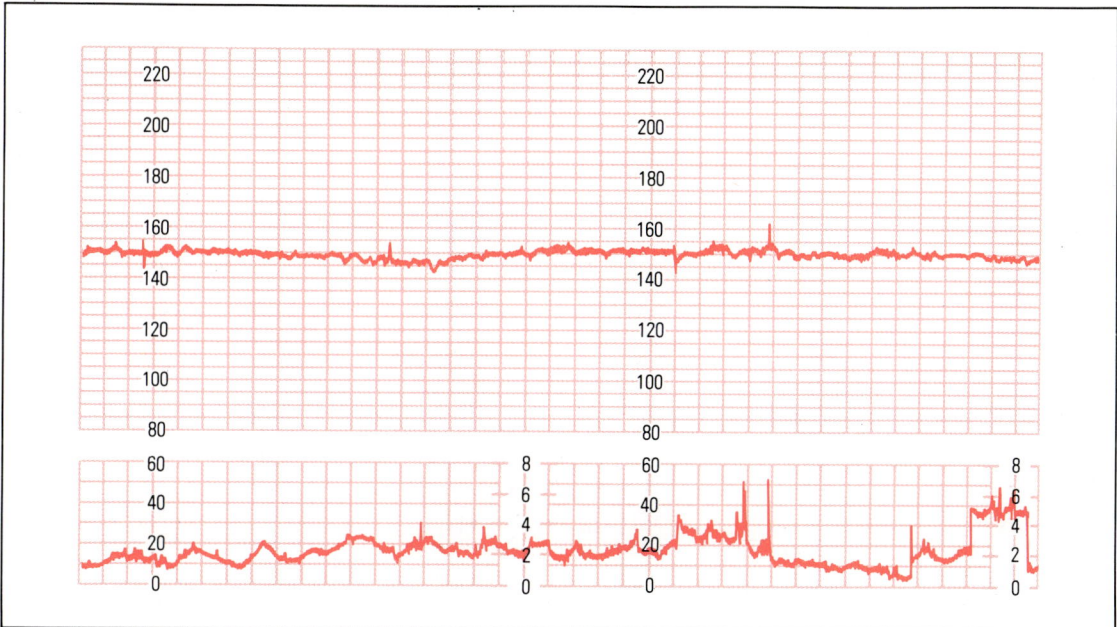

Fig.3.30 Reduced variability. The fetal heart rate is about 150 beats/min, but none of the variability seen in Fig. 3.29 exists; this is a very flat unreactive trace.

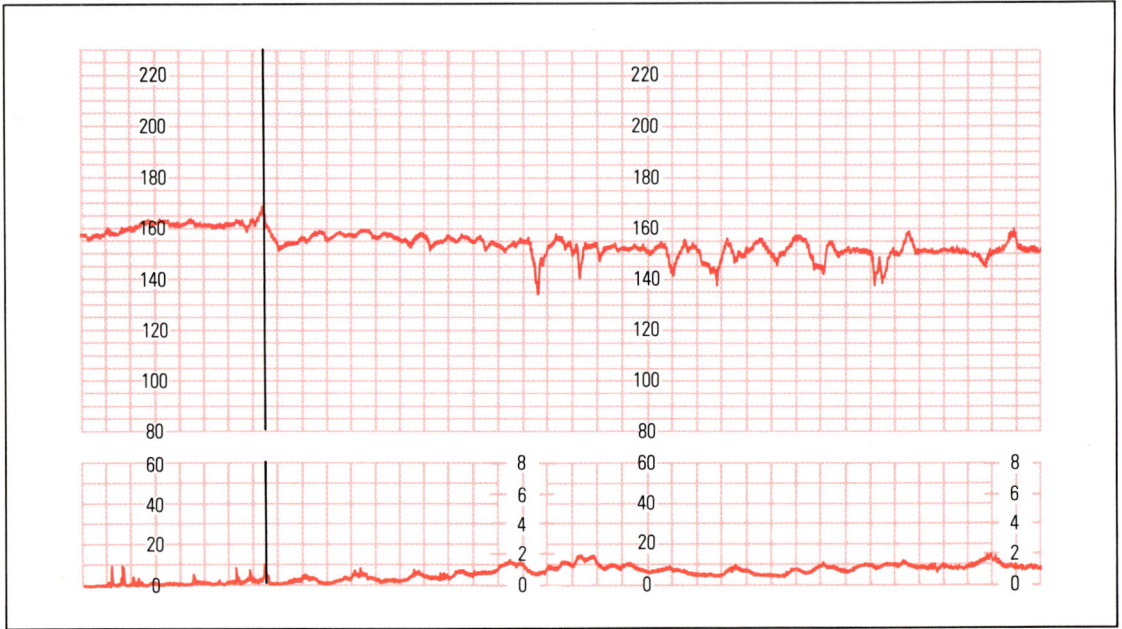

Fig.3.31 The fetus has been asleep; the left edge shows the end of a long run of a rather flat trace. In the 4th minute the fetus makes a movement (vertical bar) and wakes and the trace improves considerably thereafter, so that 10 minutes later it is a perfectly normal, reactive trace.

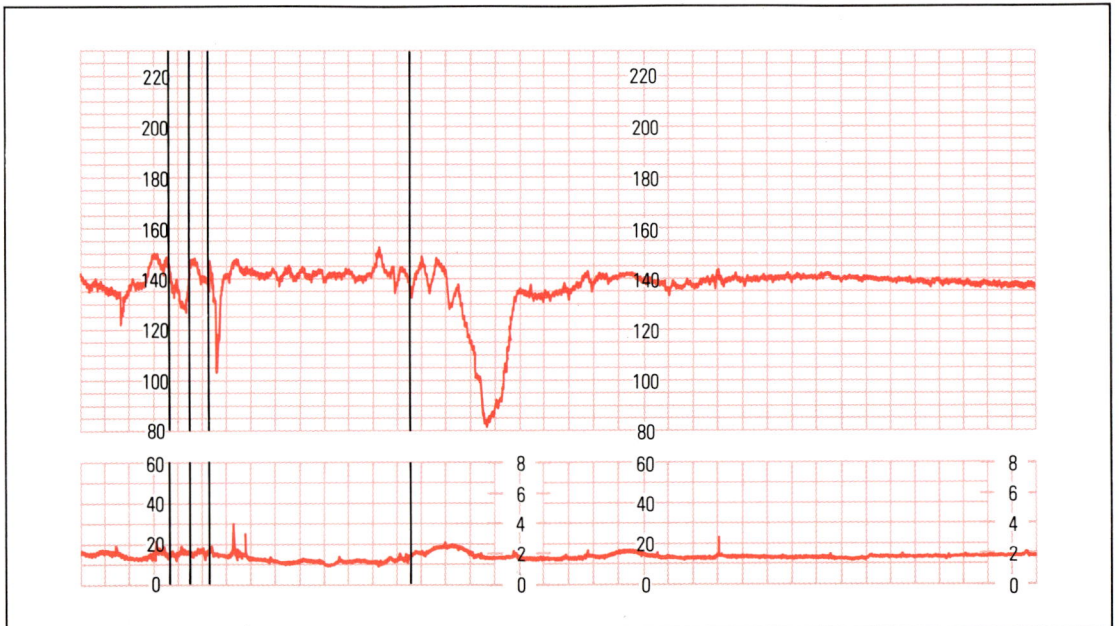

Fig.3.32 The fetal heart rate is initially about 140 beats/min with a good baseline variability. A small contraction in the 7th minute is followed by a deep deceleration to 80 beats/min, which is delayed at onset. This is a late deceleration and implies fetal hypoxia.

or early. They are a very early warning sign, but not a sinister one in itself. If there is delay in their onset, or a lag in their recovery after the end of the contraction, they are later, or non-synchronous decelerations (Fig.3.32), since they indicate a heart which is sluggish and does not respond quickly to the changes of hypoxia. Often the pattern is a complex one; variable decelerations may be a result of transient changes, for example temporary umbilical cord compression. When such a woman and her fetus are monitored for a longer period, the pattern usually becomes one of early or late decelerations, depending on whether the fetal state improves or worsens.

If there is no uterine activity for about twenty minutes during the tracing, the fetus may be stimulated by gently pressing on the abdomen. Alternatively, a trained staff member can sit with the woman and gently palpate the abdomen, noting any fetal movements which may appear on the trace.

Most women with a high risk fetus are now monitored by a series of ultrasound estimations of fetal growth and daily or twice weekly cardiotocographic measurements. Monitoring alterations in the fetal heart rate gives a more immediate assessment of the fetal state than biochemical tests, which tend to reflect past events.

Radiology

Radiology was the first method of measuring and monitoring the intrauterine fetus. It is now less commonly used, due to the hazardous effects of irradiation of the fetus. In early pregnancy, it may be teratogenic; later, it may be associated with an increased incidence of malignancy in the exposed child up to the age of ten years. Additionally, it is thought that chromosomes in the fetal gonads are more sensitive to radiation than those in the adult and exposure may thus lead to genetic mutation. However, in some circumstances, radiological examination may still be justified.

X-rays can be used to determine fetal age by examining the epiphyses for centres of ossification. These indicate that the fetus is past a certain gestational age. For example, the lower end of the femur is seen at thirty-six weeks, the upper end of tibia at thirty-eight weeks, and the calcaneum at forty weeks.

Congenital abnormalities can be spotted on X-ray using a radio-opaque element in later pregnancy. Anencephaly, hydrocephaly and spina bifida can all

be detected, but the lateness of their diagnosis often means that little can be done to prevent the baby being born.

Intrauterine death can be confirmed by examining the crumpling effects on the fetus, with overlapping of the parietal bones (Spalding's sign) and gas in the major vessels. These changes are found from two to seven days after fetal death.

X-rays can confirm the number of fetuses, and this is particularly useful in higher multiple pregnancies. If triplets, quadruplets or quintuplets are suspected, an abdominal X-ray will give a more precise picture than ultrasound.

X-rays are still of great use in assessing the maternal pelvis, since diminution of various pelvic diameters can be seen on correctly positioned X-rays.

Biological monitoring

Biological monitoring, in which fetal cells and cell products are tested, is not as widely used as biophysical methods. However, it can add useful information in the diagnosis of some fetal diseases.

Amniocentesis

At amniocentesis, amniotic fluid is withdrawn from the amniotic sac through the mother's uterus and abdominal wall. It is performed after sixteen weeks gestation, when fetal skin cells are shed into the amniotic fluid. In later pregnancy, amniotic fluid contains fetal urine and lung fluid, thus cells from the urinary and respiratory tracts may also be present. In early pregnancy, however, fetal fibroblasts are mainly used for diagnosis.

Amniocentesis is usually performed under ultrasound scanning control, so that the placenta, fetus and liquor pool can be identified. Under local anaesthesia, 10-20ml of clear fluid is withdrawn through a needle. This is easier after sixteen weeks gestation when the liquor volume increases rapidly. The increase in volume of amniotic fluid is as follows:

10 weeks	——	35ml
15 weeks	——	130ml
20 weeks	——	500ml
35 weeks	——	1000ml

There is a small risk associated with amniocentesis; less than one percent of women abort within three

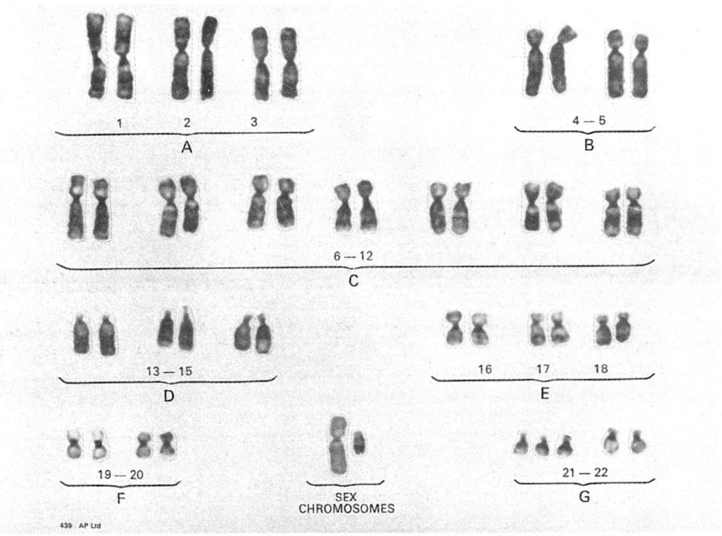

Fig.3.33 Karyotype in Down's syndrome. The chromosomes are normal, except at position 21, where there is a trisomy.

weeks of the procedure. In addition, there are other associated risks, such as rhesus immunization of a sensitized child, haemorrhage, infection, and direct damage to the fetus. In the longer term, a chronic lack of amniotic fluid, due to leakage through an unsealed punctum in the membranes, may lead to premature labour and compression of the fetus (producing hip and knee deformities). These risks can be minimized by using experienced operators, ultrasound dating of the pregnancy and localization of the sampling site. The commonly quoted figure of a one percent risk of complication is probably a high estimate.

The indications for amniocentesis in the mid-trimester of pregnancy are associated with congenital abnormalities. The alpha-fetoprotein levels in amniotic fluid can be measured as previously described. Amniocentesis is also undertaken in cases of suspected congenital abnormalities to examine fetal chromosomes. The skin cells provide a chromosome biopsy typical of the whole fetus, except in the rare incidence of a mosaic. After withdrawal, the skin cells are cultured for approximately three weeks and examined for any chromosome abnormality. The commonest is Down's syndrome, with a trisomy in position twenty-one (Fig.3.33). Amniocentesis for Down's syndrome may be offered to any woman of thirty-five years or more, since at this age the risk of the test is equivalent to the risk of having an affected fetus (Fig.3.34).

Any couple who have had a previously affected child, or a child with any chromosomal translocation, should be examined themselves and offered amniocentesis. Similarly, any couple with an X-linked disorder, for example Duchenne's muscular dystrophy, may have the fetal sex determined.

Amniocentesis in late pregnancy may be used to assess the severity of the damage to a rhesus affected fetus. The liquor is tested for bilirubin products by measuring optical density (see Fig.5.15). The amniotic fluid in late pregnancy may also be tested for fetal maturity by measuring the lecithin to sphingomyelin ratio. Both are constituents of surfactant and the amount of lecithin increases steadily to term. A fetus with ratio of two or more is unlikely to suffer respiratory distress syndrome.

Before amniocentesis is carried out, the indications for the test, procedure and possible course of action, must be discussed with the parents, for example whether termination would be considered if Down's syndrome were diagnosed.

Fetoscopy

At fetoscopy, a narrow endoscope is passed through the abdominal wall and uterus to examine the fetus. It can provide a direct view of the fetus and allow a sample of fetal blood to be taken for biochemical and haematological assessment. At present, the technique

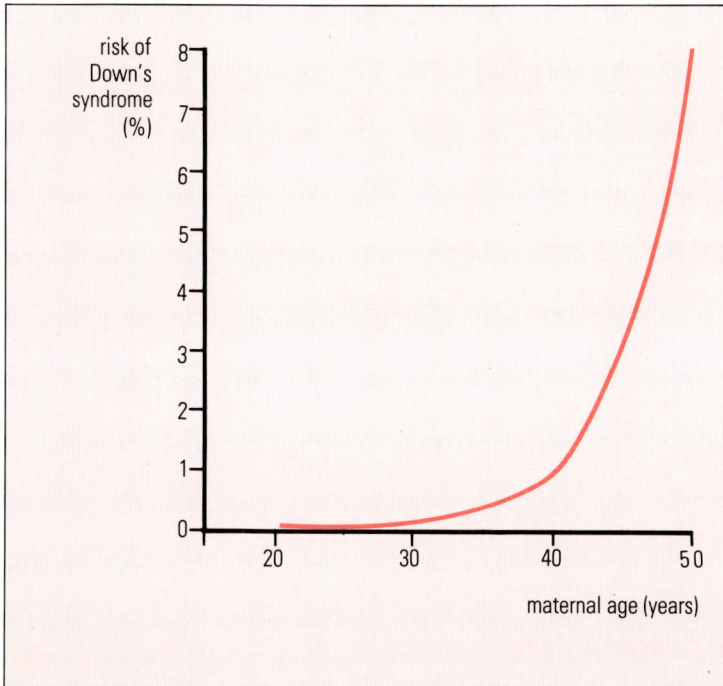

Fig.3.34 The probability of Down's syndrome increases with maternal age. Risk remains very low below 35, but increases sharply after 40 years.

is of limited use for detecting externally apparent fetal abnormalities such as hare lip, or those diseases where intrauterine diagnosis can be made by biopsy of fetal tissue.

Before embarking on fetoscopy, it is necessary that the parents fully understand what is involved in the technique, what will be investigated, the availability of results, the limitations of the test, and the course of action they would consider in view of the various possible outcomes of the investigation. In some cases, an amniocentesis prior to fetoscopy may eliminate the need for the investigation, for example investigation of haemophilia need only be done by fetoscopy if amniocentesis shows a male fetus.

The examination is performed under local anaesthetic and is usually done at eighteen weeks gestation. In some centres, fetoscopy has been replaced by ultrasound-directed fetal blood sampling from the vessels at the base of the umbilical cord. There is only minimal risk of fetomaternal haemorrhage, thus any chance of rhesus sensitization or restimulation is small because the cord blood vessel contracts.

One application of fetal blood sampling is in the investigation of the haemoglobinopathies, in particular thalassaemia, to estimate whether the fetus will suffer from a major degree of the condition. Haemophilia can be investigated by analysis of the levels of factor VIII, and in Christmas disease the amount of factor IX is assessed. In addition, chromosomal studies can be performed on leucocytes. In some centres, a prediction of chronic hypoxia can be made from measuring lactate levels and pH of fetal blood.

Fetal biopsy can be performed, for example of the skin, which may be useful in diagnosis of epidermolysis bullosa or congenital icthyosis. Liver and muscle biopsies are possible to aid in the diagnosis of disorders of these systems.

Fetal inspection can be difficult but may be indicated, for example in a couple who have had a previous child with a severe facial cleft or a severe limb defect, such as the autosomal dominant lobster claw hand. Simple operative procedures may be performed, guided by the fetoscope. With urethral and megacystis syndromes, pressure in the fetal

61

bladder can be reduced by intrauterine suprapubic catheterization.

In the future, fetoscopy may be used more often as a means of prenatal fetal treatment. At present, there is a three to five percent risk of abortion soon after the procedure but there does not appear to be any increased risk of orthopaedic or respiratory problems to the fetus, nor is there an increase in the incidence of intrauterine growth retardation. Ultrasound directed procedures, such as fetal blood sampling, may replace some of the fetoscopic investigations currently employed.

4. The Fetus at Risk

INTRODUCTION

Many of the conditions considered briefly in this chapter are described in detail elsewhere in the book. They are grouped together here to outline the idea of the fetus at high risk. The risks to the fetus can be divided into chronic and acute groups (Fig.4.1); within the former group are three major types of predisposing factor:
- Maternal
- Fetal
- Fetomaternal

Although these are all interlinked, it is useful to classify and analyse them seperately in order to quantify the hazards facing any individual fetus.

CHRONIC RISKS

Maternal factors

These factors should all be taken into account in the management of pregnancy so that any preventative measures may be implemented or necessary precautions taken to ensure successful delivery of the fetus.

Maternal age

Maternal age is a factor often associated with fetal risk in women at the extremes of reproductive age (less than twenty and over thirty-five years; see Fig.3.13). In the younger age group, girls are more

RISKS TO THE FETUS			
Chronic			Acute
Maternal factors	Fetal factors	Fetomaternal factors	
age	multiple pregnancy	intrauterine growth retardation (IUGR)	placental abruption
parity	abnormal fetus		fetal hypoxia
socioeconomic class		preterm labour	cord prolapse
race		premature rupture of membranes	
smoking		postmaturity	
diet		malpresentation	
past obstetric history		cephalopelvic disproportion	
general health			

Fig.4.1 Chronic and acute risks to the fetus. The former may be divided into maternal, fetal and fetomaternal factors.

likely to be unsupported, alone and emotionally immature. They have an increased risk of carrying a growth retarded fetus, and of having a preterm labour or premature rupture of membranes. Women over thirty-five years old have an increased risk of producing fetuses with chromosomal trisomies. They are also more likely to suffer from concurrent maternal disease, for example hypertension. Placental bed perfusion is poor in women with essential hypertension.

Parity

The parity of a woman may affect fetal risk (see Fig.3.13). Women who have not previously delivered a child (nulliparae) are untested in childbearing. It is not known whether they have a predisposition to small fetuses, or to enter preterm labour. In labour, they have a pelvis that is untested and their ability to deliver vaginally is unknown. Women of a parity greater than four have high-risk fetuses, but it is impossible to completely separate parity *per se* from other factors such as social class, as larger family size is associated with lower socioeconomic class and thus degrees of poverty. This group of women often have a rapid labour with a precipitate delivery and also have a greater chance of suffering a postpartum haemorrhage, usually due to failure of the uterus to contract efficiently.

Socioeconomic class

Socioeconomic class is an important factor when assessing fetal risk (see Fig.3.13). Women from the lower social classes are at a higher risk of having a growth retarded fetus and of having a preterm labour. It is difficult to identify the precise reason for this, but the women in these classes tend also to be at the extremes of age and parity, smoke more heavily and eat less well than women from the higher social classes. High-risk factors seem to cluster around those in social class IV and V.

Socioeconomic class is determined by the occupation of the woman's husband. If he is unemployed, in prison, or a member of the Armed Services, she is unclassifiable. Obviously, if she is unmarried, there is no husband with an occupation to classify. Hence, unmarried women are often not considered in class analyses, which is paradoxical as they constitute some of the mothers with fetuses at highest risk.

Race

Race is also an important consideration, as there are some specific risks attached to particular ethnic groups (for example thalassaemia in races of Mediterranean descent, and sickle cell haemoglobinopathies in Negroid people). As well as specific problems, many women of non-European origin, for example those from the Indian subcontinent, live in areas affected by malnutrition and chronic disease and consequently may have smaller babies. Many Negro women have a pelvis that is characteristically android in shape and therefore descent of the head is commonly delayed during labour.

Smoking

Women who smoke cigarettes place their fetuses at a higher risk and should be encouraged to stop, at least for the duration of their pregnancy. The fetus is more likely to be growth retarded (see Fig.3.11), and to become hypoxic during labour due to reduction in placental exchange.

Diet

Maternal diet is important, particularly in early pregnancy, when the opportunity to correct deficiencies still exists. Certain religions prevent some women from eating foods which contain essential elements and may also demand long periods of fasting. Vegetarians and vegans may be advised about their diet to ensure that it is more adequately suited to the needs of pregnancy; supplements of minerals or vitamins may be needed.

Past obstetric history

The past obstetric history is one of the major prognostic factors in assessing fetal risk. Reproductive patterns tend to repeat themselves and the capacity for a couple consistently to produce healthy offspring often continues from one pregnancy to another. Conversely, a previously bad obstetrical outcome may also repeat itself.

Previous uncomplicated therapeutic terminations of pregnancy in the first trimester are of little physical importance, although psychologically they may be damaging. Later therapeutic terminations may cause cervical trauma and incompetence, leading to mid-trimester abortion. However, in the majority of cases, if the termination is performed correctly, this will not occur. Spontaneous abortion in the first trimester may be associated with a slightly higher risk of placental abruption and growth retardation in subsequent pregnancies. Late spontaneous abortions are often associated with maternal chronic pelvic infection and cervical incompetence.

A woman with a previous stillbirth or intrauterine death will usually be anxious about her current pregnancy, particularly if no attributable cause was found for the previous problem. Since the patient will have a two to three times greater chance of another perinatal death, the fetus must be carefully monitored clinically, in addition to ultrasound, cardiotocographic or hormonal measurements.

A woman who has previously had a growth retarded or low birth weight infant has a high risk of recurrence. From the patient's history, the obstetrician should institute a programme of close monitoring so that any warning of this may be detected in the early stages of pregnancy. A woman with a previously abnormal fetus will need special counselling and possible investigation, depending on the nature of the abnormality. For example, if the fetus had a neural tube defect, she should be offered alpha-fetoprotein screening or a detailed ultrasound assessment.

The vast majority of women who have previously had children report a normal obstetric history. They are likely to repeat the good performance, although obviously one should not become complacent and should still be on the lookout for any possible problems. The general health of the mother and any therapy that she may be taking is very important in assessing the risk to the fetus. As well as drugs prescribed for illness, the woman may be consuming addictive drugs, for example cannabis or alcohol. The major maternal diseases and the treatments used are considered separately in Chapter 6, but they are all relevant here as they put the fetus at risk.

Fetal factors

The two principal fetal factors predisposing to chronic risk are multiple pregnancy and abnormalities in the fetus itself.

Multiple pregnancy

Multiple pregnancies occur as twins (one in one hundred births), triplets (one in eight thousand), quadruplets (one in thirty thousand), and, rarely, as higher orders. They are considered in detail in Chapter 11. In general, all the complications that can affect a single pregnancy may also affect a multiple pregnancy, but in the latter situation they tend to occur more frequently and more severely, for example maternal iron and folic acid deficiency anaemias, hypertension of pregnancy, and poly-hydramnios (particularly with uniovular twins). Preterm labour and premature rupture of the membranes occur in fifty percent of multiple pregnancies, and antepartum haemorrhage, both from placental abruption and from placenta praevia, is more common than in singleton pregnancies.

Throughout pregnancy, it is more difficult to monitor the wellbeing of two fetuses than of one, since most of the biochemical tests available are invalidated. The usual methods of monitoring are ultrasound scanning and cardiotocographic tracing, although to obtain a satisfactory trace from two fetuses requires greater expertise. In labour, malpresentations are more common, predisposing to an increased incidence of prolapse of the umbilical cord at rupture of the membranes. There can be a delay in delivery of the second twin, associated with a higher perinatal mortality rate.

Abnormal fetus

An abnormal fetus is associated with a higher risk of spontaneous abortion, of premature rupture of the membranes and of preterm labour; however growth retardation is most common. It is of vital importance to know whether a woman has an abnormal fetus, since management may be modified. Caesarean section is less strongly indicated if the fetus has a lethal anomaly, since the operation puts the mother at unnecessary higher risk for less purpose.

Many of the malformations diagnosed *in utero* are known to be fatal (anencephaly), or have a high infant mortality rate (open spina bifida), while others are not lethal (uncomplicated Down's syndrome). Between these extremes are a group of abnormalities, the risks of which are difficult to assess before birth (for example structural cardiac or renal abnormalities) and their antenatal diagnosis will pose more problems in the future.

Fetomaternal factors

Intrauterine growth retardation

Intrauterine growth retardation (IUGR) is difficult to assess as a single entity and its aetiology is not fully understood. Lack of fetal perfusion may occur due to a number of factors. Maternal health has a bearing on the supply of blood to the uterus and local factors may affect perfusion of the villae of the placenta. The placental membrane may be altered to affect transfer, or fetal circulation may be inadequate, as in the fetuses from multiple pregnancies. It is this reduced placental transfer which leads to a poorer provision of nutrients in pregnancy and so to fetal IUGR.

In labour there is an even more acute reduction in oxygen supply leading to fetal distress. Hence, the fetus that is likely to be affected by hypoxia in labour may often be predicted by the detection of poor growth in the last weeks of pregnancy.

Preterm labour and premature rupture of membranes

In the aetiology of preterm labour or premature rupture of the membranes, the cause is sometimes thought to be obvious, for example high maternal pyrexia or a multiple pregnancy, but these may not be the only contributory factors.

The low birth weight infant, whether a growth retarded or preterm fetus, is at a higher risk after birth. There is a greater incidence of respiratory distress syndrome, the infant is unable to control blood pressure satisfactorily, and temperature control is imprecise due to deficiency of brown fat. The baby sucks poorly and feeding is unsatisfactory, while absorption from the gastrointestinal tract is not well organized. The liver is immature and neonatal jaundice is more common. Problems with intraventricular haemorrhage are also more frequent in this group of infants.

Postmaturity

Postmaturity is another fetomaternal factor, the aetiology of which is not well understood. A fetus over forty-two weeks of known gestation is more likely to suffer hypoxia in association with myometrial contractions, and is therefore at risk in labour. The vessels supplying the placental bed may age, or the transfer capability of the cells of the membrane may deteriorate.

Malpresentation and malposition

Malpresentation and malposition of the fetus will place it at higher risk. The former is more common if the placenta is low-lying, thus preventing the fetus from entering the pelvis properly. These conditions increase the risk of cord prolapse, which is more likely since the presenting part of the fetus does not fit into the pelvis. There is an increased risk of injury to the fetus during operative deliveries, for example those associated with breech presentation. Malpositions are associated with longer labours and with more operative deliveries.

Cephalopelvic disproportion

Cephalopelvic disproportion occurs when the fetal presenting part is too large for the maternal pelvis through which it must travel. Disproportion is a variable feature and a woman who has it at one delivery may not have it in a subsequent pregnancy, since it depends on both the size of the fetus and the angle at which the head descends into the pelvis. A poorly flexed head is more likely to cause problems than one that is well flexed. Futhermore, the power of the uterine contractions can vary from pregnancy to pregnancy. The fetus is at higher risk if disproportion is not diagnosed, since it leads to a longer labour with a higher chance of fetal hypoxia.

ACUTE RISKS

These are chance events occurring during pregnancy which place the fetus at high risk.

Placental abruption

Placental abruption (see Chapter 5), the separation of the placenta from its bed, is associated with grand multiparity, hypertension in pregnancy, trauma, and premature rupture of the membranes, particularly in an overstretched uterus with polyhydramnios. There is a tendency for this to recur, therefore any woman who has had a previous abruption will have a higher chance of suffering another one.

This event is associated with grave risks to the mother (hypovolaemic shock, intravascular coagulopathy and renal failure) and the fetus is at immediate risk from hypoxia. The placenta separates from the placental bed with concurrent cessation of exchange over a particular area. In addition to this, vascular spasm elsewhere in the placental bed diminishes blood flow to a degree dependent upon the severity of the abruption.

Fetal hypoxia

Fetal hypoxia associated with myometrial contractions usually occurs in labour but can also occur in late pregnancy. It is more common in growth retarded fetuses and in those that are immature or postmature. It is also associated with myometrial contractions that occur too frequently or are too strong; this may be spontaneous or may follow overstimulation of the uterus with oxytocics.

Cord prolapse

Umbilical cord prolapse is associated with preterm labour and with malpositions or malpresentations, where the fit of the fetal presenting part into the pelvis is poor. In addition to prolapse, spasm of the umbilical arteries from cooling, drying and handling of the cord causes fetal hypoxia. Mechanical compression of the cord between the maternal pelvis and the presenting part of the fetus or entrapment around a limb may cause hypoxia.

CONCLUSIONS

The acute risks to the fetus are often apparent and easier to diagnose than the chronic risks. In some cases, immediate treatment of the former by delivery gives good fetal outcome. Overall, however, the diagnosis and prophylactic treatment of the chronic factors would have a more significant effect on perinatal mortality and morbidity since by altering placental transfer, the fetus is not in such a good condition to withstand any hazard that may occur in labour. Additionally, the incidence of the chronic risks is much higher than that of the acute risks.

The analysis of fetal risk should be applied individually to each woman seen at the antenatal clinic. Maternal factors should be diagnosed and quantified at the first booking visit. Fetal and fetomaternal factors should be detected through good antenatal care and managed to minimize the danger to the fetus at the time of maximum risk – delivery.

5. Complications of Pregnancy

VOMITING

Nausea or vomiting occur during the first trimester in about sixty percent of nulliparous women and fifty percent of multiparous women. Symptoms may start as early as two weeks after the missed period and may continue until the beginning of the second trimester. Nausea may occur alone or with vomiting, and whilst this is known as morning sickness, it can occur at any time of day. It is not usually associated with any metabolic upset, and most women maintain their normal food intake.

Vomiting in pregnancy is thought to be caused, in part, by the rapid rise in oestrogens and progesterone (Fig.5.1) and also by the rapid stretching of the peritoneum over an expanding uterus; there may also be a psychological element. Specific causes of vomiting, such as a urinary tract infection or reaction to medication, such as iron tablets, should be excluded.

Treatment generally consists of rest and a change in eating pattern, taking frequent small meals rather than two heavy meals a day. If the symptoms persist, an antihistamine may be beneficial but the woman should be warned of the soporific side effects of many of the drugs in this group.

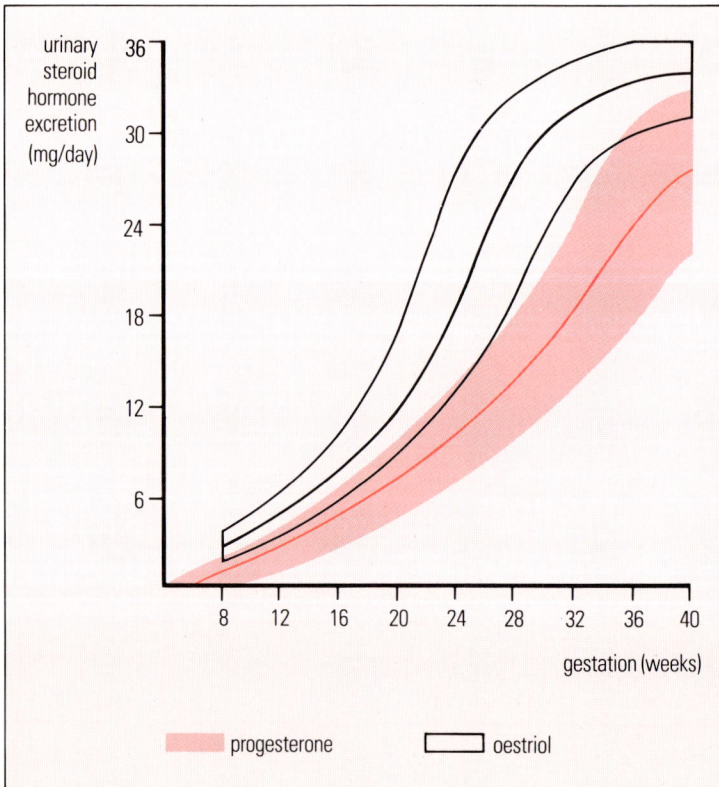

Fig.5.1 Rise in oestrogen and progesterone levels during pregnancy. The mean ±2 SD is shown for each hormone. The increase in progesterone starts first and affects the body as early as the 4th-6th week of gestation, causing a reduction in muscle tone and thus changes of pressure in the hollow muscular viscera, e.g. bladder, veins and stomach. Of the oestrogens, oestriol increases most markedly during pregnancy.

Vomiting occurs during late pregnancy in only a few women, but heartburn is common . It is due to the large mass in the abdomen pushing the acidic contents of the stomach up the oesophagus. The best advice in such cases is to maintain an upright posture and sleep with extra pillows; antacids or milk may provide symptomatic relief. Obviously, specific causes of vomiting must again be excluded.

Vomiting often occurs during labour. It may be due to oesophageal reflux exacerbated by hypotension or by drugs given for pain relief, for example pethidine. It is therefore usual to coadminister an antihistamine when giving intramuscular narcotics for pain, for example metoclopramide is given with pethidine.

Hyperemesis gravidarum

Excessive vomiting of pregnancy (hyperemesis gravidarum) is a rare condition, occurring in less than one in one thousand pregnancies in the United Kingdom. The woman suffers persistent vomiting, which is severe enough to cause metabolic imbalances. She is unable to retain adequate food or fluid and suffers from weight loss. There is haemoconcentration with electrolyte and urea disturbance and a ketosis (Fig.5.2).

The aetiology is not fully understood, but psychological and social aspects are believed to be important. Management must include exclusion of any specific causes of vomiting, such as urinary tract infection, gallbladder disease, obstructive gastrointestinal lesions, and expanding cerebral lesions.

Treatment involves admitting the woman to hospital to remove her from the home environment, maintenance of fluid and electrolyte balance with intravenous therapy, and provision of antiemetic drugs and sedation. Hyperemesis usually settles quickly with this regime. It is advisable to keep the woman in hospital for several days after the cessation of symptoms as the condition recurs readily. Termination of pregnancy is very rarely indicated if all supportive measures fail.

PRE-ECLAMPSIA

Pre-eclampsia is a disease specifically associated with pregnancy. It is characterized by the presence of two out of three major features:
- Raised blood pressure
- Proteinuria
- Oedema

The term pre-eclampsia implies that eclampsia will follow. However, since this does not always occur, some obstetricians refer to the condition as pregnancy associated hypertension (PAH).

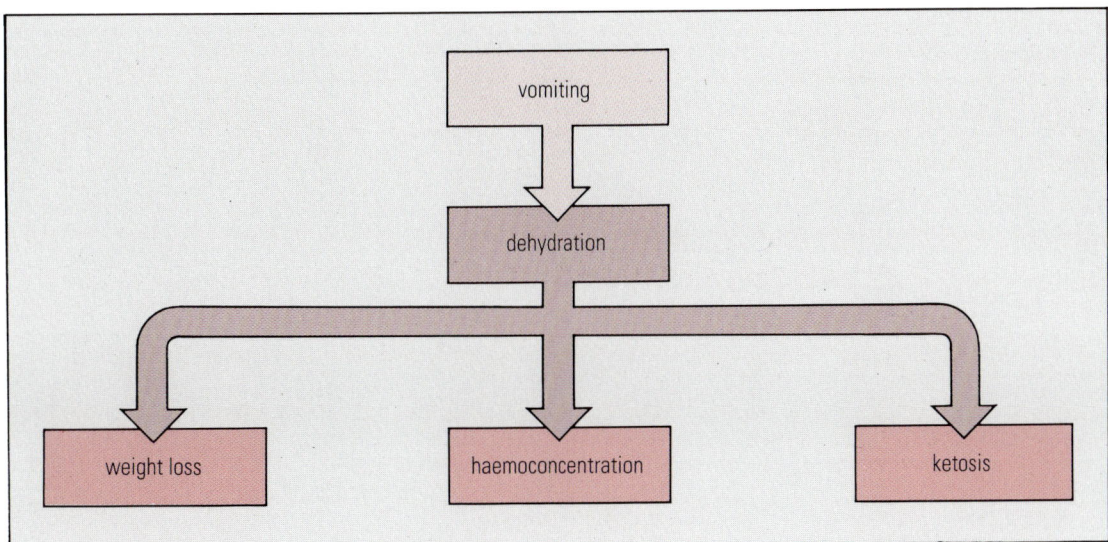

Fig.5.2 The effects of severe vomiting.

Incidence

In the United Kingdom, pre-eclampsia occurs in approximately fifteen percent of all antenatal patients. In other countries, the incidence is much lower. The incidence of the condition varies greatly within a population, but is most common in:
- Primigravidae
- Women over 35
- Multiple pregnancies
- Hydatidiform mole

Aetiology

The aetiology of pre-eclampsia is not, as yet, fully understood. However, it is probably an extension of a physiological process (Fig.5.3). In mid-pregnancy, there is an invasion of the decidua by trophoblast cells. These cells travel along the ends of the spiral arteries, eroding them and causing them to become dilated. If this trophoblast invasion does not occur, the ends of the vessels will not be opened out and so blood flow to the placental bed will be reduced.

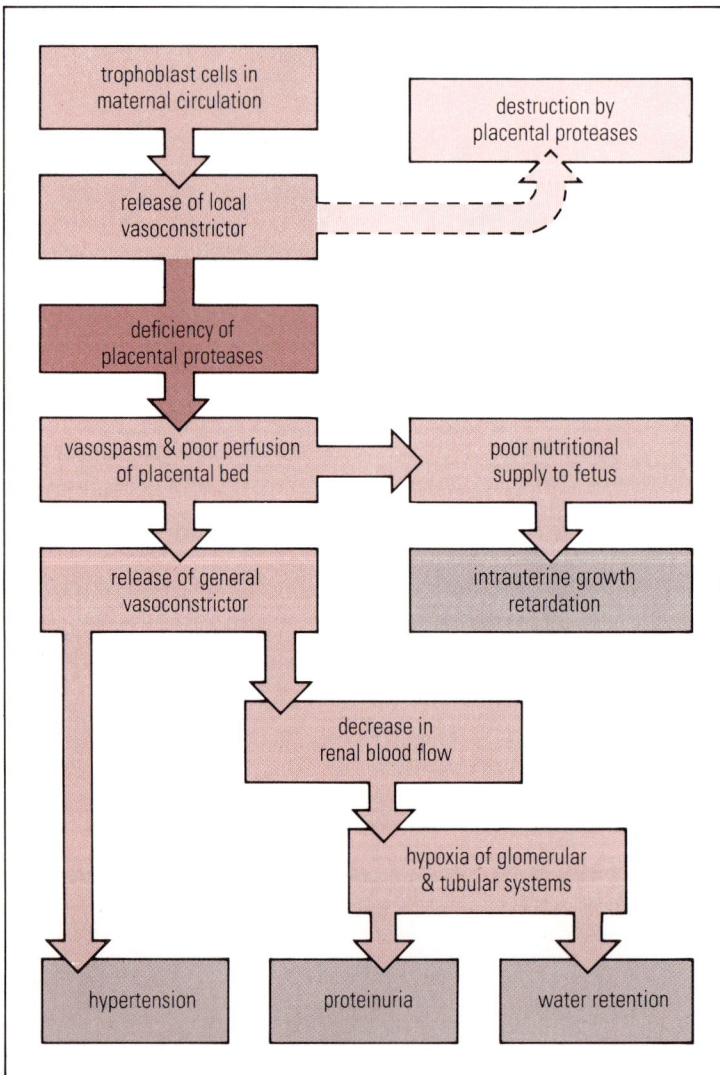

Fig.5.3 Aetiology of pre-eclampsia. It is thought that a deficiency of placental proteases is responsible for producing the clinical features of this condition.

Among women who are going to develop pre-eclampsia, there is an inhibition of trophoblast invasion. In addition, trophoblast cells may enter the maternal circulation and cause the release of local vasoconstrictors. In the normal woman these chemicals are destroyed by placental proteases, but in pre-eclampsia there is a deficiency of such enzymes. If sufficient amounts of local vasoconstrictors are released, vasospasm and poor perfusion of the placental bed occur, which may lead to intrauterine growth retardation. The subsequent release of general vasoconstrictors is associated with hypertension and a decrease in renal blood flow. This leads to hypoxia of the glomerular and tubular systems, and thus to proteinuria and retention of sodium, which results in water retention.

Clinical course

Pre-eclampsia is usually categorized as mild, moderate or severe, depending on the symptoms. In mild cases, the diastolic blood pressure does not rise above 100mmHg and proteinuria does not occur. In moderate pre-eclampsia, diastolic pressure rises to between 100 and 110mmHg, and there is occasional proteinuria. Severe pre-eclampsia is associated with a diastolic blood pressure greater than 110mmHg and with proteinuria.

A small proportion of pre-eclamptic women may be fulminating to impending eclampsia (Fig.5.4). This is characterized by frontal headaches, visual disturbances and epigastric pain. The blood pressure rises sharply with a diminution of urine production. Oedema may be present in any of the categories but is not a specific sign. The severity of the condition is determined by the other two signs.

Management

Investigations

Progress of the condition is monitored by blood pressure readings and tests for proteinuria, their frequency being determined by the severity of the problem. Weight gain may also be monitored. If the pre-eclamptic state worsens, blood pressure should be checked at intervals of up to every fifteen minutes.

In addition to the clinical observations, kidney function can be determined by monitoring the plasma urate level. This is more predictive than changes in plasma urea levels or creatinine clearance. The fetus should be carefully monitored by weekly ultrasound measurements of the cephalic and abdominal circumferences, and by daily non-stressed cardiotocographic measurements of fetal heart rate. The flow of blood to the placental bed can be estimated by Doppler measurements.

Treatment

The most important factor in the treatment of pre-eclampsia is bedrest. In this position, it is claimed that there is a relatively greater blood flow to the

SYMPTOMS AND SIGNS OF PRE-ECLAMPSIA
Fulminating pre-eclampsia
frontal headaches visual disturbances epigastric pain
Pre-eclampsia
raised blood pressure proteinuria oedema

Fig.5.4 Symptoms and signs of pre-eclampsia.

placental bed. The definitive treatment is delivery of the fetus and placenta. This can only be carried out if the obstetrician is confident that the fetus is mature enough to thrive in the paediatric facilities available. These vary greatly between different areas and from one hospital to another. A normal baby can be delivered safely from about twenty-eight weeks gestation if there is a Special Care Baby Unit available, and from about thirty-two weeks when the perinatal facilities available are part of a general paediatric service.

Other adjuncts to treatment may be used. Hypotensive agents, such as methyldopa, may improve the prognosis by allowing delivery to be delayed. In an acute phase of sharply rising blood pressure, intravenous agents, such as hydralazine, are necessary. Sedation is generally not useful, but it may be required at night to help a woman who, having rested all day, cannot sleep. Diuretics are used only when there is a very painful oedema stretching the skin, since they increase the hypovolaemia and reduce placental bed flow.

The treatment of impending eclampsia is an extension of that for severe pre-eclampsia. Hypertension must be controlled with antihypertensive agents, such as hydralazine, and with anticonvulsants, such as diazepam. All these drugs are best given intravenously. Hydralazine should be given separately from antiepileptics, so that blood pressure can be controlled independently.

If treatment is successful and the woman is brought out of the fulminating pre-eclampsia the pregnancy should be ended as soon as possible. If the fetus is viable, delivery should be performed by the most appropriate method. For the woman who is multiparous with a ripe cervix, induction and acceleration of labour is performed. If she is nulliparous or has an unripe cervix, a caesarean section should be carried out under an epidural anaesthetic.

When the obstetrician considers that the fetus is not viable, given the facilities at his disposal, he should consider transferring the woman to a hospital with an associated neonatal paediatric department which is capable of looking after the smaller baby. Transfer *in utero* is preferable to delivery of an immature baby followed by transfer in an incubator.

Prognosis

The maternal prognosis is good if eclampsia does not supervene. Death in pre-eclampsia can occur from intracranial haemorrhage, or from hepatic or renal failure (Fig.5.5). Death may also be associated with the treatment given for severe pre-eclampsia, for example anaesthesia for caesarean section. Most women with pre-eclampsia are affected for too short a time for serious permanent vascular or renal damage to occur but occasionally, pre-eclampsia does unmask a permanent essential hypertension. Postnatal investigations and follow-up are required.

CAUSES OF DEATH IN PRE-ECLAMPSIA	
Maternal	**Fetal and neonatal**
anaesthesia	intrauterine growth retardation
cerebrovascular accident	reduced placental bed blood flow
hepatic failure	low birth weight
renal failure	hypoxia

Fig.5.5 Maternal and fetal and neonatal causes of death in pre-eclampsia.

The fetus is at increased risk because of reduced placental bed blood flow. This may lead to hypoxia in labour and should be watched for carefully by intrapartum monitoring. The fetus is also at higher risk of being of low birth weight, both because of intrauterine growth retardation and because he may be delivered early as a part of the treatment of pre-eclampsia.

The perinatal mortality rate increases in proportion to the severity of the condition. However, rates are often lower among those with mild pre-eclampsia than among the background population because the mothers and fetuses in the former group receive greater care.

ECLAMPSIA

Eclampsia is one of the most dangerous complications of pregnancy. It is a state of coma associated with convulsions and usually occurs in late pregnancy, commonly preceded by pre-eclampsia. It is rare in the United Kingdom because of efficient antenatal care and thorough treatment of the pre-eclamptic state.

Incidence and aetiology

The incidence is difficult to determine, but is estimated to be approximately one in every three thousand women delivered. There is severe local cerebral vasoconstriction which leads to cerebral hypoxia. Among women who develop eclampsia

there may be an underlying cerebral dysrhythmia which is then triggered by hypoxia.

Clinical course

Eclampsia often occurs unexpectedly, especially when it develops in early pregnancy (before thirty-two weeks gestation). However, it is usually associated with a worsening of the pre-eclamptic state. Approximately fifty percent of eclamptic fits occur during pregnancy, the remainder occurring during labour or in the puerperium (Fig.5.6).

The eclamptic fit is similar to an epileptic fit, with tonic and clonic phases, and fits are often repeated at frequent intervals.

Management

Treatment aims to keep the patient alive during a fit, and to prevent further fits. During a fit, the woman should be turned on her side and an airway maintained by either holding up the chin or, it possible, inserting a mechanical airway to hold up the tongue. She should be stopped from falling or biting her tongue. Further fits should be prevented by heavy sedation; as a first aid measure, barbiturates or even morphia may be used. Most hospitals now use an intravenous mixture of chlorpromazine, promethazine and pethidine, 50mg of each in 500ml of five percent dextrose. The rate of infusion is titrated against the woman's level of consciousness and blood pressure readings. When the woman is out of

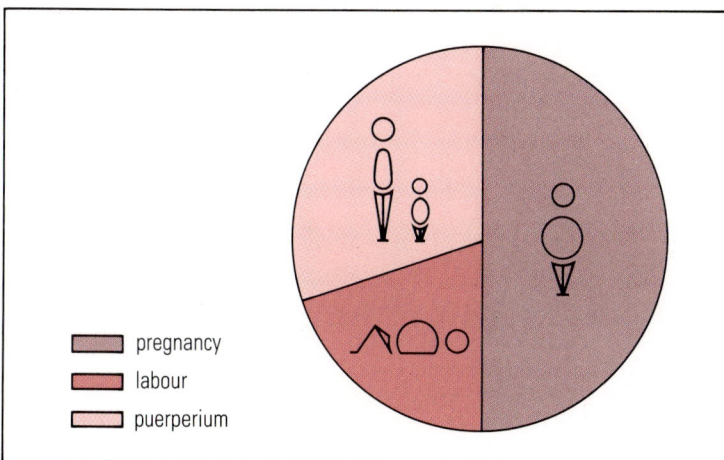

Fig.5.6 Incidence of eclampsia. Eclamptic fits commonly occur in the antenatal period (after 28 weeks). About 20% occur in labour and the remaining 30% in the puerperium, usually in the first 48h after delivery.

pregnancy
labour
puerperium

73

danger and fits have stopped, the condition may be reversed with intravenous frusemide, diazepam and hydralazine. The latter should be infused separately from the anticonvulsant, so that blood pressure can be controlled independently.

A woman who has just had an eclamptic fit remains semiconscious or unconscious and requires careful nursing. She should be kept on her side and turned every hour to prevent hypostatic pneumonia. An indwelling urinary catheter is helpful, as it prevents her being stimulated by a filling bladder; it also provides a convenient way of measuring urinary output and proteinuria.

Administration of a long-acting antibiotic is advisable to prevent infection of the urinary and respiratory tracts. If, after a few hours, there are no further fits, delivery of the fetus should be considered. As in pre-eclampsia, the obstetrician must evaluate the viability of the fetus. Delivery should then take place by the most appropriate method.

If the fetus is considered to be not yet viable, the obstetrician may allow the pregnancy to continue once the eclamptic process has been stabilized and the pre-eclampsia has been controlled. However, this is a risky option since the eclamptic process may recur. It is also possible that the fetus might not grow much more because of the extreme constraints put on the placental bed. If the hospital does not have full neonatal facilities, this extra time should be used to transfer the mother to a larger, better-equipped unit.

Prognosis

The mother's prognosis depends upon the speed with which the fits are controlled. In general, prognosis is good if management has been thorough. The outlook in future pregnancies is also good as eclampsia is unusual in subsequent pregnancy, possibly because of the extra care taken of any woman who has a history of the condition.

Fetal outlook is poor and depends upon both the stage of gestation at which eclampsia occurs and the management of the mother. If the pregnancy is past thirty-two weeks gestation, the fitting process can be controlled and delivery is prompt, the outlook is good. At earlier gestations, or when the woman has been unconscious and hypoxic for a long time, the prognosis is poor. Perinatal death occurs due to hypoxia during the fits or because of immaturity.

RHESUS INCOMPATIBILITY

The problem of rhesus incompatibility has been largely overcome in recent years by prophylactic treatment. Nevertheless, some women in the United Kingdom will have affected children and in some parts of the world it is still a major problem because of inadequate facilities for cross-matching blood.

Humans can be divided into two groups based on the presence or absence of an antigen on the erythrocytes, similar to that found in the rhesus monkey. If this antigen is present, the person is rhesus positive (Rh-positive), and if absent, rhesus-negative (Rh-negative). The Rh-negative trait is a recessive characteristic and can only be transmitted if two gametes carrying the Rh-negative gene fuse to form the homozygous recessive genotype. Heterozygotes can be Rh-negative carriers but are phenotypically Rh-positive.

The genes for the rhesus antigen are probably carried on a pair of chromosomes. It is supposed that there are six main genes for the antigen (C,D,E,c, d,e), the genes being transmitted in groups of three on each chromosome, so that each individual carries six genes in three pairs. Older theories consider that a single gene locus is responsible, and this has never been disproved. On each chromosome, the three loci can be occupied by C or c, D or d, and E or e; the most common genotypes are shown in Fig.5.7. The important alleles are D and d, which determine whether a person is Rh-positive or Rh-negative. Presence of the D allele in the genotype produces a Rh-positive phenotype, which is inherited dominantly.

The phenotypes of children will depend upon the genotypes of their parents (Fig.5.8). If the mother is homozygous Rh-positive (DD), all the children will be Rh-positive, irrespective of the father's genotype, since the D allele is phenotypically dominant. If the mother is heterozygous Rh-positive (Dd), the phenotype of the children will depend upon the genotype of the father. If the mother is homozygous Rh-negative (dd), the phenotype of the children will again depend upon the genotype of the father. If he is homozygous Rh-positive (DD), all the children will be Rh-positive. If he is heterozygous Rh-positive (Dd), there is an equal chance of producing a Rh-positive or Rh-negative child. If he is homozygous Rh-negative (dd), all the children will be Rh-negative.

Rhesus incompatibility occurs in a Rh-positive fetus if a Rh-negative woman has been immunized by Rh-positive red cells. The red cells may have passed

RHESUS GENOTYPES		
Genotype	**Frequency (%)**	**Phenotype**
cde/cde	15	negative
CDe/cde	32	positive
CDe/CDe	17	positive
cDE/cde	13	positive
CDe/cDE	14	positive
cDE/cDE	4	positive
Other genotypes	5	positive

Fig.5.7 Rhesus genotypes. In the UK, 85% of the population is Rh-positive and 15% is Rh-negative. These proportions differ in other parts of the world, for example in Kenya 5% is Rh-negative, while in the Far East this percentage is even smaller.

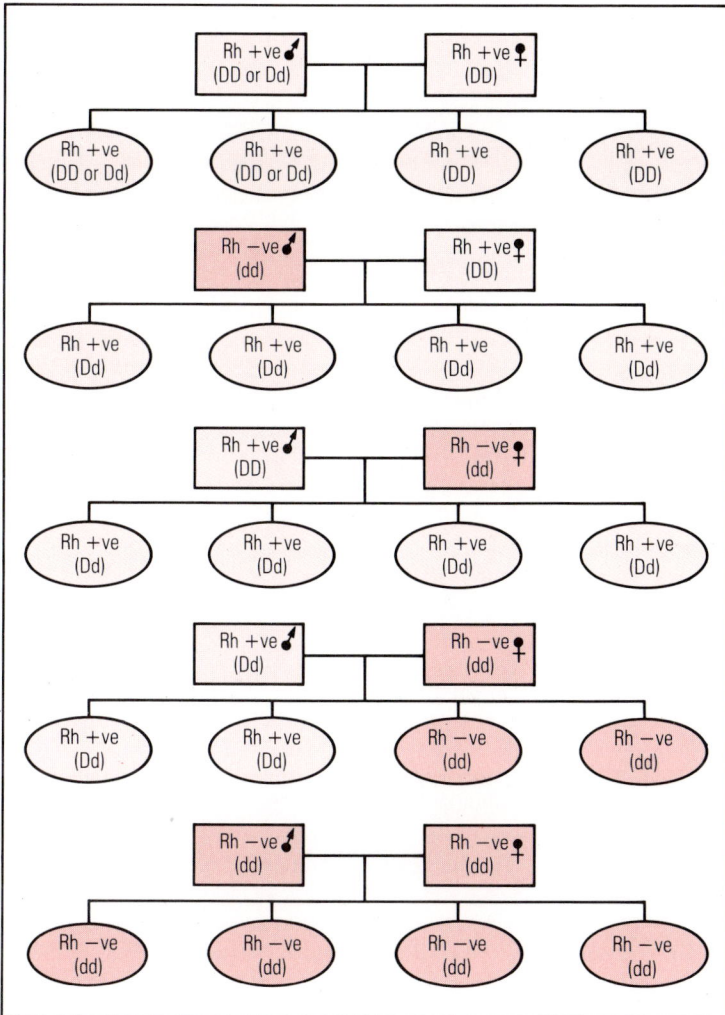

Fig.5.8 Rhesus phenotypes. The potential phenotypes of children from 5 sets of parents with different Rh genotypes. The Rh-positive individuals may be homozygous (DD) or heterozygous (Dd). Rh-negative individuals are always homozygous (dd).

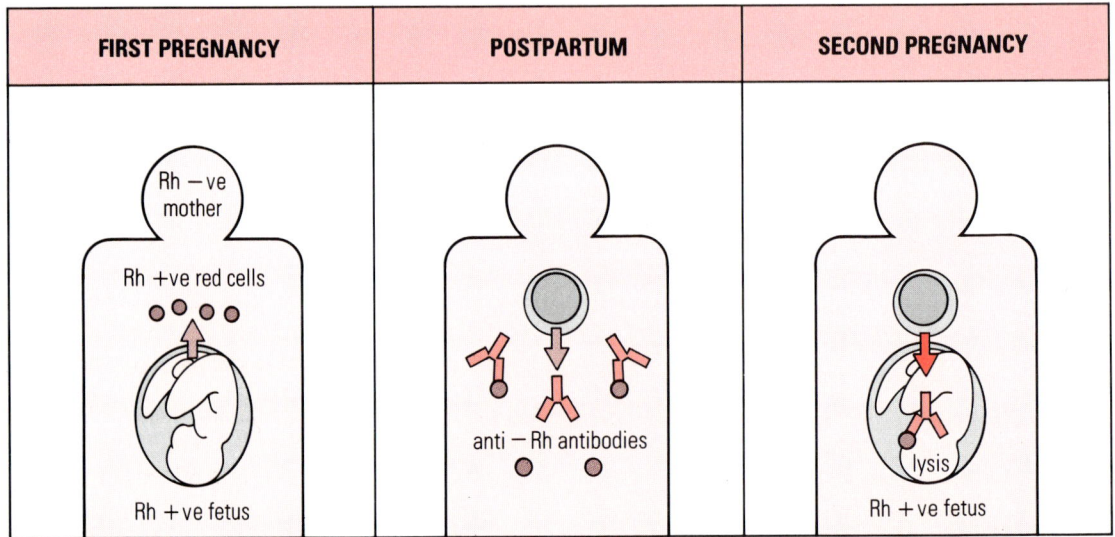

| FIRST PREGNANCY | POSTPARTUM | SECOND PREGNANCY |

Fig.5.9 Rhesus incompatibility. Left: a Rh-negative woman can be sensitized by a Rh-positive child when fetal red cells bearing the Rh-antigen cross the placenta into her circulation. Middle: the largest perfusion of fetal red cells occurs at delivery of the placenta but the response comes later, by which time the first fetus is already delivered. Right: in the second pregnancy, only very few fetal Rh-positive red cells need cross the placenta to produce a large increase in the antibody titre; this often happens in middle and late pregnancy. Haemolysis of fetal Rh-positive red cells results. Modified from Roitt, I. M. et al (1985) *Immunology*. Churchill Livingstone/Gower Medical Publishing.

into her bloodstream during a badly cross-matched blood transfusion or from a previous Rh-positive fetus across the placenta (Fig.5.9). Fetal red cells cross the placental bed in nearly all pregnancies, irrespective of the rhesus state; they cause no problem unless there is incompatibility. Transfer of red cells most often occurs during delivery of the placenta, thus the first baby born to a Rh-negative woman is rarely affected. However, the establishment of an immune response will affect subsequent pregnancies with Rh-positive fetuses. A similar effect may occur with a spontaneous or therapeutic abortion if fetal red cells enter the maternal circulation. The effect then usually comes when a second infusion of Rh-positive red cells enters the maternal circulation, during either another pregnancy or at blood transfusion.

Clinical consequences of the rhesus effect

Rhesus antibodies generated in the mother's reticuloendothelial system cross the placenta easily and, if present in a high enough concentration, cause specific pathological responses in the fetus. Depending on the speed at which this occurs and the degree to which antibodies break down the fetal red cells, anaemia may result. If the haemoglobin level drops below 4g/dl, heart failure leads to oedema, which may develop in extreme cases, to hydrops fetalis (Fig.5.10). The accelerated rate of red cell breakdown causes a great increase in bilirubin level in the serum. While the fetus is in the uterus, this diffuses across the placenta and is excreted by the maternal liver and biliary system. After birth, placental transfer ceases, the neonatal liver cannot cope with the high concentrations of bilirubin, and, as a consequence, jaundice appears rapidly and can become severe (icterus gravis neonatorum).

For a short time after birth, residual rhesus antibodies circulate in the baby's bloodstream and cause continuing haemolysis of red cells. If serum bilirubin levels rise above 120μmol/litre, metabolic damage to the basal nuclei in the brain (kernicterus) may occur. This damage is associated with staining of the tissue by bilirubin. Kernicterus used to be one of the common causes of chronic mental retardation but is now less frequent in the United Kingdom.

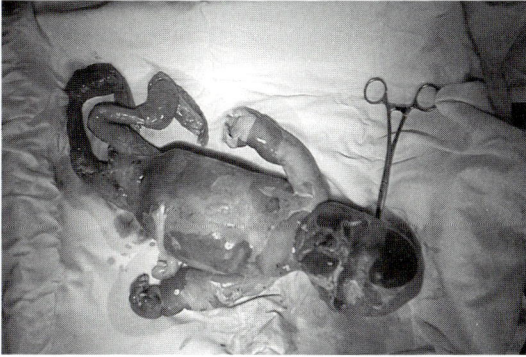

Fig.5.10 Hydrops fetalis. The baby is grossly oedematous with fluid in all body compartments. This produces typically bloated features and causes embarrassment to the heart after birth.

Management

Rhesus prophylaxis

In the developed world, use of anti-D gammaglobulin (anti-D) has produced outstanding results (Fig.5.11). It is wise to give 250–500IU of anti-D gammaglobulin to all Rh-negative women with Rh-positive fetuses. Furthermore, all Rh-negative women should receive anti-D gammaglobulin after therapeutic or spontaneous abortion, amniocentesis or ectopic pregnancy, as the blood group of the fetus is not known in these cases. As a further precaution, a Kleihauer test may be performed to check the presence of fetal red cells in the mother's blood; if they are present in excessive amounts, an additional dose of anti-D gammaglobulin may be given.

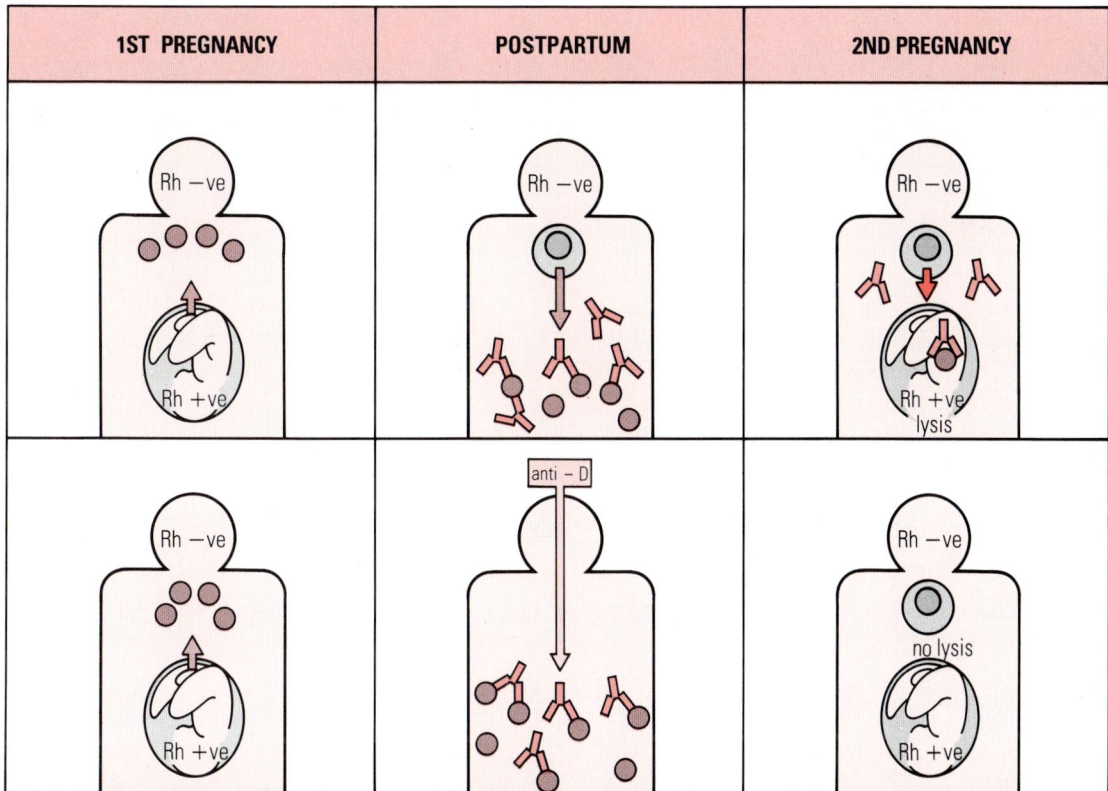

Fig.5.11 Rhesus prophylaxis is performed by giving anti-D gammaglobulin to the Rh-negative mother immediately after delivery. This adheres to the fetal Rh-positive red cells so that no recognition can be made by the maternal immune system. Thus maternal antibodies, which would attack the red cells of subsequent Rh-positive fetuses, are not generated. Modified from Roitt, I. M. et al (1985) *Immunology*. Churchill Livingstone/Gower Medical Publishing.

Anti-D gammaglobulin is usually given within seventy-two hours of delivery as most fetal blood transfer occurs during separation and delivery of the placenta. About one-third of women who should receive therapy in the postnatal period do not present for treatment. Anti-D may also be given in the antenatal period, with the advantage that all women are under supervision at this time. However, two injections are necessary for antenatal administration, and large quantities will be required if this policy is to be implemented nationally.

Early detection

HISTORY

Rhesus incompatibility should be suspected if a Rh-negative woman has a past obstetrical history of:
- Jaundiced babies
- Exchange transfusions
- Hydrops fetalis
- Unexplained stillbirths or neonatal deaths

ANTENATAL TESTS

All women should have their rhesus status identified at the booking visit and all Rh-negative women should be checked for the presence of antibodies. If initially negative, the woman should be rechecked later at about twenty-eight and thirty-four weeks gestation. If a positive result is obtained, more frequent checks will be needed.

If the indirect Coombs' test for antibodies rises above 40IU/ml by twenty weeks, amniocentesis should be performed with ultrasound localization of the placenta and fetus. The bilirubin level in the amniotic fluid is determined and compared with Lilely's risk graph (Fig.5.12), which permits prediction of the risk to the rhesus affected fetus by relating the optical density of the amniotic fluid to the week of pregnancy. Thus, from a precise knowledge of the woman's date of gestation and the optical density of the amniotic fluid, the obstetrician can decide whether it is best to keep the fetus in the uterus or to deliver the baby, either by induction or caesarean section.

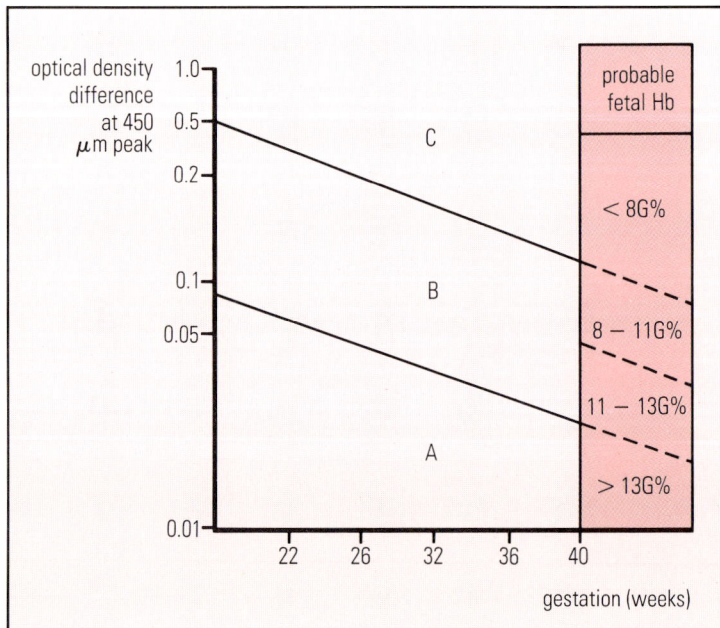

Fig.5.12 Liley's risk graph. The optical density difference represents the amount of bilirubin breakdown products. At the lowest difference values (zone A), there is almost no risk of intrauterine death at any stage of gestation. However, increasingly in zones B and C, greater elevations of optical density are associated with increasing bilirubin breakdown products and therefore greater risk of fetal death.

Cord blood tests

The baby's rhesus status should be determined immediately after birth by examination of cord blood. If Rh-negative, other investigations can be carried out without urgency. However, if the baby is Rh-positive, the haemoglobin level must be checked immediately and an indirect Coombs' test carried out. The serum bilirubin level should also be measured as a baseline, but it is rarely raised at birth.

Treatment

Treatment of affected fetuses can start during pregnancy. If a severe degree of haemolysis is detected by a high amniotic fluid bilirubin level, intrauterine transfusions may keep the fetus alive until it is mature enough for delivery.

INTRAUTERINE TRANSFUSIONS
Using the same precautions as in amniocentesis, a soft plastic catheter is introduced via a needle into the peritoneal cavity of the fetus. Fresh Rh-negative blood (70ml/kg estimated fetal weight) of the same ABO group as the mother is introduced. This transfusion may have to be repeated until the fetus is viable.

INDUCTION OF LABOUR
Delivery should be timed carefully, balancing the risks of immaturity against the risks of continued exposure to rhesus antibodies. Fresh Rh-negative blood and a competent paediatric neonatal service must be available at delivery. This may mean transferring the mother to another hospital since, with the decreased incidence of rhesus disease, not all obstetric and paediatric units are fully equipped to deal with this problem.

When the risks have been assessed and the paediatrician has been consulted, either labour is induced (if the cervix is ripe and the past obstetrical history favourable) or elective caesarean section is performed. At birth, cord blood should be examined and exchange transfusion carried out if required.

LATER TREATMENT
Biliburin levels in the baby may rise rapidly after birth and should not be allowed to increase above 120μmol/litre. Furthermore, since antibodies are still present in the fetal blood, continued red cell lysis may occur. Consequently, both haemoglobin and serum bilirubin are measured every six hours in the first days of life. Emergency exchange transfusions or topping-up transfusions may be required and the necessary equipment and staff must be available.

BLEEDING IN EARLY PREGNANCY

The four commonest causes of vaginal bleeding before twenty-eight weeks gestation are:
- Spontaneous abortion
- Ectopic pregnancy
- Hydatidiform mole
- Lower genital tract causes

It is important that any woman experiencing vaginal bleeding in early pregnancy has her blood group checked. If she is Rh-negative, anti-D immunoglobulin should be given to prevent rhesus sensitization.

Spontaneous abortion

This is the most common cause of vaginal bleeding in early pregnancy, occurring in about twenty percent of women; the aetiology is usually unknown. Spontaneous abortion may be threatened, inevitable, incomplete, complete, or septic.

Threatened abortion

A patient with a threatened abortion may have a history of uterine contractions, but lower abdominal pain is usually not severe. Vaginal blood may be red or dark red but the bleeding is not profuse. On examination, the woman is not shocked and the lower abdomen may be slightly tender on palpation. On bimanual examination, the cervix is closed (Fig.5.13 left) and the uterine size is equivalent to that expected for the gestational age. If pregnancy is far enough advanced (ten to twelve weeks), the fetal heart may be detected with a Doppler monitor. An ultrasound scan will show an amniotic sac and fetus, and the fetal heart can be seen pulsating if the pregnancy is past seven to eight weeks gestation.

Treatment consists of rest, usually at home, and reporting to hospital only if any increased abdominal pain or bleeding occurs.

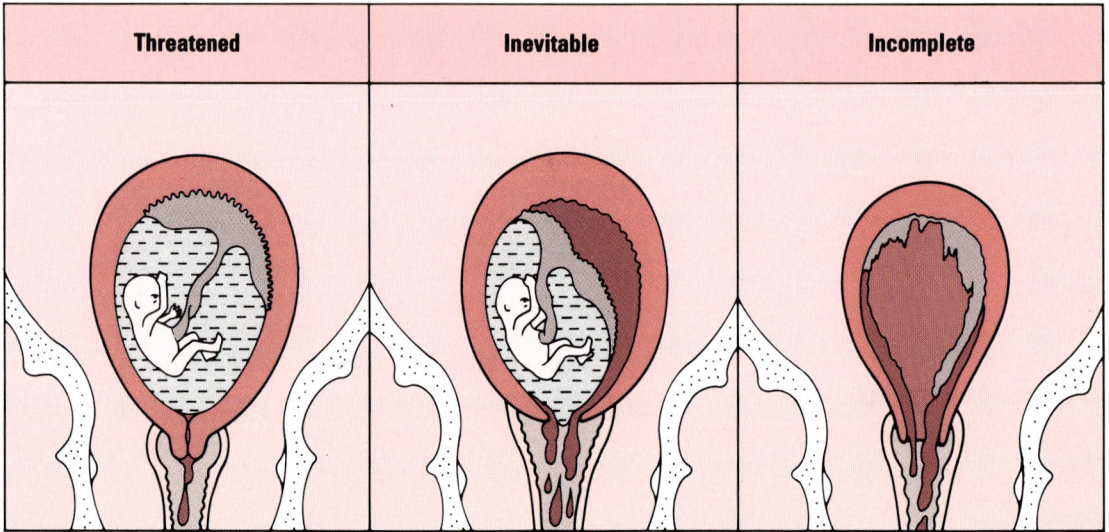

Fig.5.13 Spontaneous abortion. Left: in a threatened abortion, the cervix is closed and there is only a small amount of vaginal bleeding. Middle: in an inevitable abortion, the cervix is open and the bleeding is more profuse; the pregnancy will not continue. Right: in an incomplete abortion, the fetus and amniotic fluid are passed vaginally but some parts of the membrane or placenta are retained. This can lead to severe bleeding.

Inevitable abortion

An inevitable abortion (Fig.5.13 middle) has the signs and symptoms of an incomplete abortion (see below). The cervical os will be open and the abortion will take its course. Treatment is the same as that for an incomplete abortion.

Incomplete abortion

A woman with an incomplete abortion (Fig.5.13 right) will have a history of lower abdominal pain similar to dysmenorrhoea, which persists and often becomes worse. There is vaginal bleeding and passage of clots or tissue. On examination, the patient may be in a stable condition, or may be shocked if blood loss has been excessive. On abdominal palpation, there will be suprapubic tenderness and on bimanual pelvic examination, the uterus will be equivalent to the size expected for the gestational age; the cervical internal os will be open. Products of conception may be felt in the os or in the vagina. The fetal heart will not be detected with a Doppler monitor and an ultrasound scan may show retained products of conception but no viable fetus. The pregnancy test may take several days to become negative as any viable fragments of trophoblastic tissue will secrete sufficient hCG to give a positive result.

Management consists of treating the shock with intravenous plasma expanders and blood transfusion, administration of oxytocics to stop uterine bleeding, and suction currettage under anaesthesia to evacuate the retained products of conception.

Complete abortion

A woman with a complete abortion will have a history of much more lower abdominal pain that that which accompanies a threatened abortion. There is usually vaginal bleeding, and probably, passage of clots. On examination, the patient is usually well, but may be shocked if excessive blood loss has occurred. Abdominal examination may show a swelling or tenderness, but on bimanual assessment the uterus will be smaller than expected for the gestational age and the cervical os closed. No fetal heart sounds are heard with a Doppler monitor, and ultrasound scanning shows an empty uterus. The pregnancy test is not very helpful as it takes several days to become negative.

If the symptoms settle and there is minimal vaginal bleeding, the patient should be advised that the pregnancy has probably been lost and that she

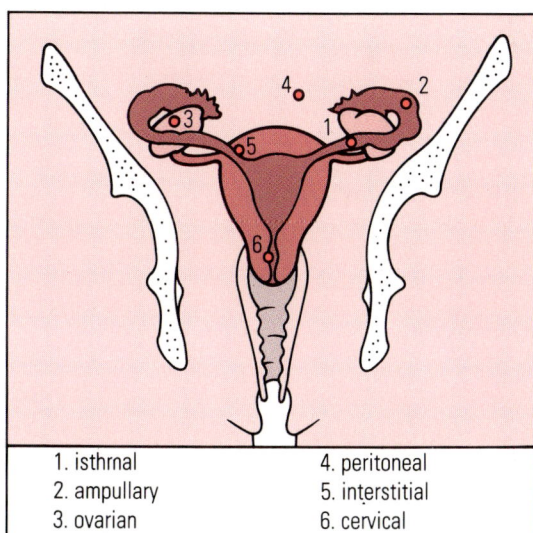

1. isthrnal	4. peritoneal
2. ampullary	5. interstitial
3. ovarian	6. cervical

Fig.5.14 Possible sites of ectopic pregnancy. Ampullary pregnancy is by far the commonest type of ectopic pregnancy, whilst cervical is the most rare.

should return if the pain or bleeding recurs. If bleeding is more pronounced, the woman should be admitted to hospital and given an oxtocic drug (for example, Syntometrine) to reduce uterine bleeding. A transfusion may be necessary. Curettage is not required if the abortion is complete.

Septic abortion

A septic abortion is one in which infection occurs, commonly following an incomplete induced abortion. The woman may present with lower abdominal pain and intermittent vaginal bleeding. On examination, she will be unwell, pyrexial with a tachycardia, and may have septic shock. The lower abdomen is tender and on bimanual examination the uterus is found to be tender and enlarged, although smaller in size than expected for the gestational age. There is tenderness in both fornices.

Management starts with admission to hospital and the treatment of any shock with intravenous plasma expanders. Sepsis should initially be treated with broad-spectrum antibiotics. When bacterial sensitivities are known from the vaginal swabs, specific antibiotic agents may be administered. There is a danger that infections may spread through the uterus

to the parametrium, up the fallopian tubes to the peritoneum, along the uterine veins, or into the urinary tract. The woman should be kept under close observation in case septic shock is followed by renal shutdown. Any retained products of conception must be evacuated under anaesthesia. This is best delayed for six to twelve hours to allow the tissue concentration of antibiotics to reach a therapeutic level.

Therapeutic abortion

A therapeutic abortion may be perfomed after two independent doctors agree that the risks of the pregnancy proceeding are greater than the risk of termination. Indications for therapeutic abortion are:

● To save the mother's life.
● To preserve the mother's health.
● To prevent ill health occurring in other children in the family.
● To prevent the birth of a severely congenitally abnormal child.

If performed before fourteen weeks gestation, a cervical dilatation and suction evacuation under anaesthesia is the usual technique.

Ectopic pregnancy

In an ectopic pregnancy, the blastocyst implants outside the cavity of the uterus. Among the endemic British population it occurs in one in three hundred pregnancies. While the blastocyst may implant anywhere outside the uterus (Fig.5.14), the commonest site is the fallopian tube (ninety-nine percent of ectopic pregnancies), either in the isthmus, or, more often, at the ampullary end. In an ampullary pregnancy, the embryo may squeeze out of the lateral end of the tube and secondarily attach itself to either the ovary or elsewhere in the general peritoneal cavity. Occasionally, the blastocyst may settle in the corneal part of the tube, producing an interstitial ectopic pregnancy, and even more rarely, it travels down through the uterus to implant in the cervix.

Factors predisposing to an ectopic pregnancy include past pelvic inflammation, tubal surgery, or the presence of an intrauterine contraceptive device. However, the majority of women presenting with an ectopic pregnancy have none of these. There is

81

usually a history of amenorrhoea and lower abdominal pain which may be localized on one side; this may be followed by intermittent light vaginal bleeding. If the ectopic pregnancy has caused the tube to rupture, the woman will be shocked with a rigid abdomen. If the tube has not ruptured, she will not be shocked and there will be tenderness and guarding in the affected iliac fossa. Bimanual examination reveals a normally sized uterus with tenderness in one fornix and often pain on moving the cervix. An ultrasound scan frequently shows an empty uterus and may show a pregnancy sac behind the uterus if the former has not already ruptured. Blood may be seen in the pouch of Douglas.

Rupture of an ectopic pregnancy at the isthmal end of the tube characteristically occurs suddenly at six to eight weeks gestation, causing severe shock with much loss of blood, which is expelled intraperitoneally. An ampullary ectopic pregnancy leaks blood from the far end of the tube into the pouch of Douglas. This presents later (eight to ten weeks gestation). The symptoms are not so traumatic and the degree of shock is not very great.

The diagnosis of a leaking, unruptured ectopic pregnancy can be very difficult. It is aided by an ultrasound scan showing an empty uterus along with a positive hCG test, which indicates the presence of some trophoblastic tissue in the body. Often, the ordinary pregnancy test is not sensitive enough to detect the low levels of hCG found in ectopic pregnancy, and a test for the β subunit is required.

Treatment of a woman with a ruptured ectopic pregnancy is based on control of the shock by intravenous plasma expanders and blood transfusion, accompanied by urgent laparotomy and haemostasis. This is usually achieved by salpingectomy, although occasionally, a more conservative approach to the tube is possible. Where the pregnancy has not yet ruptured, or if the diagnosis is in some doubt, the woman must be admitted to hospital; with cross-matched blood available, a diagnostic laparoscopy is performed, proceeding to laparotomy if necessary.

Hydatidiform mole

A hydatidiform mole is a cystic mass of vesicles derived from the chorionic villi. The mole originates from a conceptus where the embryo has either died and been absorbed at an early stage, or where the embryo was never formed. The villi swell and can develop into a rapidly growing tumour. The stretching of the decidua produces much bleeding. Hydatidiform mole occurs in less than one in two thousand pregnancies in the endemic British population; the incidence varies in different parts of the world, occurring in up to one in one hundred pregnancies in the Philippines.

The woman may give a history of exaggerated symptoms of early pregnancy, with extreme nausea and breast tenderness, often associated with intermittent loss of dark vaginal blood. On examination, the uterus is larger than expected. The cervix is closed but occasionally, molar vesicles may be seen in the vagina. At investigation, hCG levels are extremely elevated and an ultrasound scan shows a characteristic snowstorm appearance (Fig.5.15). Treatment is by suction evacuation of the molar tissue under general anaesthesia and oxytocin cover. Severe blood loss can occur during this operation and at least four units of blood should be available.

In the United Kingdom, approximately ten percent of hydatidiform moles progresss to a malignant choriocarcinoma. To prevent this occurring, any woman who has had a mole should be followed up at a centre specializing in trophoblastic disease, where hCG levels are checked at monthly intervals until they return to normal. If this does not happen within two months, the woman should be admitted for cytotoxic treatment. Once hCG levels are normal, she should be followed up for two years to ensure that any recurrence is detected.

Lower genital tract causes

Bleeding in early pregnancy may follow cervicitis and vaginitis, cervical erosion, a cervical polyp or, occasionally, carcinoma of the cervix.

Cervical erosions usually occur at the site of a split cervical os in a multiparous woman. There is an accumulation of columnar epithelium, which normally lines the canal of the cervix. The epithelium grows downwards and replaces an area of desquamation on the ectocervix, which would normally be covered by stratified squamous epithelium. Erosions are quite common in pregnancy and have no malignant potential.

Vaginal infections, such as moniliasis, may be so severe as to cause spotting of blood or a brown discharge, but this is unusual. A cervical polyp or erosion may be associated with painless slight bleeding. On examination, the uterus is the correct

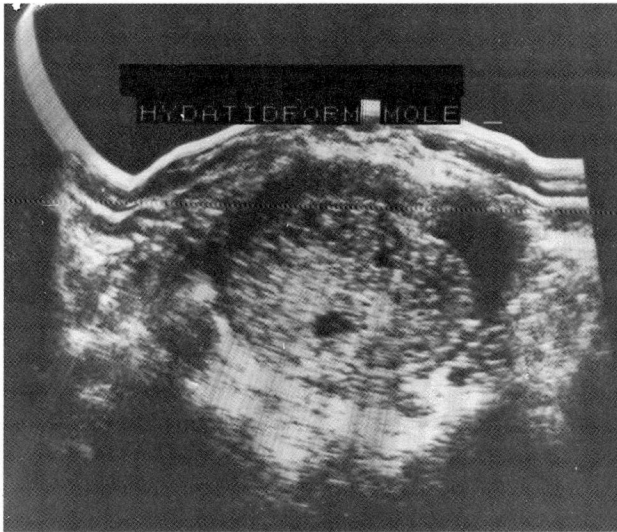

Fig.5.15 Hydatidiform mole. An ultrasound scan reveals echoes from all the reflecting surfaces of the vesicles. This produces a characteristic picture described as the snowstorm effect. Courtesy of Dr. R. Patel.

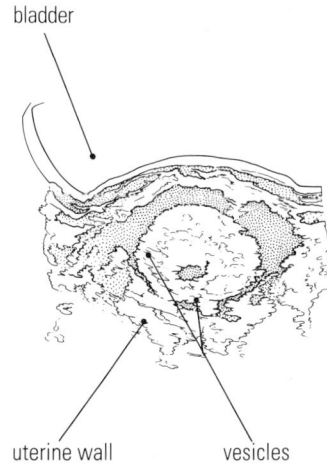

size for the stage of gestation and the polyp or erosion may be seen by exposing the cervix with a speculum. In most cases, no treatment is necessary.

It is important to exclude carcinoma of the cervix; this can be done by taking a Papanicolaou smear at the antenatal booking visit. The diagnosis of carcinoma of the cervix in pregnancy must always be confirmed by biopsy; the subsequent treatment depends on the maturity of the fetus and the stage of spread of the disease. It is also important to exclude bleeding from the rectum or the urethra in early pregnancy, as these can be wrongly reported as vaginal bleeding.

BLEEDING IN LATE PREGNANCY

Antepartum haemorrhage is defined as bleeding from the genital tract after the twenty-eighth week of gestation and before the onset of labour. It occurs in three percent of pregnancies. There are three main causes:
- Placental abruption (35% of cases)
- Placenta praevia (28% of cases)
- Causes in the lower genital tract (1% of cases)

A definitive diagnosis is not made in forty percent of cases of antepartum haemorrhage. Some are probably due to a stripping off of the membranes from the lower segment of the uterus as it is pulled up in later pregnancy. A small amount of bleeding then comes from the decidua.

Placental abruption

Bleeding from the placental bed due to partial separation of a normally situated placenta is termed placental abruption (abruptio placentae). Spasm of the blood vessels around the periphery of the clot causes a sudden and severe cut-off of oxygen supply to the fetus. The bleeding may be concealed or revealed (Fig.5.16). If concealed, there is almost no bleeding externally; if revealed, there is vaginal loss of some of the blood that has been shed.

The cause of placental separation is not known, but the condition is commonly associated with grand multiparity, hypertension, folate deficiency, trauma (including external cephalic version), or an overstretched uterus (for example, due to poly-hydramnios), especially if sudden decompression occurs at rupture of the membranes. It is also more common after a previous abruption.

Clinical signs and symptoms

The symptoms depend on the severity of bleeding and separation of the placenta. If very severe, the woman will be unconscious and collapsed with no immediately available history. In a less severe case, she may appear well. Classically, there is a history of sudden onset of moderately severe lower abdominal pain; this is different from any pain the woman may have had with uterine contractions. She may have noticed some vaginal loss of dark red blood. However, the amount of blood lost to the exterior does not relate to the severity of the abruption, as a large amount is pushed into the myometrium.

On examination, the woman may be collapsed, pale and sweating, with a rapid thready pulse, even though the blood pressure is within normal limits (for example, 110/70mmHg). The blood pressure may not be helpful in judging the clinical status, as it tends to fluctuate between hyper- and hypotensive values. It is therefore better to assess the pulse rate and central venous pressure rather than the peripheral arterial blood pressure.

The uterus is tense and hard; it does not relax between contractions (if present), and there is often tenderness in one localized area. It is difficult to assess the lie or presentation as the fetus cannot be felt through the uterine hardness. The condition of the fetus varies with the severity of the abruption but fetal death is not uncommon. As well as separation of the placenta from the placental bed, there is spasm of many of the spiral arteries that bring maternal blood to the placental bed.

Vaginal examination may yield some old dark blood and the cervix may be dilated as abruption commonly precipitates the onset of labour. Vaginal examination is the best way to assess the presentation of the fetus and is easier than abdominal examination. A fetal scalp electrode may be attached to the fetus to determine whether it is alive. In some cases, ultrasound scanning can show a clot in the retroplacental space.

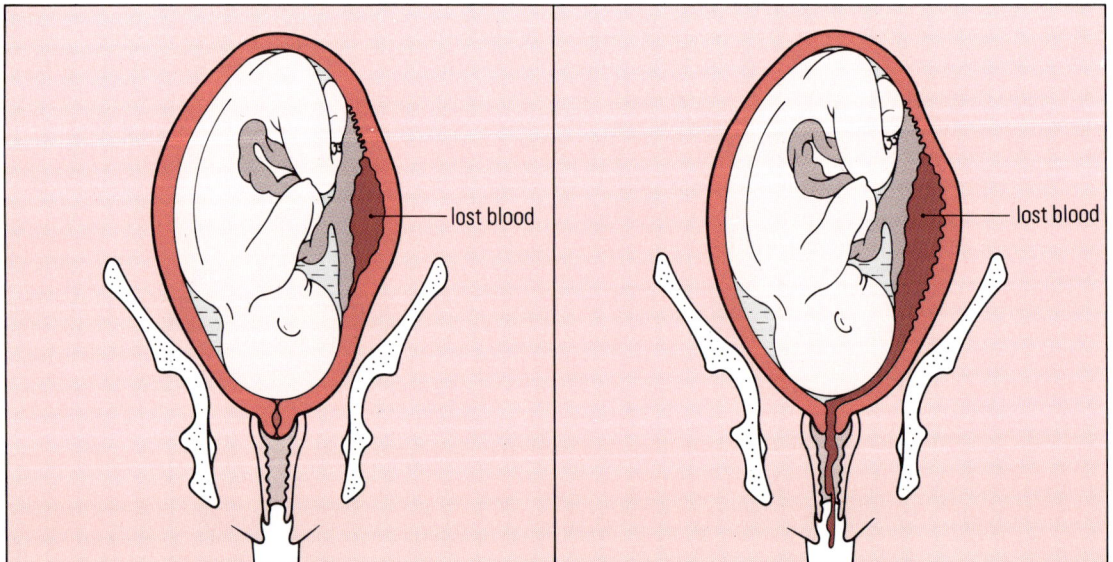

Fig.5.16 Placental abruption. Left: in a concealed abruption, lost blood remains within the uterus. Right: in a revealed abruption the blood leaks around the edge of the placenta, between the membranes and the decidua, and is lost through the cervix.

Management

Management consists of regular observations of the mother's conscious state, pulse, arterial blood pressure and central venous pressure. Urine output and clotting function may deteriorate and must be monitored carefully. The woman must be treated for shock with intravenous plasma expanders and blood as soon as it is available. When the woman is admitted to hospital, her haemoglobin level should be assessed and a minimum of four units of blood cross-matched urgently. Clotting function should be measured, particularly fibrinogen levels, as hypofibrinogenaemia may result from a large abruption.

If the fetus is dead and the woman not in active labour, contractions can be induced with oxytocics once the maternal condition is stable. If the fetus is alive and reasonably mature and the woman not in active labour, labour can be induced with oxytocics as soon as the mother's condition stabilizes, provided the cervix is ripe. After myometrial stimulation, it is common for labour to start and to proceed rapidly and uneventfully. However, this procedure is risky and any deterioration in fetal condition would necessitate a caesarean section. Surgical intervention is becoming the preferred method of delivery of a woman not in labour whether the cervix is favourable or not.

Placenta praevia

Placenta praevia is defined as a placenta implanted wholly or partly in the lower segment of the uterus. The lower segment does not contract before or during labour and is only passively stretched. It forms the cervix and isthmus of the uterus prior to pregnancy. There are four grades of placenta praevia, dependent upon the position of the placenta in the lower segment (Fig.5.17):

- Grade I. The placenta extends into the lower segment, but does not reach the cervical os.
- Grade II. The placenta implants in the lower segment and extends to the internal cervical os, but does not cover it.
- Grade III. The placenta implants in the lower segment and lies across the internal os. When cervical dilatation starts, however, the os is not completely covered.
- Grade IV. The placenta implants centrally in the lower segment, covering the os at all stages of dilatation.

Aetiology

The cause of placenta praevia is unknown. There is an increased association with multiparity and with multiple pregnancies. There is evidence that ovulation early in the menstrual cycle may be associated with early fertilization which, by allowing more time for the ovum to travel, leads to implantation lower in the uterus.

Clinical signs and symptoms

The woman generally complains of a small amount of vaginal bleeding that is not associated with abdominal pain. The blood is often bright red (being fresh) and the bleeding recurrent. The condition of the woman is dependent upon the severity of the bleeding; she is usually in a stable condition unless bleeding has been severe, in which case she will be shocked. The uterus is usually soft and not undergoing contractions. The fetal lie may be oblique or transverse but if longitudinal, the presenting part is usually high and not engaged within the pelvic brim.

If a placenta praevia is suspected, a digital vaginal examination must never be performed. The woman must be admitted to hospital, where a gentle examination with a speculum may be carried out when she is in a stable condition. This will allow any pathology of the cervix, for example cervical polyp, to be seen. However, even if a polyp is found, it must not be assumed that this is the cause of the bleeding; a placenta praevia must be excluded.

Initially, blood should be sent for estimation of haemoglobin and for cross-matching. The fetal condition is best assessed by checking the fetal heart rate with a cardiotocograph. Estimation of the position of the placenta should be made in the ward with a real-time ultrasound scan prior to the availability of formal ultrasound or angiography.

Management

Management begins with admission to hospital. As long as heavy vaginal bleeding does not persist, delivery should be delayed until the fetus is mature (usually after thirty-six weeks). The route of delivery will depend upon the placental site.

If, despite definitive ultrasonic investigation, there is still doubt about the placental position, a thorough

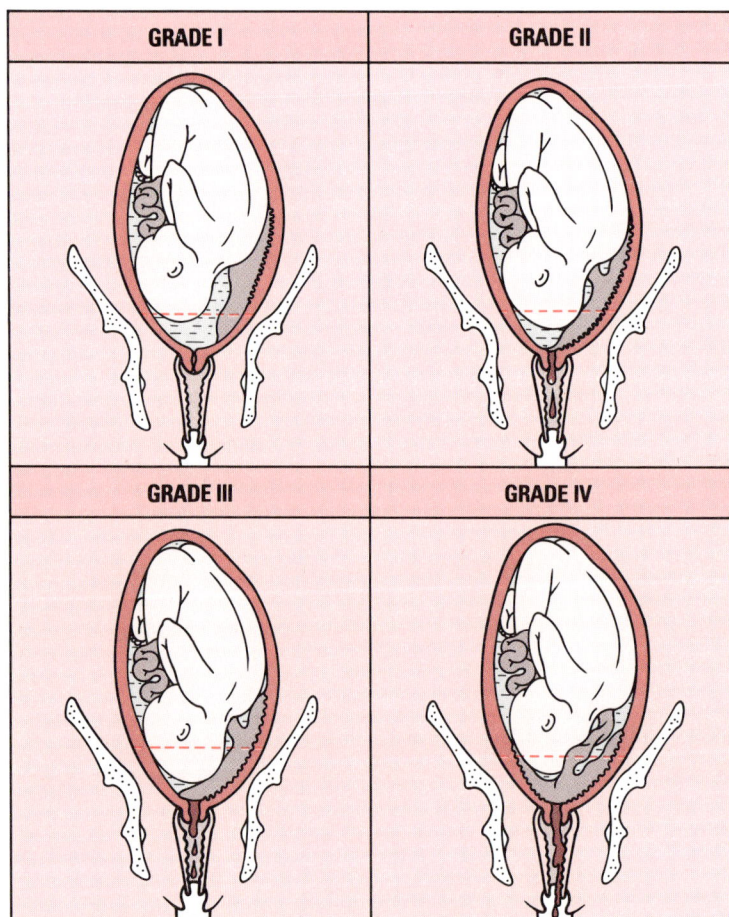

Fig.5.17 The grades of placenta praevia. The area below the dotted line is the lower segment of the uterus.

pelvic examination should be performed in theatre, under anaesthetic, after thirty-six weeks, with all the back-up necessary for emergency caesarean section. If a grade III or IV placenta praevia has been localized with ultrasound, an elective caesarean section should be performed without any preceding examination in theatre. Some cases of grade II placenta praevia will deliver vaginally, provided the placenta is located anteriorly. Most of the grade I cases can be delivered vaginally.

If a woman is found to have a placenta praevia grade II, III or IV during her antenatal period, she is usually admitted for the last few weeks of pregnancy. If it is grade I, the woman is informed of the situation and warned to come in to hospital immediately should bleeding occur.

Any woman who has had a placenta praevia is at higher risk of having a postpartum haemorrhage. This is because the lower uterine segment contracts less efficiently than the upper segment after childbirth and the placental bed may continue to bleed.

Lower genital tract causes

Other causes of vaginal bleeding in late pregnancy are the same as those outlined in the section on vaginal bleeding in early pregnancy. The identification of an apparent local cause, for example a cervical polyp, does not mean that abruption or placenta praevia is not also present. The more serious conditions must be excluded before the bleeding can be attributed solely to a local cause.

ABDOMINAL PAIN IN PREGNANCY

Abdominal pain is common during pregnancy; the uterus stretches rapidly, exerting pressure on surrounding organs and pulling on its ligamentous supports, particularly the round ligaments. The peritoneum over the organ becomes stretched and other intra-abdominal organs are displaced. Further-more, any existing adhesions, due to previous inflammation, are also stretched and may cause pain. Additionally, any fibrous areas (old scars) of the anterior abdominal wall may cause pain due to stretching.

Diagnosis

The diagnosis of abdominal pain in pregnancy depends upon:
- History of the pain
- Nature of the pain
- Severity of the pain
- Timing, frequency and radiation of the pain
- Association with urinary or bowel habit
- Timing and character of the last normal menstrual period
- Vaginal bleeding with the pain
- Changes in the pattern of fetal movements
- Any past history of abdominal pain or previous abdominal and pelvic operations
- Any relevant past obstetrical history

Examination

The doctor should examine the whole body, looking for anaemia or jaundice and assessing the woman's general bearing in relation to the pain, which may give some indication of its severity. The spine, chest and lungs should be checked.

The abdomen should be inspected for scars and localized swelling. It should then be palpated, gently at first, to localize the pain, and then more deeply, to elicit any areas of guarding and to check for the presence of masses. A bimanual pelvic examination should be carried out to assess the size, shape and tenderness of the pelvic organs and the state of the cervix. If there is any suspicion of placenta praevia (which is not usually associated with pain), the pelvic examination should not be carried out. Finally, if the pain is related to the pouch of Douglas or to the lower abdomen, a digital rectal examination will be helpful in localizing the problem.

Investigations

The diagnosis of acute abdominal pain rests principally on the history and examination. Other investigations are performed to determine the exact cause of the pain. These may include haemoglobin estimation or a white cell count if anaemia or infection is suspected. The urine may be checked for the presence of bacteria and cells to confirm a urinary infection. High vaginal swabs may be taken to check the bacteriology of that area. In the first trimester, a laparoscopy may be required if a specific source of pain is noted in one area and if there is any suspicion of a serious condition, for example an ectopic pregnancy.

Some of the causes of abdominal pain during pregnancy are dealt with elsewhere in this book, but the headings are grouped here under the physio-pathology of pain. To facilitate analysis, the causes of pain are divided into those associated with pelvic organ dysfunction and those from other regions. Whilst the former are the direct concern of the obstetrician, the latter are common in pregnancy and need diagnosis and treatment.

Pain in early pregnancy

Pelvic causes

ABORTION
Spontaneous abortion can be painful because of uterine contractions. An incomplete abortion may produce pain either from the stretching of the cervix, or from contraction of the uterus on trapped contents, such as blood clots or products of conception.

ECTOPIC PREGNANCY
Pain in ectopic pregnancy may be due to stretching of the peritoneum over the fallopian tube, particularly in the isthmal region, or to bleeding into the peritoneal cavity. In a ruptured ectopic pregnancy, sudden pain is caused by irritation of the peritoneum by blood loss into the pouch of Douglas and peritoneal cavity. Less acute pain is caused by slow

leakage of blood from the lateral end of the fallopian tube into the peritoneal cavity. Both types of blood loss produce a different pattern of pain.

RETROVERTED IMPACTED UTERUS

Pain originates from the bladder, trapped in the abdomen by the uterus. The urethra is stretched resulting in retention of urine and bladder filling (see Chapter 6).

STRETCHING OF THE ROUND LIGAMENTS

Pain arises from tension on the round ligaments, which contain very little elastic tissue and therefore have limited elasticity. Very occasionally, blood vessels within the ligaments rupture, producing a localized area of pain. Such pain commonly radiates

down to the pubic tubercle where the ligament is inserted. Tenderness is usually located over the course of the round ligament.

FIBROIDS

Fibroids may produce pain in mid-pregnancy (about fourteen to twenty weeks) when small blood vessels rupture inside their engorged substance. Degeneration of the tumour is marked by the formation of soft red areas due to necrosis and oedema — red degeneration (Fig.5.18). Treatment is conservative. Very rarely, torsion of a fibroid may occur.

OVARIAN TUMOURS

Pain may be caused by rupture of an ovarian tumour with spillage of its contents into the peritoneal cavity, but this is quite rare. Twisting of an ovarian tumour upon its pedicle is also rare in pregnancy (although common in the puerperium). Bleeding into an ovarian cyst commonly causes pain due to the stretching of the ovarian substance.

Suprapelvic causes

APPENDICITIS

This is a common condition in young women and is no less frequent in pregnancy. The classical pattern of a shift of the pain from the peri-umbilical region to the iliac fossa is sometimes altered by pregnancy, and pain may arise *de novo* in the right side. The increasing size of the uterus pushes the caecum and the base of the appendix upwards. By twenty-four weeks, the appendix is often located above the level of the umbilicus, and pain and tenderness may occur in this area.

Appendicitis is more serious in pregnancy because the cortisol levels are raised, resulting in a poor inflammatory response. Furthermore, the appendix is pushed upwards into the general abdominal cavity, hence the omentum does not circumscribe the inflamed tissue, localizing it into a corner of the lower abdomen, as it would in a non-pregnant woman.

Appendicitis in pregnancy has always had a bad prognosis for both the mother and the fetus, possibly because it is underdiagnosed or, having been diagnosed in late pregnancy, there is a fear that abdominal operation might put the fetus as risk. Yet in most cases the fetus and mother will suffer much

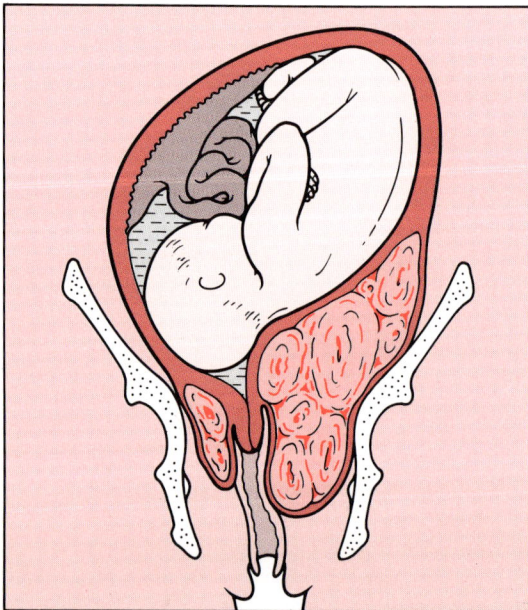

Fig.5.18 Red degeneration of a fibroid. Blood has leaked into the spaces between the fibrous whirls of the tumour and necrosis has occurred.

more from continuing appendicitis than from a properly conducted appendectomy.

The treatment of appendicitis in early pregnancy is the same as in the non-pregnant. The surgeon must perform a laparotomy and remove the inflamed appendix.

URINARY INFECTION

Most urinary infections in pregnancy occur in the bladder base and urethra, producing increased frequency and dysuria rather than intra-abdominal pain. However, occasionally there is an ascending infection with inflammation of the ureter or kidneys. Urinary infection involving the upper urinary tract can produce unilateral pain in the abdomen but it is more likely to be accompanied by backache in the renal angles caused by pyelonephritis. Rarely, uretitis or the formation of a calculus in the ureter can produce abdominal pain; cellular and bacteriological investigations of the urine are helpful in diagnosis.

VOMITING

Many women vomit in early pregnancy and excess retching can cause an ache in the abdomen. The pain is non-specific tiredness of the rectus abdominis and oblique muscles and is best treated with antiemetics.

Pain in late pregnancy

Pelvic causes

LABOUR

Labour contractions can occur before the expected date of delivery and can be very painful. Recurrent cramping pains, moving from the back to the suprapubic region, are characteristic of uterine contractions. Palpation of the uterus over several minutes will assist with this diagnosis.

ABRUPTIO PLACENTAE

When a normally sited placenta becomes separated, blood fills the space between the placenta and its bed and is forced between the fibres of myometrium, tearing them apart. This is very painful and produces shock. It is associated with a high perinatal mortality rate and a not insubstantial maternal mortality rate. Once diagnosed, the condition should be treated

with antishock therapy, pain relief and expeditious delivery.

RUPTURED UTERUS

This is rare and typically follows previous surgery, particularly a classical caesarean section, but can occur in an unscarred organ.

Rupture of the upper segment of the uterus usually occurs in late pregnancy or early labour. There is sudden pain with great shock. On examination, the abdominal wall is rigid and nothing can be felt through it; fetal parts cannot be distinguished and no fetal heart can be heard. Fetal death invariably results. The pain is due to muscle damage and peritoneal irritation by blood. Dehiscence of the lower segment tends to be less painful and may give minimal symptoms. Treatment is by immediate laparotomy accompanied by rapid blood transfusion.

POLYHYDRAMNIOS

Excessive amniotic fluid in late pregnancy causes overstretching of the uterus and can be very painful. The cause of polyhydramnios must be diagnosed and appropriate treatment implemented. Very rarely, an amniocentesis is required to relieve the symptoms. Diuretics are not helpful.

Suprapelvic causes

PRE-ECLAMPSIA

Pre-eclampsia worsening towards eclampsia causes epigastric and right hypogastric pain due to stretching of the peritoneum over the oedematous liver. The treatment is the same as that for the total pre-eclamptic process.

PEPTIC ULCERATION

Low grade gastric and duodenal ulcers generally involute in pregnancy. The pain is similar to that outside pregnancy and is due to acid irritation of submucosal tissues.

CHOLECYSTITIS

Cholecystitis is one of the most common causes of upper abdominal pain in women with high-fat diets. In pregnancy, it occurs in association with stretching and inflammation of the gallbladder. Pain occurs usually in the upper abdomen, commonly under the right rib margin and over the tip of the ninth rib. Treatment is conservative in the first instance, with antibiotics and intravenous therapy. Later, surgery may be necessary.

APPENDICITIS

As already discussed, this is still one of the commonest causes of abdominal pain, even in late pregnancy. The incision for an appendectomy rises as gestation proceeds (Fig.5.19). Should appendectomy have to be performed in very late pregnancy (after thirty-seven weeks) it is wise not to perform a caesarean section at the same time, but to allow the woman to recover. A normal labour and vaginal delivery are possible as early as two or three days after appendectomy.

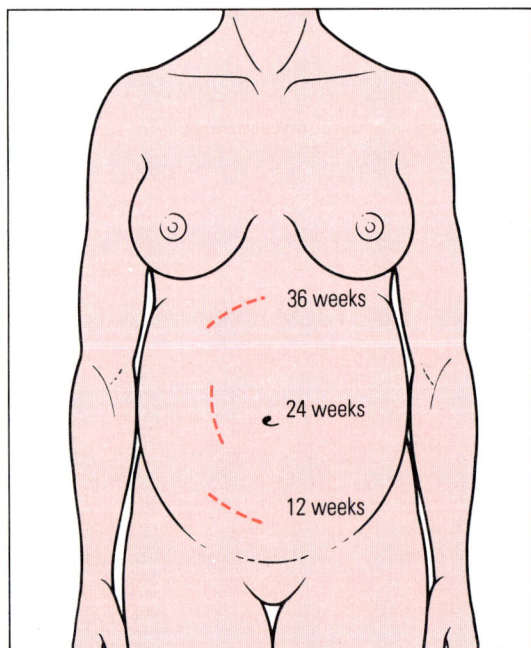

Fig.5.19 Appendicitis in pregnancy. The site of incision for an appendectomy rises as gestation proceeds. The surgeon should mark the point of maximum tenderness at the preoperative examination, so that he may later make an incision over this point. A McBurney incision of the right iliac fossa is useless in later pregnancy.

RECTUS HAEMATOMA

As the rectus muscle and its surrounding tissues are stretched, rupture of the venae comitantes of the deep inferior epigastric artery may occur. These vessels rupture where they pass from the protection of the posterior rectus sheath to the unprotected peritoneum, about 10cm below the umbilicus. The onset of pain is sudden, starting as a bout of coughing or straining, and is acute, being fairly well localized to one small area of the abdomen. Conservative treatment is best but if a laparotomy is performed and a rectal haematoma is found, it should be evacuated. The bleeding point is often difficult to localize.

Management of abdominal pain

Management of abdominal pain depends upon the diagnosis, which must be made clinically and promptly. If conservative treatment is appropriate, the woman should be observed under controlled conditions in an antenatal ward. If the surgeon is in doubt, he may wish to observe for a few hours. As in the non-pregnant woman, this should be a limited observation period with re-examination by the same surgeon.

Those who are less familiar with pregnancy, working in general surgery, should remember that a laparotomy is not a forbidden operation, but is as essential as it would be out of pregnancy. Any fetus in a woman with an abdomen which is affected by acute inflammatory disease will stand a better chance of surviving if the disease process is dealt with promptly.

6. Pregnancy and Intercurrent Disease

URINARY DISORDERS IN PREGNANCY

During pregnancy, increased progesterone levels are associated with relaxation of the smooth muscle of all organs, including the ureters. In the urinary tract, relaxation causes dilatathion and kinking, both of which encourage urinary stasis; this in turn increases the likelihood of infection.

Asymptomatic bacilluria

This occurs in approximately four percent of pregnant women and can only be detected by finding bacilli in significant number (>10,000/ml) in a midstream specimen of urine (MSU). In such women, there is a higher incidence of superimposed symptomatic urinary tract infection and pyelonephritis. Structural abnormalities of the urinary tract are also associated with asymptomatic bacilluria in pregnancy, and there is a weak association with megaloblastic anaemia and pre-eclampsia. For this reason, an MSU is checked by a nitrozine test early in the antenatal care of all patients. If this is positive, another MSU should be tested for bacteria. If this is also positive, long-term treatment with an antibiotic or a urinary antiseptic to which the organism is sensitive is indicated, despite the absence of symptoms. If the infestation continues, treatment must be continued using three rotating antibiotic agents consecutively, each for two weeks; the sensitivity of the organisms should be checked after each cycle of six weeks.

An intravenous urogram is essential at about three to four months after delivery for all women with persistent bacilluria; this will show urinary tract abnormalities in about a quarter of such cases.

Acute pyelonephritis

Symptomatic urinary tract infection occurs in about two percent of pregnant women. There is usually a history of dysuria, increased urinary frequency and sometimes associated backache, vomiting and rigors. On examination, the woman may be pyrexial, dehydrated and tender over either one or both renal angles. An MSU should be immediately examined by microscopy to detect the presence of pus cells, and then cultured for growth of the organism and its sensitivity to antibiotics.

Management includes admission to hospital for bedrest and a high consumption of fluids. If vomiting is persistent, parenteral therapy should be considered, giving five percent dextrose alternating with 0.9 percent sodium chloride. Antibiotic therapy with a broad-spectrum agent should be started after the urine sample has been taken and before sensitivity results are available. As with any febrile illness, labour may start and so it is important to institute treatment of urinary tract infection without delay. If the attack occurs in early pregnancy, the woman should be checked carefully at antenatal visits since recurrence is common. Similarly, postpartum urinary infection may follow and this also requires prompt action.

Chronic pyelonephritis

Chronic pyelonephritis may recur in pregnancy following renal damage in childhood or in a previous pregnancy. It may also be associated with renal structural abnormality, for example disorganized calices and a shrunken cortex. On examination, the woman may be hypertensive with a prepregnancy hypertension rather than hypertension which has begun in pregnancy. Examination of the urine may show pus cells and casts; proteinuria is often present.

The main complications during pregnancy are an increased incidence of superadded acute attacks of pyelonephritis, and hypertension of pregnancy in addition to any pre-existing condition. There may also be an associated intrauterine growth retardation of the infant.

In the management of such a woman, it is important to treat any acute exacerbation of pyelonephritis without delay. In some centres, a woman with a history of chronic renal disease is treated continuously with antibiotics throughout her pregnancy. She should be seen often, have her blood pressure checked, and have an MSU cultured on each occasion. Renal function tests are performed frequently, paying particular attention to plasma urate levels; fetal growth must be monitored serially. After delivery, investigations of renal function and an intravenous urogram must be performed.

Renal failure

This is usually due to either tubular or glomerular necrosis. The former may be reversible if the woman can be kept alive long enough for repair to occur; the latter is irreversible.

In obstetrics, the commonest cause of renal failure is acute hypovolaemia associated with a large blood loss at either abortion, abruption of the placenta, or postpartum haemorrhage. Renal failure may also follow septicaemia, particularly from anaerobic infection following a septic abortion, puerperal sepsis or pyelonephritis. A further cause of renal failure is haemolysis, which may follow severe trauma, abruption, or an incompatible blood transfusion.

The history usually details one of these events and, in careful management of the patient, renal failure is noted by measuring all fluid intake and output. Oliguria is diagnosed when urine production is less than 750ml/24 hours and anuria when production is less than 400ml/24 hours.

Management starts with treatment of the primary condition, for example restoring the blood volume or correcting the septicaemia or haemolysis. The urine output, its osmolarity, and both blood and urine biochemistry should be checked. Renal perfusion must be maintained, usually by treating the primary condition, restoring blood volume and replacing fluids to maintain the central venous pressure. However, this is a coarse guide and it is important not to overload the circulation with fluids. After treatment of the initial condition, the fluid intake should be limited to 500ml/24 hours plus a volume equivalent to the urine that has been passed.

Dialysis, by the peritoneal or venous routes, should be considered early in the management of renal failure, before irreversible biochemical changes take place. The main indications for dialysis are a steadily rising blood urea, plasma potassium approaching 7mmol/litre, severe metabolic acidosis and pulmonary oedema.

During recovery from renal failure, there is usually a diuretic phase during which much urine is passed.

Plasma biochemistry must be monitored carefully during this stage, as substantial sodium and potassium losses follow; supplements may be required in addition to parenteral fluids.

Pregnancy after renal transplantation

With the increase in the number of successful operations, more women are living normal lives and becoming pregnant following renal transplantation. To achieve pregnancy implies successful acceptance of the donated organ, and renal function is usually normal.

Some women may be receiving long-term immunosuppressive drugs to maintain the transplant; these could potentially affect fetal development, but few cases of abnormalities have actually occurred. The transplanted kidney is often sited low in the abdomen at the pelvic brim. Passage of the fetus may then be impeded, necessitating caesarean section. Generally, however, a transplant recipient who is well enough to become pregnant will deliver a healthy baby.

Urinary retention

This is a rare occurrence, and is usually associated with an incarcerated retroverted uterus at the end of the first trimester (Fig.6.1). By this stage, the uterus is usually growing out of the pelvis and becoming an abdominal organ. If it is retroverted, the fundus may be caught under the sacral promontory and the woman will present with acute discomfort, unable to pass urine. On examination of the abdomen, the bladder will be full and the uterus will not be palpable.

Management consists of passing an indwelling catheter and allowing the urine to drain for several days. The woman should be advised to rest, in bed face down, as much as possible so that the uterus can come forward. After the fourteenth week of pregnancy, the uterus has usually settled into an anteverted position in the abdomen; it is no longer a pelvic organ and there are no further problems.

Rarely, the uterus is bound down in the pelvis by old adhesions. Further growth longitudinal to the axis of the uterus is prevented and so the pregnancy either aborts, or it continues with anterior sacculation.

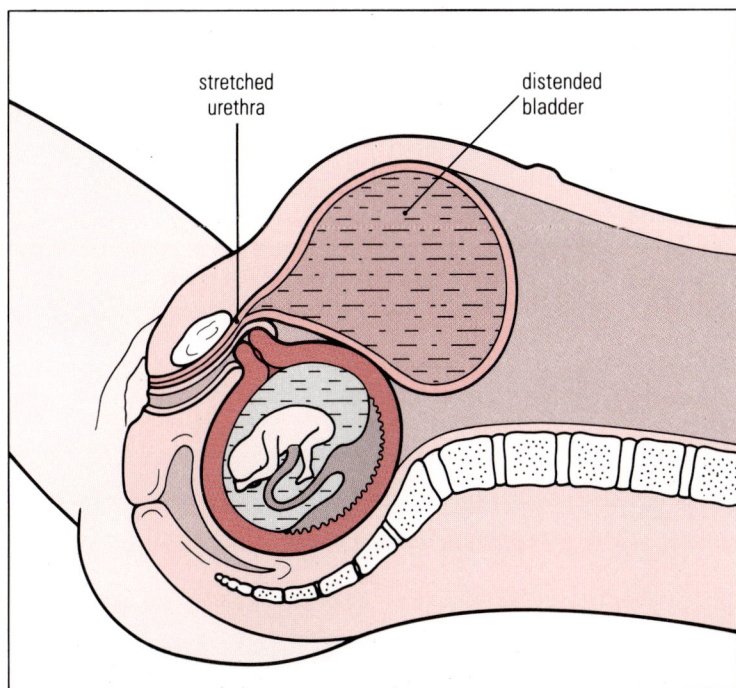

Fig.6.1 Acute retention of urine in pregnancy. The impacted retroverted uterus is trapped below the sacral promontory. The urethra is stretched and uterine growth causes further stretching, which often leads to retention.

ENDOCRINE DISEASE IN PREGNANCY

The greatly increased oestrogen levels in pregnancy affect all endocrine glands in the body and, consequently, the hormone balance. Only pathological changes will be dealt with in this section.

Diabetes

Diabetes is a disorder of protein, fat and carbohydrate metabolism due to hypofunction of pancreatic β cells, which produce insulin. Consequently, the body is less capable of coping with wide variations in amino acids, free fatty acids and glucose absorbed from the alimentary tract.

Incidence

About one percent of women in the pregnancy age group have diabetes and about two percent are potential diabetics; a further one percent may have latent diabetes:

- Potential diabetes. A normal glucose tolerance test is produced, but the woman is at increased risk of developing diabetes because of a past history of babies weighing over 4000g at birth, or of an overweight stillbirth, or a first degree family history of diabetes.
- Latent diabetes. A diabetic type of glucose tolerance test is produced when the woman is stressed, but is normal when non-stressed. A common stress is pregnancy; another could be the administration of steroids.
- Subclinical diabetes. No symptoms or signs of diabetes are evident. There is nothing in the past history to suggest diabetes, but an abnormal glucose tolerance test occurs persistently, both in and out of pregnancy.

Prediabetes is a traditional term, which refers to the period of a person's life before they developed diabetes. It can only be diagnosed in retrospect and should not be used for a woman who shows biological or biochemical features prospectively. The terms listed above are much more accurate descriptions.

Women with potential, latent, or subclinical

diabetes are more likely to develop diabetes in later life. More germane to the obstetrician is that all of these conditions are associated with a higher perinatal mortality rate than that which is present in the background population. Consequently, one should check for the presence of these conditions and, if found, the woman should be monitored as carefully as one would a diabetic.

Diagnosis

Of those women diagnosed as having diabetes in the antenatal period, about ninety percent know that they have the condition and will already be receiving treatment with insulin or will be on a special diet. Other cases may be suspected from a history of unexplained stillbirth or neonatal death, particularly of large babies, a first degree family history of diabetes, or a past history of babies weighing over 4000g. During pregnancy, the urine is checked for glucose at each antenatal visit; recurrent glycosuria

may lead the obstetrician to suspect diabetes. The diagnosis is confirmed by checking blood sugar levels. This is most efficiently done as a glucose tolerance test, but may be truncated to a two-point glucose tolerance test, which measures the blood sugar level once during fasting, and then again two hours after the patient has received a measured load of glucose. A single determination of the fasting blood sugar concentration is insufficient. Pre- and postprandial blood sugar estimations are best used for management and control, rather than for diagnosis.

A raised blood sugar level affects glycosylated haemoglobin HbA1. Thus, a raised HbA1 indicates poor diabetic control in the preceding weeks and although this is not a precise measurement, it is still a useful agent to monitor during pregnancy.

Effects of diabetes

The effects of diabetes on the fetus, mother and neonate are summarized in Fig.6.2.

EFFECTS OF DIABETES		
Effects on fetus	**Effects on mother**	**Effects on neonate**
spontaneous abortion	increasing instability of diabetes	big baby
abnormal fetus	polyhydramnios	hypoglycaemia
intrauterine death	infection	respiratory distress syndrome
	exacerbation of pre-existing hypertension	congenital abnormalities
	pregnancy hypertension	
	retinopathy	
	renal disease	
	vascular disease	

Fig.6.2   The possible effects of diabetes on the fetus, the mother and the neonate.

THE FETUS

Amongst diabetic mothers, the abortion rate is increased, particularly if the woman's diabetic balance is unstable. Such a metabolic disturbance may be reflected in the fetus.

Later in gestation, placental exchange is restricted so that the risks of hypoxia to the fetus are greater, especially if pregnancy is also complicated by a placental abruption, raised blood pressure, or a prolonged labour. The incidence of congenital abnormality is increased, particularly if the diabetes affects the maternal vascular system. Fetal sacral agenesis may also be associated with maternal diabetes.

The fetus of a diabetic mother may be larger than normal, and there may be difficulties in delivery, such as cephalopelvic disproportion, prolonged labour, or shoulder dystocia.

THE MOTHER

During pregnancy, the mother's diabetic balance often becomes unstable and more difficult to control, particularly around twelve weeks and towards the end of pregnancy. Most women increase their insulin dosage substantially, although a small number will have an unchanged or even decreased requirement. The maximum increase in insulin requirement may occur at any time and so repeated monitoring is needed throughout the pregnancy. The mother's diabetic balance should be monitored very carefully immediately after delivery since insulin requirements return to prepregnancy levels within days.

The serious complications of diabetes are retinopathy, renal disease and vascular disease. These are greatly ameliorated if diabetes is managed properly during pregnancy. The prevalence of pre-eclampsia amongst diabetics is approximately double that of normal women. Furthermore, diabetic women who do develop pre-eclampsia often have a worse course, particularly if there is an increased weight gain. This too will affect insulin requirements.

Due to the increased size of the fetus and the mother's potential instability, operative delivery is often needed, which may cause additional problems to the mother.

THE NEONATE

The baby of a diabetic mother is often larger than would be expected from its gestational stage since the organs and skeleton are larger than in normal fetuses; there is also some water retention. Despite this, the baby is relatively immature for the stage of development, which increases the risk of respiratory distress syndrome occurring in the first few days.

Hypoglycaemia may occur in the first few days, particularly if maternal diabetic control has been poor, since the fetal pancreas is accustomed to high blood sugar levels and thus produces large amounts of insulin. After delivery, the blood sugar levels are nearer normal, but the circulating insulin may cause temporary hypoglycaemia. Blood sugar must be carefully monitored and extra glucose given as necessary.

Management

PREGNANCY

Diabetes should be diagnosed early. Fortunately, many women are aware of their condition when they first attend the antenatal clinic. The pregnant diabetic woman should be seen at a special clinic by both an obstetrician and a diabetic physician in consultation. Management of the condition with oral hypoglycaemic agents is inappropriate in pregnancy, as these may cross the placenta; all women should be transferred to insulin, administered as a morning and an evening dose of soluble insulin rather than, or in addition to, the slower absorbing preparations. The former regime allows finer control of the blood sugar.

Blood sugar is best monitored using a blood glucose meter with capillary blood samples; intravenous samples should be kept for special testing and not used for routine balancing. Urine testing is unreliable since the renal threshold of glucose is reduced in pregnancy. Pre- and postprandial capillary samples, taken half an hour before and after each of the three major meals of the day, provide an excellent way of checking control.

Vomiting in a diabetic pregnant woman must be treated promptly to prevent a reduction in carbohydrate intake. Infections must be diagnosed and treated quickly; urinary tract infections should be excluded since they can rapidly upset the insulin control.

The diabetic woman should be seen more frequently at the antenatal clinic and should be monitored for pre-eclampsia. Most cases used to be admitted to hospital from thirty-two weeks for the last stages of pregnancy, but obstetricians now usually advise staying at home, provided the pregnancy is proceeding normally and close and frequent control can be maintained by a combination of home and antenatal clinic visits.

LABOUR

Delivery may be performed before full term if there are obstetric indications, or if the diabetic control is poor and getting worse. However, the conventional idea of delivery at thirty-seven weeks no longer applies routinely, and each woman must be judged individually.

Caesarean section, both elective and emergency, is performed more frequently to deliver diabetic women, since they are already a high-risk group. However, not every diabetic woman requires a caesarian section, and a normal vaginal delivery is obviously preferable.

If labour is allowed to proceed, it should be monitored carefully with continuous fetal heart rate monitoring, externally at first, and then by scalp clip once the membranes have ruptured. Diabetic control should be meticulous during labour, usually with intravenous dextrose and insulin and regular capillary sampling. Oxytocin may be used if required, and it is best to avoid a prolonged labour. If advance is not brisk in the second stage, one should be prepared to assist with a forceps delivery.

Shoulder dystocia during delivery of a large baby is one of the major problems which may occur in the diabetic or potentially diabetic mother. The head delivers and rotates into the transverse position, but stays at the outlet. Due to the wide bisacromial diameter, the fetal shoulders jam in the anteroposterior diameter of the mid- or lower cavity of the pelvis. If this happens, the woman should be put immediately into a lithotomy position, preferably with her buttocks lifted off the bed. The deliverer then takes the delivered head and presses it firmly down towards the mother's anus (Fig.6.3) to release the anterior shoulder. If this manoeuvre is successful, the posterior shoulder usually slips out fairly easily afterwards. Syntometrine should not be given until the anterior shoulder has been released from under the symphysis pubis.

It is too late to consider an episiotomy when shoulder dystocia is diagnosed because it is not possible to get the scissors into the perineum. Consequently, a good episiotomy is often performed prophylactically with vaginal delivery of a diabetic mother when the head is pressing on the perineum.

A paediatrician should always be present at the delivery of a diabetic mother for resuscitation of the baby, if necessary, immediate observations, and to deal with any variation in the neonatal blood sugar level.

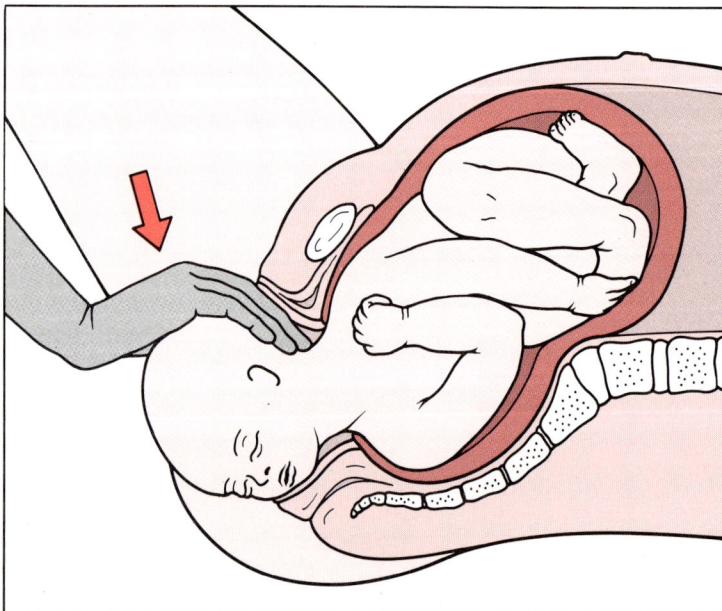

Fig.6.3 Management of shoulder dystocia. The woman should be brought to the edge of the bed, so that her buttocks overhang it, and a firm, even pressure should be applied with the flat of the hand on the side of the fetal head, pushing it towards the mother's anus. By this means, it should be possible to draw the anterior shoulder under the symphysis pubis.

PUERPERIUM

After delivery, the woman is given insulin in her prepregnancy doses, which may require adjustment. After a caesarean section, intravenous dextrose and insulin are used until the woman is drinking and eating, after which insulin may be given in prepregnancy doses. Infection is more common in diabetic women and must be watched for.

The patient should later be advised about contraception and limitation of her family; it is probably wise to avoid oral contraception because the oestrogens affect carbohydrate handling, making control of the diabetic mother difficult. The intrauterine device is very useful in these cases.

Outcome

The perinatal mortality rate in diabetes has decreased sharply over the years so that it is now little above that of other women, when standardized for age and parity. However, this has only been achieved by meticulous monitoring and careful management of these women and it would be wrong to consider that diabetes is not still a major problem for the pregnant mother and her fetus.

Thyroid disease

Pregnancy is potentially a hyperthyroid state. At a very early stage, there is a reduction in the renal tubular absorption of iodine, so that excretion of this element increases. Plasma levels fall and the thyroid gland triples its uptake of iodine from the blood. The gland hypertrophies and manufactures increased amounts of the thyroid hormones, thyroxine (T4) and tri-iodothyronine (T3). Much of T4 is protein bound and so not all pregnant patients become hyperthyroid, but a proportion do exhibit mild symptoms (Fig.6.4).

Thyrotoxicosis is difficult to diagnose for the first time in pregnancy, for there is normally a hyperdynamic state and the boundary between normal and abnormal physiology is difficult to delineate. If a woman is hyperthyroid before pregnancy, previous treatments should be continued. Carbimazole and propylthiouracil may be used but the dose may have to be increased.

. If the disease becomes increasingly difficult to control, thyroidectomy may be required in the middle trimester but one should remember that the hyperdynamic condition may be only temporary and the woman may return to her normal state once pregnancy is over. It is wise to avoid radioactive iodine

THYROID FUNCTION TESTS		
	Pregnancy	Thyrotoxicosis
Heart rate	↑	↑
Basal metabolic rate	↑	↑
Protein bound T4	↑	↑
Protein bound T3	↑	↑
Free T4	normal	↑
Free T3	normal	↑
Thyroid-binding globulin	normal	↑

Fig.6.4 Comparison of alterations in thyroid function tests in pregnancy and in thyrotoxicosis.

testing in pregnancy because of pick-up by the fetal thyroid. All antithyroid drugs are excreted in breast milk and thus breast feeding is generally contra-indicated.

Hypothyroidism is rare in pregnancy since without treatment, women with this condition do not usually become pregnant. However, with the wider use of thyroxine, pregnancy rates have increased. Re-placement therapy with thyroxine should be con-tinued throughout pregnancy and infants of all mothers with thyroid disease should be checked by a skilled pediatrician. Neonatal thyrotoxicosis is rare if maternal control has been good, but in severe cases of Graves' disease, long-acting thyroid stimulator (LATS) antibodies may cross the placenta and cause neonatal thyrotoxicosis.

Postpartum hypothyroidism may, paradoxically, be proceeded by an episode of postpartum hyper-thyroidism. This can be due to an increased quan-tity of thyroid antibodies produced at pregnancy with a rebound phenomenon after the immuno-suppression factors of pregnancy have been removed. Hence, treatment with thyroxine should be only short-term. However, such women should be watched in later life for they may develop a deficient thyroid function.

Parathyroid disease

Hyperparathyroidism in pregnancy is usually di-agnosed by the chance finding of asymptomatic hypercalcaemia. It is associated with maternal and fetal bone disease, and with an increased perinatal mortality. The high plasma calcium levels in the mother are reflected by parathyroid suppression in the fetus. After birth, the fetus may be hypocalcaemic for some weeks, but usually recovers. Most women with hyperparathyroidism who become pregnant proceed normally. If treatment is required during pregnancy, operative procedures are best performed in the second trimester.

Hypoparathyroidism in the reproductive age group usually follows inadvertent surgical removal of the parathyroid glands at thyroidectomy. Rarely, the condition might be a part of an autoimmune disorder, in which there are antibodies against many other endocrine glands, such as the thyroid and ovaries. The fetus may also be hypoparathyroid because of the untreated maternal condition. Treatment is with oral vitamin D and calcium. This prevents the worst effects of the fetus. Tetany may occur during pregnancy and

acute necrosis of the maternal femoral head has been reported, possibly because of the observation of the femoral head on pelvic X-rays.

Adrenal disease

The level of circulating cortisol is raised in pregnancy following the increased metabolism of the adrenal cortex and the decreased breakdown of glucocor-ticoids and mineralocorticoids, most of which are bound to globulin and are inactive.

Hypoadrenalism is usually associated with atrophy of the adrenal cortex. Few untreated cases become pregnant. If a woman has been diagnosed and is treated with replacement cortisol, she should have a normal pregnancy. The dose of cortisol may have to be increased, particularly in times of stress, such as labour.

It should be remembered that many women with incidental diseases, such as Crohn's disease or asthma, are treated with cortisol. They too may experience some suppression of adrenal function and require cortisol supplementation in times of stress. However, their maintenance dose may be reduced, due to the natural increase in corticosteroid production that occurs in pregnancy.

Untreated hyperadrenalism is rarely associated with pregnancy, since ovulation is usually depressed. However, it may occur due to hypersecretion of adrenocorticotropic hormone (ACTH), which causes the adrenal gland to become hyperplastic and produce excess quantities of corticosteroids (Fig.6.5). The treatment, paradoxically, consists of giving more corticosteroids to stimulate negative feedback and so suppress ACTH production. Therapy with prednisolone or fludrocortisone should be continued and the woman should be watched carefully for hypertension, which may need active hypotensive therapy. Occasionally, changes in bone growth in earlier life may have led to pelvic malformations and so to cephalopelvic disproportion.

ANAEMIAS

Anaemia may be due to either a decrease in production or an increase in loss of red blood cells, as summarized in Fig.6.6. Decreased production (haemopoietic anaemia) is commonly due to iron or folate deficiency. Increased blood loss is generally due to haemolytic or haemorrhagic anaemia. Haemolytic

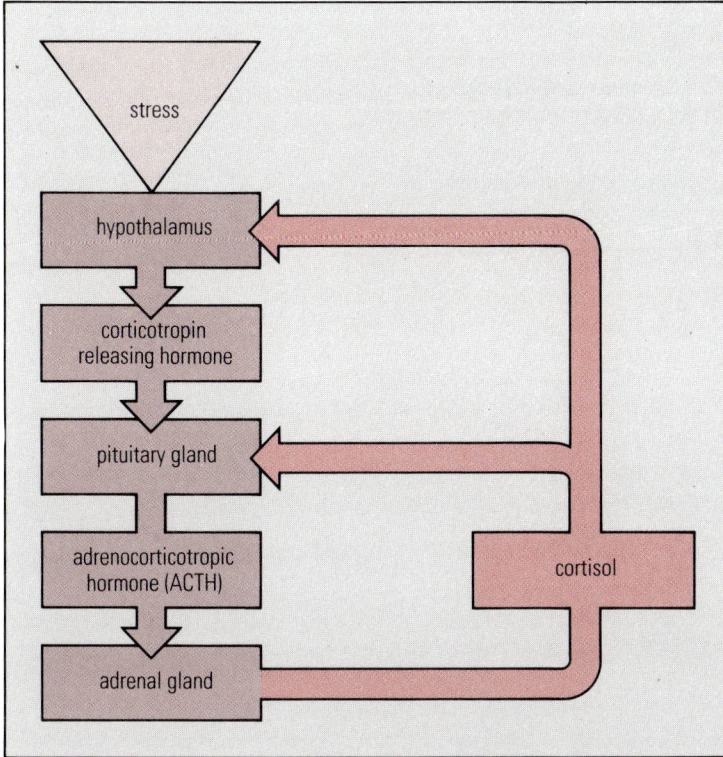

Fig.6.5 The effects of stress on the adrenal gland and the positive feedback of increased levels of cortisol in pregnancy.

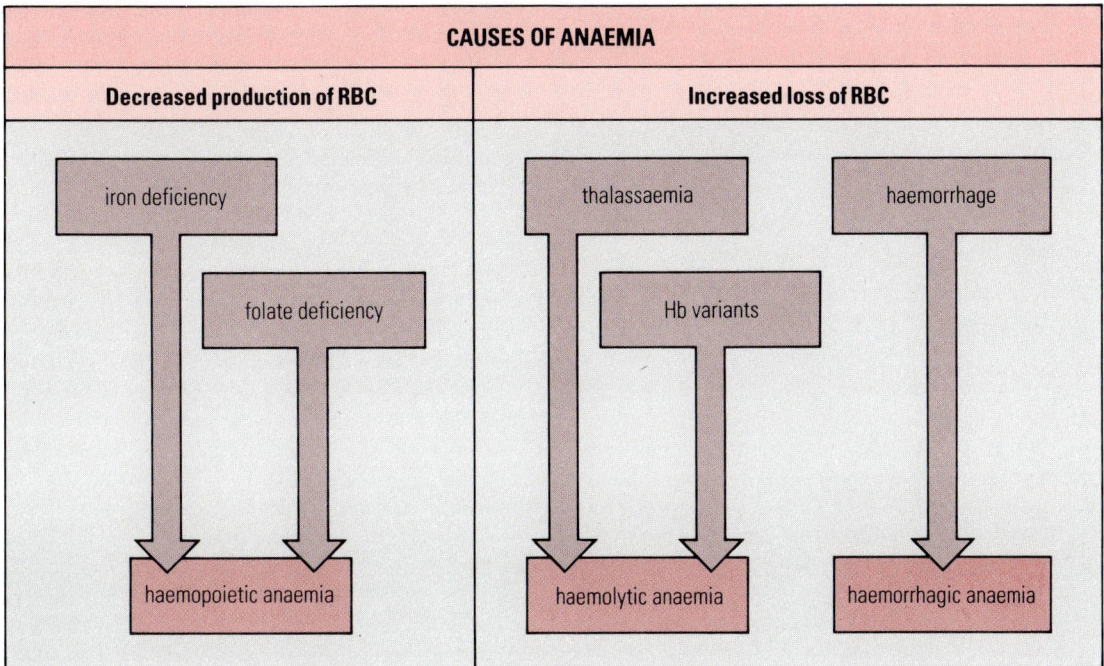

Fig.6.6 Causes of anaemia.

| CAUSES OF IRON DEFICIENCY ANAEMIA ||
Reduced intake	Increased requirements
dietary deficiency	increased maternal RBC & fetal Hb
poor absorption	multiple pregnancy
poor utilization	frequent pregnancies

Fig.6.7 Causes of iron deficiency anaemia. This may be due to a reduced intake of or increased requirement for iron.

anaemia may be due to thalassaemia or to haemoglobin variants. In the United Kingdom, anaemia due to chronic haemorrhage is very rare; the most common cause is gastrointestinal bleeding.

During pregnancy, there is a physiological haemodilution, with the increase in plasma volume being proportionally greater than the increase in red cell mass. The maximum fall in haemoglobin concentration would be 1.5g/dl at thirty-four weeks gestation. During pregnancy, a haemoglobin level of less than 10.5g/dl is generally taken to indicate anaemia.

Iron deficiency anaemia

The causes of iron deficiency anaemia are summarized in Fig.6.7. The condition may follow a reduction in iron intake or an increase in iron requirement. Diminished iron intake may be a result of a dietary deficiency, persistent vomiting or poor absorption of the dietary iron. Ingested iron may also be poorly utilized, for example in women suffering chronic infection.

The increase in iron requirement is caused by an increase in the maternal red cell mass and fetal haemoglobin, especially in the last weeks of gestation. This increased requirement is greater in women with a multiple pregnancy, or in those who have have had many pregnancies, particularly if in close succession.

The diagnosis of iron deficiency anaemia may be made clinically when a woman is tired and has pale conjunctivae. In most instances, however, women are asymptomatic and the diagnosis is made by haematological investigations (Fig.6.8). The haemoglobin level is usually checked at least three times during pregnancy, at twelve, twenty-eight and thirty-six weeks gestation. A level below 10.5g/dl should be investigated; whilst this may be merely a physiological response because of an increase in the plasma volume, it may also be due to anaemia. A drop in the haemoglobin level can be a relatively late event in iron deficiency anaemia. Other haematological indications include a decreased mean corpuscular volume (MCV), resulting in microcytic cells, and a decrease in both the mean corpuscular haemoglobin (MCH) and the mean corpuscular haemoglobin concentration (MCHC). The blood film may be unhelpful, as hypochromia is present only in severe iron deficiency and usually only if the woman enters pregnancy in this state. The total iron-binding capacity (TIBC) is increased. The serum ferritin level is decreased, and serves as a good indicator of the level of iron stored. The most rapid test for iron status would be an examination of marrow aspirate, but this is rarely required. When stained, the marrow shows if

SIGNS & SYMPTOMS OF IRON DEFICIENCY ANAEMIA	
Clinical	Haematological
tiredness	↓ Hb (<10.5g/dl)
pale conjunctivae	↓ MCV (<80x10^{-9} litres)
	↓ MCH (<27 pg/dl)
	↓ MCHC (<30%)
	↓ serum iron (< 14 mmol/litre)
	↑ TIBC (> 80 mmol/litre)
	↓ serum ferritin (< 15μg/litre)

Fig.6.8 Signs and symptoms of iron deficiency anaemia. The condition may be diagnosed by clinical methods or by haematological investigations.

iron is being incorporated into the haemoglobin in normoblasts.

The management of iron deficiency anaemia can be preventative or curative. Preventative measures include early recognition of women at high risk, for example, those with multiple pregnancies and those with a poor diet. These women should be offered regular iron supplements of at least 100mg of elemental iron daily. It is necessary to check repeatedly that the woman is taking this prophylactic therapy. If anaemia still develops, one should consider whether it is not being absorbed or not being utilized.

Curative therapy depends upon the severity of the anaemia and the stage of gestation. Mild anaemia can usually be controlled with oral therapy. If the dose has to be increased or if the woman is unable to swallow tablets, liquid preparations should be given. If the anaemia still does not improve and the gestational stage is less than thirty-six weeks, parenteral iron therapy can be given. Intravenous iron dextran is given in appropriate dosage according to the woman's body size, so that 250mg produces a rise in haemoglobin of about 1g/dl. It is vital that a very small dose be given first to rule out hypersensitivity. Intramuscular therapy may also be used, giving iron dextran on alternate days; however, the injections can be painful and may cause staining of the skin.

Severe iron deficiency anaemia (Hb < 8g/dl) after thirty-six weeks gestation is usually treated by admitting the woman to hospital and giving a blood transfusion, since there is little time left to make red blood cells. Careful checks should be made throughout the rest of the pregnancy to ensure that the improvement is maintained and that anaemia does not recur.

CAUSES OF FOLATE DEFICIENCY ANAEMIA	
Reduced intake	**Increased requirement**
dietary deficiency	manufacture of DNA
vomiting	multiple pregnancy
malabsorption	frequent pregnancies
	chronic infection
	rhesus problem

Fig.6.9 Causes of folate deficiency anaemia. This may be due to reduced intake of or increased demand for folate.

Folate deficiency anaemia

The causes of folate deficiency anaemia are summarized in Fig.6.9. The condition may follow a reduced intake of or an increased demand for folate. The former may be a result of dietary deficiency (folate in vegetables is destroyed by prolonged cooking), vomiting or malabsorption syndromes. There is an increased folate requirement during pregnancy since it is necessary for DNA manufacture in both the fetus and the enlarging maternal organs. The increase is even greater in multiple pregnancy (one of the commonest causes of folate deficiency anaemia in the UK), among grand multiparae (particularly if pregnancies occur close together), in women suffering chronic infection, and in women with a rhesus problem where increased fetal haemolysis makes greater demands for folate.

The diagnosis of folate deficiency may rarely be made clinically when the patient complains of tiredness, breathlessness and oedema. In more severe cases, there may be other signs of malnutrition. Diagnosis may depend upon laboratory investigations (Fig.6.10). The FIGLU test (for formir inoglutamate in the urine) is unreliable during pregnancy.

Haemoglobin levels may be very low but this is a late change. The erythrocytes occasionally show macrocytosis, while the leukocytes demonstrate beading of their nuclei. Both serum and red cell folate levels are unreliable for diagnostic use during pregnancy.

The most reliable way of diagnosing folate deficiency during pregnancy is to examine a bone marrow aspirate from the iliac crest. Megaloblastic changes are found with even mild degrees of folate deficiency, whereas macrocytes are not seen in the peripheral circulation until the deficiency is severe.

Management may be prophylactic or curative. Prophylactic oral folate, 300g/day in combination with an iron supplement, is usually given to pregnant women, particularly in the last twenty weeks. Curative treatment for mild folate deficiency consists of oral therapy at 500–1000g/day. In more severe deficiency, parenteral therapy must be used, since megaloblastic changes in the gut impair absorption of oral folate.

If very severe folate deficiency anaemia occurs late in pregnancy, transfusion may be needed. It is important to remember that prolonged breast feeding and a poor diet may result in folate deficiency manifesting for the first time in the postnatal period.

SIGNS & SYMPTOMS OF FOLATE DEFICIENCY ANAEMIA	
Clinical	**Haematological**
tiredness	↓ Hb (<10g/dl)
breathlessness	↑ MCV (> 100×10^{-9} litres)
oedema	↓ MCH (<27 pg/dl)
	↓ MCHC (<30%)
	↑ megaloblasts in bone marrow aspirate

Fig.6.10 Signs and symptoms of folate deficiency anaemia. The condition may be diagnosed clinically or by haematological investigations.

Thalassaemia

In thalassaemia, production of the globin chain of haemoglobin is defective. Women with this condition often originate from Mediterranean areas and have an inherited defect in the synthesis of the α or β globin chain of adult haemoglobin A. Only the heterozygous, or carrier, form is important during pregnancy; the homozygous form is usually lethal.

The diagnosis of thalassaemia may be suspected in a woman who originates from the Mediterranean or who has a family history of the condition. The haematological indices include a low haemoglobin level and an inadequate MCHC. The red cells show increased fragility and the serum iron is raised. Definitive diagnosis of thalassaemia is obtained by electrophoresis, when the various haemoglobins are separated by the electrophoretic process.

The management of anaemia due to thalassaemia includes oral iron supplementation, despite the fact that the serum iron level is already raised, in conjunction with extra folate, since there is an increased marrow turnover. If the anaemia is severe, parenteral folate should be given. Transfusion may be indicated in severe anaemia near to term or in haemolytic crisis. Management in labour is based on the prevention of crises by reducing stress and hypoxia.

It is important to remember that the partner's blood should also be examined by electrophoresis; if he too is a thalassaemia carrier, there is a chance that the fetus may be homozygous. Such couples are the main users of a service of prenatal fetal blood sampling or chorionic villous biopsy (see Chapter 3) for the diagnosis of thalassaemia.

Haemoglobinopathy

Haemoglobinopathies occur due to genetically determined alterations of the amino acids in the globin chain of adult haemoglobin A (HbA). There are several substitutions known, but only four are important during pregnancy and all are chain substitutions:
- HbS is found in Negro populations of African origin, and in some Southern European and Middle Eastern individuals.
- HbC is commonest in Ghanaians.
- HbD$_{Punjab}$ occurs in people of that area.
- HbE is found in people of South-East Asian origin.

All of these variants are inherited and all may exist in either a hetero- or homozygous form.

The alteration in the globin chain allows the red cells to break down much more easily, producing a histological picture of flattened or sickled red cell envelopes. A sickling crisis may be prompted by a lowered oxygen tension together with acidosis. This in turn blocks the capillaries, causing stasis, which leads to further hypoxia and acidosis, causing further sickling. Thus, a vicious circle is created.

Diagnosis of haemoglobinopathy should be suspected in any women from the relevant areas, in those with a family or past history of the condition, or in those with bone marrow infarcts or sudden abdominal pains. Haematological investigations show a reduced haemoglobin level, while a blood film may show target and sickle cells. Electrophoresis demonstrates an abnormal haemoglobin pattern in both the heterozygous and homozygous forms. It is important to detect which form of haemoglobin variant is present, since spontaneous sickling occurs mostly in the HbS subgroups HbSS, HbSc and HbS thalassaemia. Spontaneous sickling does not usually occur with sickle cell trait (HbAS), but can be prompted by anoxia.

The management of such a patient includes early detection of the problems, folate supplements (2mg/day), and the prevention of conditions leading to a crisis, for example hypoxia, dehydration or trauma. If a crisis should occur, the haemoglobin level should be checked every four to six hours and transfusion should be considered.

Management of the subgroups of HbS disease is according to one of the following regimes, depending on the severity of the condition and the speed of deterioration during pregnancy.

HbSS disease

Any one of the following regimes may be used:
• Regular transfusions should be given throughout pregnancy to convert the woman into a carrier, i.e. to raise the circulating HbA level so that it is higher than the circulating HbS level.
• An exchange transfusion should be given at 36 weeks gestation followed soon afterwards by a caesarean section.
• Treat conservatively. With close antenatal supervision of haemoglobin levels, the maternal and fetal condition is maintained and no prophylactic transfusion should be given unless there is an additional indication.

HbS thalassaemia

This behaves in the same way as HbSS disease and any of the three treatments may be used.

HbSC disease

This requires close clinical supervision to avoid any stimulus to a crisis, such as hypoxia, dehydration or trauma. This particularly applies immediately after delivery. In HbSC disease, the haemoglobin level is often within normal limits and unless electrophoresis is performed, the condition may go undetected.

Sickle cell trait (HbAS disease)

This requires no special treatment, but stimuli to a crisis should be avoided.

Haemorrhagic anaemia

This refers to chronic haemorrhagic states, the two commonest causes of which are gastrointestinal pathology in the form of ulceration, and gastrointestinal bleeding caused by infestation with tapeworms or hookworms. The diagnosis may be made clinically, and if the patient is not already taking iron therapy, the colour of the stool is relevant.

On haematological examination there is a low haemoglobin level, although the erythrocytes will appear normal. Stool specimens should be analysed for blood content and also for signs of infestation with worms and larvae. Peptic ulceration during pregnancy is not common in the United Kingdom but if present, it may improve during this time, so that endoscopical investigation is often not needed. X-ray studies should be avoided in pregnancy.

The management of a patient with haemorrhagic anaemia consists of treating the cause of ulceration or infestation and correcting the anaemia with iron and folate supplements; transfusion may be useful if there is a severe anaemia in late pregnancy.

CARDIOVASCULAR DISEASE IN PREGNANCY

Heart disease

The incidence and severity of heart disease encountered during pregnancy is decreasing. The most common cause is acquired heart disease due to rheumatic fever, however, the incidence of this condition has decreased since its treatment has become more effective. Congenital defects are encountered relatively more often due to the improved survival rate of children with such defects. However, the proportion of rheumatic to congenital lesions is still five to one in general hospitals.

Physiology

The effects of pregnancy on the cardiovascular system include an increase in blood volume of approximately thirty-five percent, or 1500ml (Fig.6.11). This is due mainly to an increase in plasma volume (of approximately forty percent) and also to an increase in erythrocytes (of around twenty percent). The maximal increase in blood volume generally occurs by about sixteen to twenty weeks gestation.

There is also an increase in cardiac output (Fig.6.12), from about 5 to 7 litres/min, due mainly to an increased stroke volume which occurs at a similar time in gestation. There is a further increase during labour, particularly in the first stage.

Maternal and fetal complications of heart disease are summarized in Fig.6.13.

Maternal complications

Pre-existing heart disease may be exacerbated by anaemia or cardiac arrhythmia, and heart failures induced. Any febrile illness or infection, in particular respiratory infection, can precipitate heart failure, as can severe pre-eclampsia. Multiple pregnancy causes further increase in the blood volume and cardiac output, and thus increases the chance of heart failure occurring. Any pregnant woman with a known heart lesion who is working hard physically is also at increased risk.

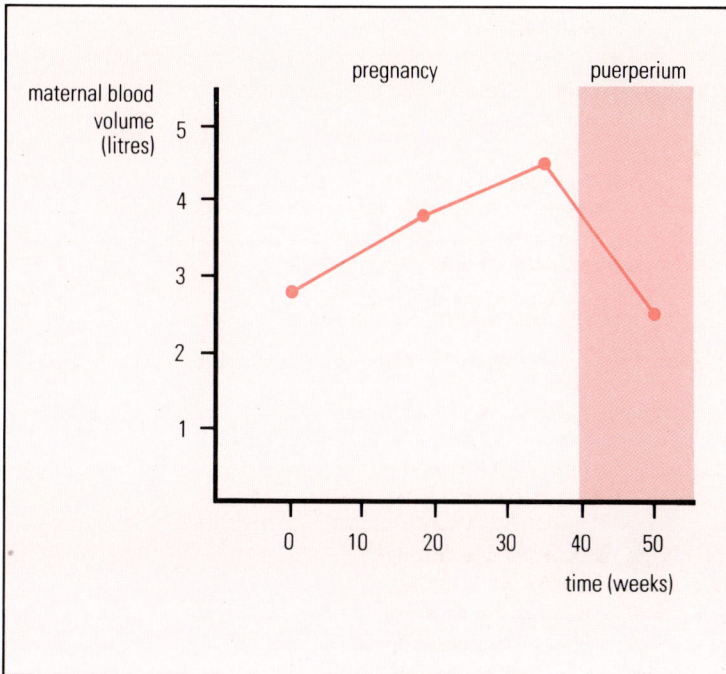

Fig.6.11 Blood volume is increased by up to 40% in pregnancy, thus increasing the load on the heart.

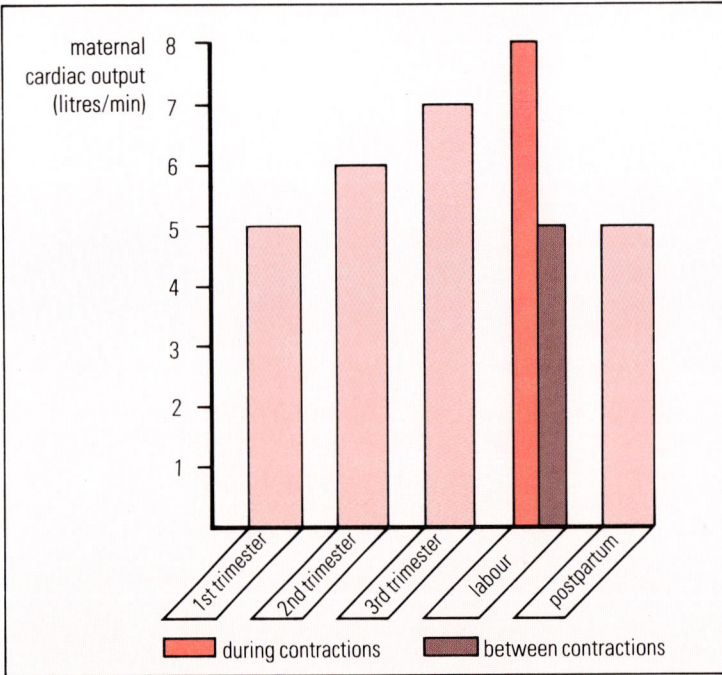

Fig.6.12 Cardiac output during pregnancy. Modified from Whitfield, C. R. (editor) (1986) *Dewhurst's Textbook of Obstetrics and Gynaecology for Postgraduates (4th edition)*. Oxford: Blackwell Scientific Publications.

COMPLICATIONS OF HEART DISEASE IN PREGNANCY	
Fetal	**Maternal**
preterm delivery	anaemia
intrauterine growth retardation	arrhythmia
	pre-eclampsia
	recrudescence of rheumatic disease
	congestive cardiac failure (CCF)
	acute bacterial endocarditis

Fig.6.13 Complications of heart disease in pregnancy.

Fetal complications

The effects of heart disease on the fetus include a slightly increased incidence of preterm delivery and of intrauterine growth retardation. The incidence of these correlates with the severity of the heart disease.

The greater degrees of hypoxia, as noted with cyanotic heart disease, are associated with severe reduction in placental bed blood flow with resultant poor growth.

MANAGEMENT OF HEART DISEASE IN LABOUR

ensure blood availability

antibiotic cover (if necessary)

use oxytocin not Syntometrine

ensure adequate analgesia

minimize effort of 2nd stage

spontaneous labour & vaginal delivery preferable

ensure availability of drugs for CCF

Fig.6.14 Management of a woman with heart disease in labour.

Management

MANAGEMENT DURING PREGNANCY
Awareness of the existence of a heart lesion is critical and early diagnosis should be made by taking a careful history and performing a chest examination. Appropriate investigations include an ECG, chest X-ray and echocardiogram. The severity of the lesion should be assessed in conjunction with the cardiac physician, who should share the management of the woman. Functional cardiac impairment may be graded according to the exercise tolerance of the patient:
• Grade 1: no limitation on exercise.
• Grade 2: some decrease in exercise tolerance.
• Grade 3: shortness of breath with slight exertion.
• Grade 4: shortness of breath at rest.

It may be a useful marker to management to assign patients to a particular grade, but their condition can easily alter during pregnancy, so that placement in grade 1 or 2 does not imply that the woman is not at risk – by thirty weeks gestation she may be short of breath at rest and require urgent treatment.

Other equally important prognostic features include the woman's age, the duration of the rheumatic carditis, if present, and the degree of structural change in the heart, for example myocardial scarring or stenosis of two valves.

The woman should be advised to rest as much as possible and may need to give up work earlier than other women, particularly if she has a multiple pregnancy. She must be advised that infection should be treated early, and women who suffer with chronic bronchitis should be given antibiotics so that they can start treatment immediately, should the infection occur. Dental extractions or other potential infecting incidents should be covered by prophylactic antibiotics to prevent bacterial endocarditis.

To avoid anaemia, prophylactic iron and folate are given. The woman should be seen frequently during the antenatal period, paying particular attention to the heart rate and rhythm, and to the avoidance and treatment of any incidental infection, in addition to her full antenatal care.

MANAGEMENT DURING LABOUR
A checklist for the management of heart disease in labour is presented in Fig.6.14. In general, a spontaneous onset of labour with vaginal delivery is preferred. Induction or caesarean section should only be performed for strong obstetric indications.

During the first stage, extra work must be reduced. This is generally achieved with good analgesia, by either epidural block or systemic analgesia. Blood should be cross-matched and available, since any sudden haemorrhage and anaemia may precipitate heart failure. Antibiotics should be given if there is a congenital lesion or prosthetic heart valve, but otherwise the first stage should be managed normally.

107

During the second stage, unnecessary work must again be prevented. In most women, a quick spontaneous delivery is usually achieved with minimal expulsive effort. If this does not occur, elective vacuum extraction or forceps delivery should be performed.

During the third stage, it is usual to avoid use of Syntometrine, since this may cause peripheral vascular constriction in addition to uterine muscle contraction. This increases the central venous pressure rapidly and may precipitate pulmonary oedema. Oxytocin may be given, since it causes uterine muscle contraction without increasing the peripheral resistance, so there is no increase in central venous pressure. A diuretic may be used prophylactically during the third stage to help counteract the effects of the sudden increase in blood volume. Antibiotics may be needed, especially if the woman has experienced cyanotic episodes.

MANAGEMENT IN THE PUERPERIUM

Special attention must be paid to the avoidance of deep vein thombosis, pulmonary embolus and infection. It is important to check that the woman has adequate help at home, so that she will not become overworked, causing decompensation of her cardiac function. Contraceptive advice is given before the woman leaves hospital, since a pregnancy occurring too soon after the previous one places an extra strain on the cardiovascular system.

If heart failure should occur at any stage during the pregnancy or labour, it must be treated with admission to hospital, bedrest, and the administration of digitalis for an arrhythmia. Oxygen may be required, and a diuretic may be necessary if there is much oedema; morphine relieves tension, and aminophylline may be needed to relieve bronchospasm if the condition is severe.

Hypertension

Hypertension may be pre-existing or may be due to pregnancy (pre-eclampsia). It is important to distinguish between the two, as they have different implications for the woman and the fetus.

Pre-existing hypertension may be due to:
- renal disease
- coarctation of the aorta
- phaeochromocytoma
- essential hypertension
- primary aldosteronism
- Cushing's syndrome

Of these, the first four are by far the most commonly found in the pregnancy age group. Renal disease may be evident from a history of repeated urinary tract or renal infections before pregnancy; the urine may contain protein, casts, cells and organisms. Coarctation of the aorta is usually known to the woman prior to pregnancy. To exclude this as a cause of hypertension, the obstetrician should examine the femoral artery pulses at the booking visit. A phaeochromocytoma is a rare occurrence in pregnancy, and may be excluded by examining the urine for vanillylmandelic acid. If these three causes have been excluded, the woman is usually considered to have essential hypertension.

Any of the above features will cause the blood pressure to be raised at the initial booking visit and this will persist throughout the pregnancy. Hypertension of pregnancy (pre-eclampsia) does not generally occur before twenty-four weeks gestation and the woman often has no history of hypertension; pre-existing hypertension may be complicated by superadded pregnancy hypertension.

Management

A woman with pre-existing hypertension is seen more frequently at the antenatal clinic to ensure that the condition does not suddenly worsen. Careful monitoring is made of fetal growth by ultrasound, and later, of fetal wellbeing by cardiotocography. Antihypertensive therapy instituted prior to pregnancy is generally continued; however, a beta blocker is commonly replaced with methyldopa, which probably has less effect on fetal growth. This is best done in consultation with a physician.

The management of pre-eclamptic women is dealt with in Chapter 5.

Prognosis

The prognosis for the fetuses of hypertensive mothers is worse than for those of pre-eclamptic mothers.

The immediate prognosis for the mother is good if care is meticulous. It is likely that the prevalence of pre-existing hypertension will increase with successive pregnancies and the advancing age of the woman, hence contraceptive advice and family limitation is very important.

GENITAL TRACT INFECTIONS IN PREGNANCY

During pregnancy, the incidence of upper genital tract infection is usually reduced, partly because women with such infections do not easily become pregnant. Lower genital tract infection of the vagina is much more common in pregnancy due to the altered vaginal environment and cervical secretions.

Syphilis

This is a rare condition in the United Kingdom. It may present clinically with one or more primary chancres of the genital tract. In pregnancy, syphilis is most often diagnosed from routine serological tests made at the booking visit. It is common to perform a Wasserman reaction (WR) as a screening investigation, but more specific immunological tests are required to make a diagnosis since the WR can be positive for reasons other than syphilis (for example yaws). Immunological diagnosis may be based on tests such as the *Treponema pallidum* immobilization test or the fluorescent treponemal antibody test.

The fetus may be infected across the placenta, the infection leading to stillbirth or congenital syphilitic lesions such as a depressed bridge to the nose or Hutchinson's teeth later in life (Fig.6.15).

Syphilis diagnosed in pregnancy should be treated vigorously as the fetus can be cured at this time. Intramuscular penicillin (one to two million units daily for five days) will cure most cases of syphilis in the pregnant woman. The tests should be repeated at monthly intervals and, if necessary, a repeat course of penicillin should be given. The newborn should be tested and if positive, he too should be treated with penicillin. If the mother is allergic to penicillin, erythromycin may be used.

Among certain populations where syphilis is more common, it may be wise to repeat the testing later in pregnancy, to detect those who become infected during the course of pregnancy.

Gonorrhoea

Women with chronic gonorrhoea rarely become pregnant. If an acute attack arises in pregnancy, it usually affects the urethra and trigone of the bladder, producing persistent severe burning at the beginning

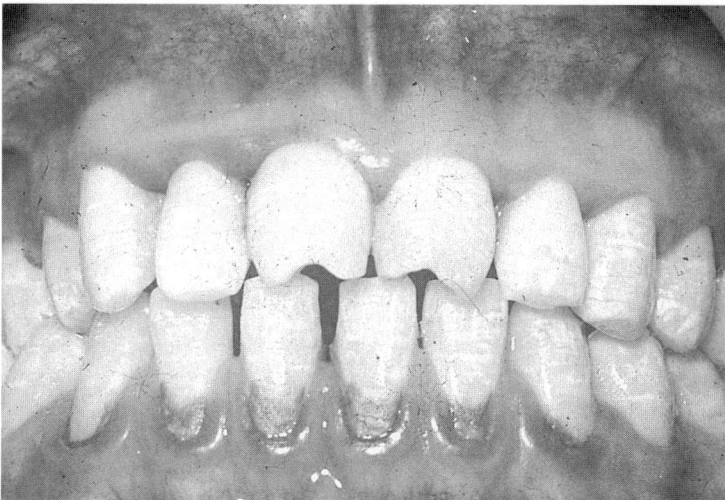

Fig.6.15 Hutchinson's teeth develop following syphilitic infection. They are characteristically barrel shaped with notches at their edges. Courtesy of Dr J. S. Bingham.

and end of micturition. The vulva and vagina may be affected more commonly in the pregnant than the non-pregnant, and an irritant discharge may be found.

The diagnosis is confirmed by taking swabs from the urethra and endocervical regions. These should be transported in Stuart's medium, as the gonococcus is sensitive to drying and would not survive on an ordinary swab.

The gonococcus is a sensitive organism and treatment with one million units of penicillin intramuscularly for two days is sufficient. However, the results of the swabs may show a penicillin-resistant organism and therefore other antibiotics may be required.

The WR reaction of any woman with gonorrhoea should be checked before starting therapy, since some will have also contracted syphilis. The lower dose of penicillin used to treat gonorrhoea could mask, but not cure, the effects of syphilis.

Treatment for gonorrhoea during pregnancy usually cures the mother and fetus. If the fetus should be born through a genital tract affected with gonorrhoea, ophthalmia neonatorum may follow (Fig.6.16). Consequently, it is wise to swab the eyes of babies who are born from affected mothers. Cloramphenicol ointment (one percent) is the best treatment for the condition.

Herpes genitalis

Herpes infections have spread rapidly in America and, to a lesser extent, in the rest of the developed world. They are associated with irritant vesicles of the clitoris, labia and cervix (Fig.6.17), and possibly with a thin vaginal discharge. Diagnosis is confirmed by gently scraping the base of the vesicle and preparing a smear for virological examination. Viral culture can be performed but special culture media are required in which so send the scrapings from the outpatients' clinic to the laboratory. Herpes antibodies may be present in the blood but these are not always indicative of a current infection, since once a woman has been infected, the titre will persist.

If herpes is discovered in early pregnancy, it is worth treating the woman with antiherpes agents, which at least cut down the infectiveness and prevent spread of the organism. Acyclovir, 200mg five times a day for five days, is the conventional course.

If herpes is discovered in late pregnancy (after thirty-four weeks), the route of delivery of the child should be considered. Herpes can affect the newborn (particularly the neurological system) and if active infection is present in the genital tract, it is probably wise to perform a caesarean section to avoid contamination. Intrauterine infection of the fetus is unusual.

Chlamydial infection

Chlamydiae are non-motile rickettsiae which appear in two forms: a small infectious extraceullular elementary body, and a large initial body. Both grow in the cytoplasm of host cells and may be found colonizing the upper vagina without producing any symptoms.

Chlamydiae can cause conjunctivitis in the new-

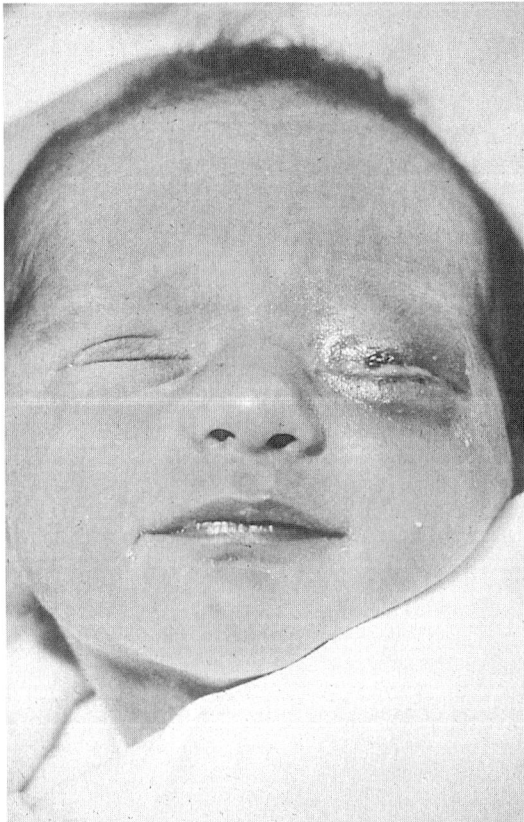

Fig.6.16 Ophthalmia neonatorum, caused by gonorrhoeal infection, has produced marked ophthalmic oedema in this neonate. Courtesy of Dr C. S. Nicol.

born delivered through the vagina of an infected mother. Consequently, it is wise to treat either the mother with erythromycin before delivery or her baby with tetracyline eyedrops, possibly substantiated by erythromycin if the infection seems not to be responding.

Acquired immunodeficiency syndrome (AIDS)

Although this used to be considered a disease of homosexual males, AIDS can be transmitted to women. Blood transfusion from the infected donor and shared needles used in intravenous heroin addiction are both routes of infection which can affect either sex. In addition, the virus may be transmitted

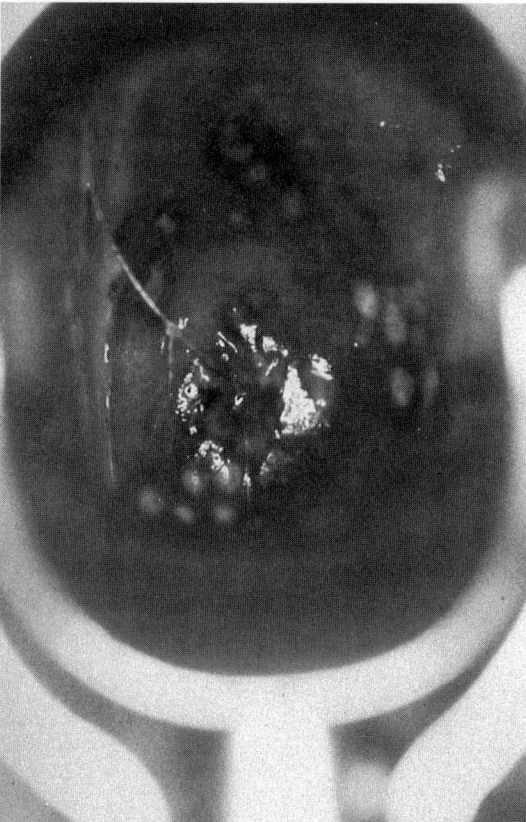

Fig.6.17 Herpetic vesicles and erosion on the cervix. The tail of an intrauterine device is visible. Courtesy of Dr J. S. Bingham.

via semen from an affected male. Although this is more common during a homosexual act, the virus entering through minute breaks in the mucosa of the anal canal, it can also be transmitted during heterosexual acts through similar breaks in the integrity of the cervix or vagina.

The condition manifests as poor resistance to a series of first minor, and then major infections. Neurological conditions such as Alzheimer's disease may occur. Treatment is symptomatic at present, although research into the development of vaccines is proceeding. Trisodium phosphonoformate seems potent against the virus and other antiherpes agents are currently being tested.

AIDS, caused by human immunodeficiency virus (HIV), is becoming more common in the developed world. If a woman has AIDS when she is pregnant, there is a fifty percent chance that her fetus will become infected. Since there is no cure for AIDS at present, that baby, when born, has a high chance of being severely diseased. Transmission can probably also occur through milk. Management of such cases is supportive at the moment.

Testing all pregnant women for HIV antibodies is not practical at present, but many countries are testing women whose partners have AIDS or, at a lesser risk, women whose partners are haemophiliacs on active treatment or who have had a condition which required blood transfusion. The next level of testing should logically be screening of women whose partners have slept with men, although it would be difficult to elucidate that part of the history. Consequently, total population screening at antenatal clinics may be introduced.

Candidiasis

Candidiasis is much more common among pregnant than non-pregnant women. It is caused by *Candida albicans*, a fungus which spreads rapidly in moist, warm areas. During pregnancy, the vagina becomes slightly more alkaline, which facilitates growth of the fungus.

Candidiasis presents with a thick, irritant, offensive discharge, often with solid pieces being passed. It may be accompanied by a little bleeding from the broken vaginal skin. The vagina may need mechanical cleaning with saline baths, but douching should be avoided in pregnancy. Nystatin pessaries (100,000 units twice a day) are effective in most cases. If this does not work, miconazole in a two percent cream is helpful. Econazole is also useful for resistant cases.

The fetus may be affected by passing through a vagina infected with *Candida*. Skin infection is the most common manifestation, although gut or fatal lung infections occur rarely. These are also treated with nystatin.

Trichomoniasis

This vaginal infection is also common in pregnancy. It is caused by a flagellate protozoan which spreads very rapidly in the vagina.

Trichomoniasis is characterized by a thin, offensive, irritant discharge, which may be secondarily infected with pyogenic organisms to produce a thicker discharge. It is best treated with oral metronidazole (200mg three times a day for seven days) and saline baths to remove the mucopurulent discharge from the vagina. A course of metronidazole should also be offered to the partner, for this condition can be passed back and forth between sexual partners, with the male often being asymptomatic and unaware that his urethra is infected with the protozoan.

The fetus delivered through an area infected with *Trichomonas* sometimes develops a skin infection. This can be treated with metronidazole either locally or systemically.

7. Normal Labour

THE STAGES OF LABOUR

Labour is the process during which the fetus, membranes and placenta are expelled from the uterus. It is conventionally divided into three stages (Fig.7.1).

First stage

This stage begins with the onset of labour and finishes when the cervix is fully dilated to 10cm. The onset of labour is often difficult to diagnose, and depends upon the woman herself being able to recognize it; if she has not been told what to expect, she will probably be uncertain whether or not it has begun. Labour usually commences with regular painful contractions of the uterus, which occur initially every half hour. They are first felt in the small of the back, just above the buttocks, and then radiate round to the suprapubic area. Less frequently, the onset of labour is signalled by a show of bloody mucus, or by rupture of the membranes with escape of amniotic fluid. The first stage is very variable in length and may last for many hours.

Second stage

This stage begins with the full dilatation of the cervix and ends following complete delivery of the baby. It is termed the expulsive stage of labour and usually lasts for less than two hours.

Third stage

This stage commences after the baby is born and continues until the full expulsion of the placenta and membranes. This is the shortest of the three stages and lasts for only a matter of minutes.

PHYSIOLOGY OF NORMAL LABOUR

Maternal physiology

Labour is hard work and the woman can become de-hydrated. The alimentary tract is static during labour and fluid accumulates in the stomach, intestine and large bowel. This will be either absorbed or passed on when labour is over, but pooling in the stomach may lead to vomiting.

Most labours do not last for many hours but the woman will need support. She may breathe too quickly and deeply in the first stage of labour which can cause a rapid fall in $P\text{CO}_2$ and a relative alkalosis in the blood. If this becomes excessive it can lead to carpopedal and other muscle spasms. However, most overbreathing and maternal distress can be prevented by properly educating the woman before she reaches labour and by providing reasonable analgesia.

Psychology should be considered a part of the normal physiology of labour. Labour is basically a normal event, which is usually eagerly anticipated by the woman and her partner. For them, it is perhaps one of the biggest moments of their lives and the attendant should remember this. He or she is but a helper, the most important person being the woman, supported by her partner.

Physiology of the uterus

The contents of the uterus are moved downwards by the action of the myometrium. Regular waves of contraction pass from two centres on either side of the uterine fundus, causing the muscle to contract. These centres might be considered analogous to the sino-atrial pacemakers of the heart. Uterine pacemakers cannot be demonstrated structurally in the human, although they can be seen in other species. The impulse spreads over the uterus like a ripple passing downwards (as occurs over the atria of the heart), rather than travelling along preformed pathways (as occurs along the bundle of His). Individual myometrial cells are activated by the passage of this impulse along their cell membranes.

The uterine musculature consists of an outer thin longitudinal layer and areas of inner circular muscle around the two cornua and the internal and external sphincters of the cervix. However, most uterine muscle is in the form of spiral fibres (see Chapter 2); these complete between two to two and a half turns

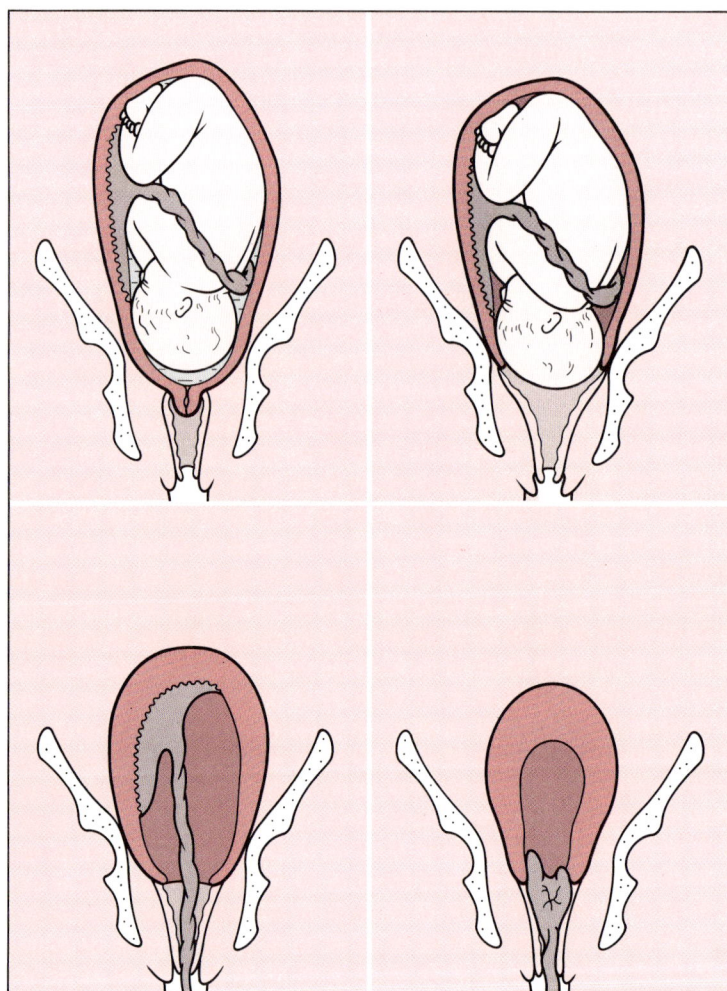

Fig.7.1 The stages of labour. The first stage is from the onset of labour (upper left) to the full dilatation of the cervix (upper right). The second stage is from full dilatation of the cervix (upper right) to delivery of the baby (lower left). The third stage is from delivery of the baby (lower left) to delivery of the placenta and membranes (lower right).

around the uterine cavity, with blood vessels situated between each turn. If the fibres contract in a co-ordinated way, they bring the fundus closer to the cervix and slightly narrow the lumen of the cavity.

Contractions initially occur about once every thirty minutes, each lasting for half a minute. The frequency then increases so that by the time the active stage of labour is reached, they are occurring every two to three minutes and lasting for forty-five to sixty seconds. Contractions become painful, probably due to hypoxia of the muscle caused by the strength and duration of the contraction.

The cervix is dilated by descent of the presenting part. The more the presenting part is pushed down,

and the more the uterine muscle pulls upon the cervix, the wider the dilatation.

The pressure in the myometrium, and therefore inside the amniotic cavity, reflects muscle activity during uterine contractions, and these changes may be measured: they can be felt by the experienced examiner's hand on the abdomen during labour; they can be shown by the use of an external tocograph, which reflects the upward pressure on the back of the anterior abdominal wall; or, more accurately, they can be measured internally by a tube led into the uterine cavity through the cervix. Both external and internal methods can be connected with a strain gauge to measure changes and the results can then be printed

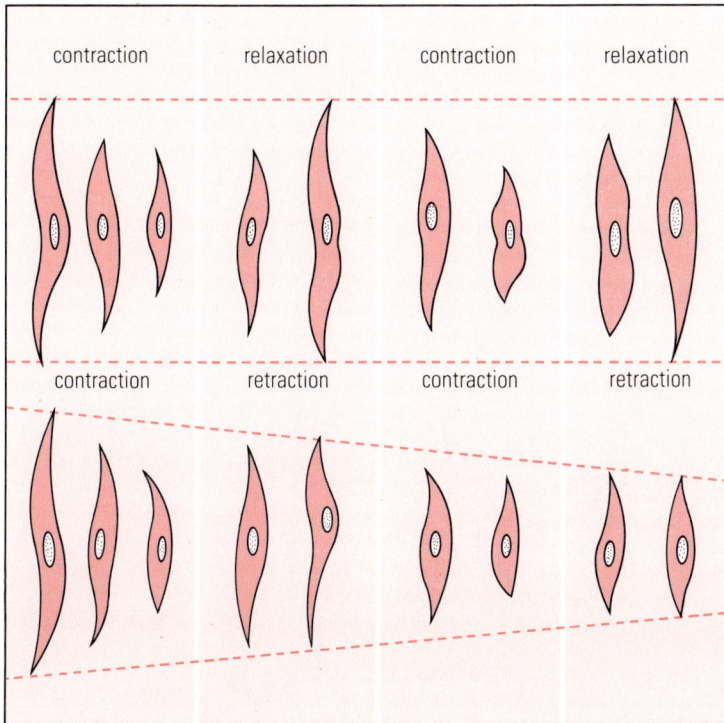

Fig.7.2 Muscle contraction. Upper: most muscle fibres become shorter when they contract; at relaxation, they return to the same length as before. Lower: muscle fibres of the myometrium contract and retract; with each contraction the fibres become a little shorter.

out for examination. Uterine contractions are spontaneous and self-perpetuating. If a strip of uterine muscle were removed from the body, thus isolating it from its nerve supply, and placed in a bath of warmed and oxygenated electrolyte solution, it would keep contracting for many hours. Contractions probably start after dihydroandrosterone, released from the fetal adrenal, stimulates increased bursts of oxytocin secretion from the maternal pituitary gland. These stimulate the increased production of prostaglandin PGE_2 and PGF_2 from the amniotic membranes and the myometrium. An increase in free calcium ions then combines with myocin in the muscle cells to initiate contraction. Thus, the stimulus to initiate labour contractions comes from outside the myometrium, whilst that which stimulates the continuance of contractions emanates from within the tissue.

During labour uterine muscle fibres contract and retract; they do not return to their original length after contraction as do most muscle fibres (Fig.7.2). Thus

there is a heaping up of fibres, particularly in the upper segment of the uterus, whilst the lower segment becomes thinner and more stretched.

The cervix is pulled up, the cervical canal is effaced and its length diminishes; after further contractions the cervix is pulled open. It is occasionally difficult for a woman to distinguish between the contractions of late pregnancy and those of labour. The former are identified as Braxton Hicks contractions and are said to be pain-free, but in some women one type merges into the other.

PROGRESS OF NORMAL LABOUR

First stage

During the course of labour, the fetal head is passed down the birth canal. The widest diameter of the bony pelvis at the inlet is the transverse but at the outlet it is the anteroposterior. Hence the fetus, having little clearance as it passes through the pelvis, progresses best if it rotates to accommodate these changes (Fig.7.3).

The head usually engages in the brim of the pelvis in the occipitotransverse position and an increase in

contractions makes the head flex, so that the fetal chin is tucked against the chest (Fig.7.4), thus allowing still more descent. The pelvic floor is a gutter comprised of the two sheets of the levator ani. This gutter slopes downwards and forwards, so that when the well flexed head impinges upon one side, it will move down

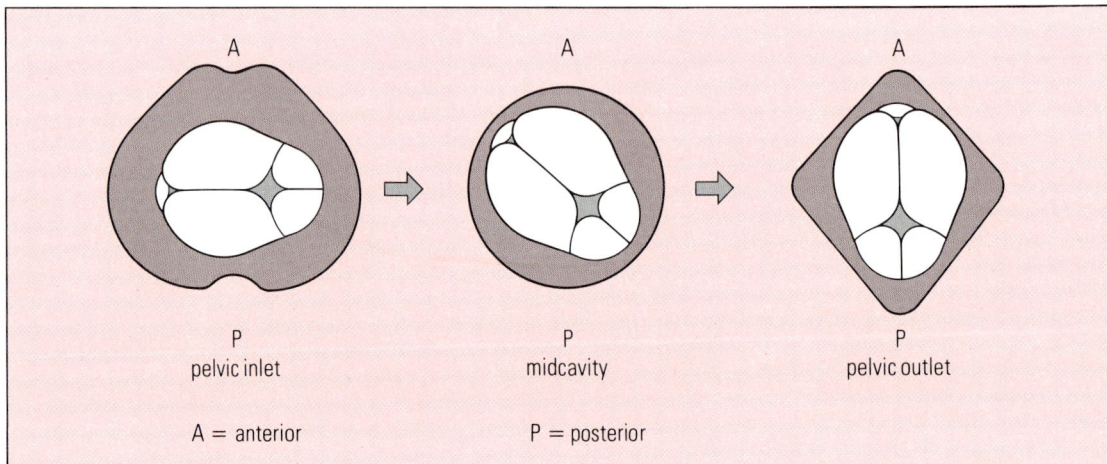

pelvic inlet

midcavity

pelvic outlet

A = anterior

P = posterior

Fig.7.3 Rotation of the fetal head. The occiput usually moves forwards so that the longest diameter of the fetal head passes through the widest diameter of the pelvis in its different planes.

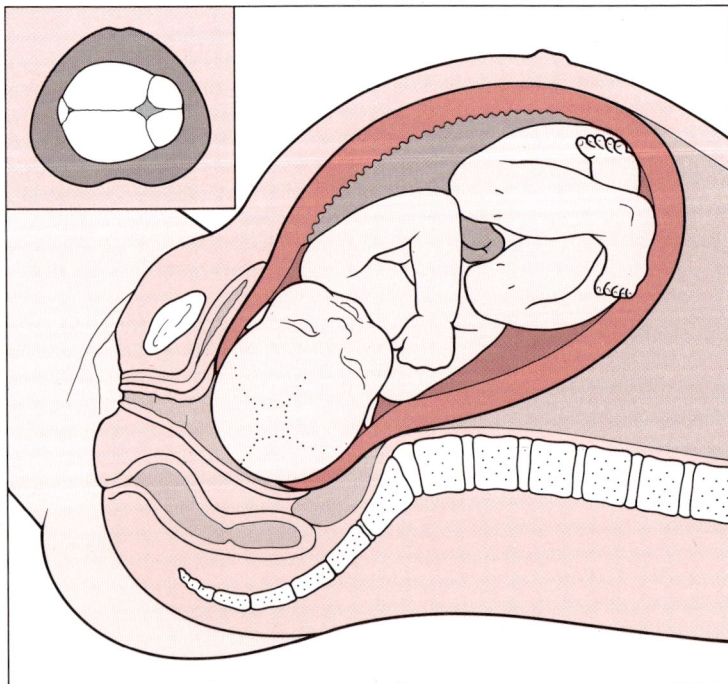

Fig.7.4 The fetal head is engaging in the inlet of the pelvis with the head in the transverse diameter. The head is well flexed, with the chin tucked against the chest.

116

the gutter. Thus, the occiput rotates forwards (Fig.7.5), under the symphysis pubis, and is able to pass into the lower pelvis. Should there be any abnormality of the pelvis, such as a flat or prominent sacrum, this rotation cannot take place in the midcavity and arrest will occur.

Second stage

The second stage of labour begins when the cervix is fully taken up and dilated. The lower uterine segment, the cervix and the upper vagina form a continuous tube. The well flexed head, now in the occipito-anterior position, proceeds down this curved tube (Fig.7.6), pushed on by uterine contractions from above; some of this work is assisted by the woman's voluntary efforts.

As the head descends it distends the vulva more and more and becomes visible from the outside. It is still in an occipitoanterior position and moves downwards, so that the occiput is under the pubic arch. Further progress leads to crowning of the fetal head, when the maximum cephalic diameter is past the vulval entrance. Extension allows delivery of the top of the head, followed by the forehead and the face in turn (Fig.7.7).

Soon afterwards the head, now in the outside environment, rotates through 90° so that the occiput is facing laterally. Meanwhile the shoulders have entered the brim of the pelvis in the transverse position, so that the widest diameter of the shoulders (the bisacromial) is in the transverse diameter of the pelvic inlet. The shoulders rotate so that they present at the outlet in the anterior position. Usually, the head of the baby is led gently backwards by the attendant towards the mother's anus; this allows the escape of the anterior shoulder from under the symphysis pubis. The head is then lifted towards the mother's abdomen to allow the posterior shoulder to escape. This man-oeuvre should be performed very gently since considerable damage can occur to the posterior wall of the vagina. Delivery of the rest of the baby follows easily because the greatest diameters, those of the head and the shoulders, are now out of the vagina.

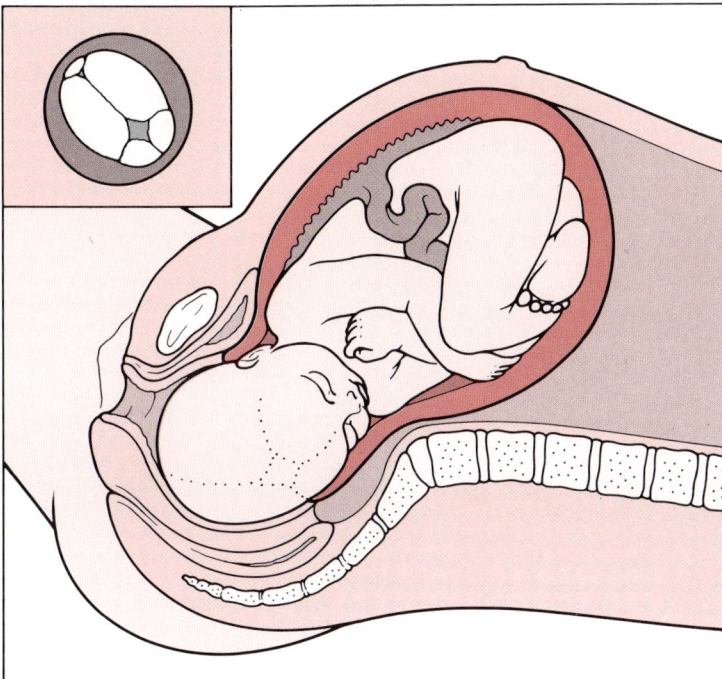

Fig.7.5 The fetal head rotates in the midcavity of the pelvis so that the occiput moves forwards. The head is still well flexed, thus presenting the smallest diameter of the head to the pelvis.

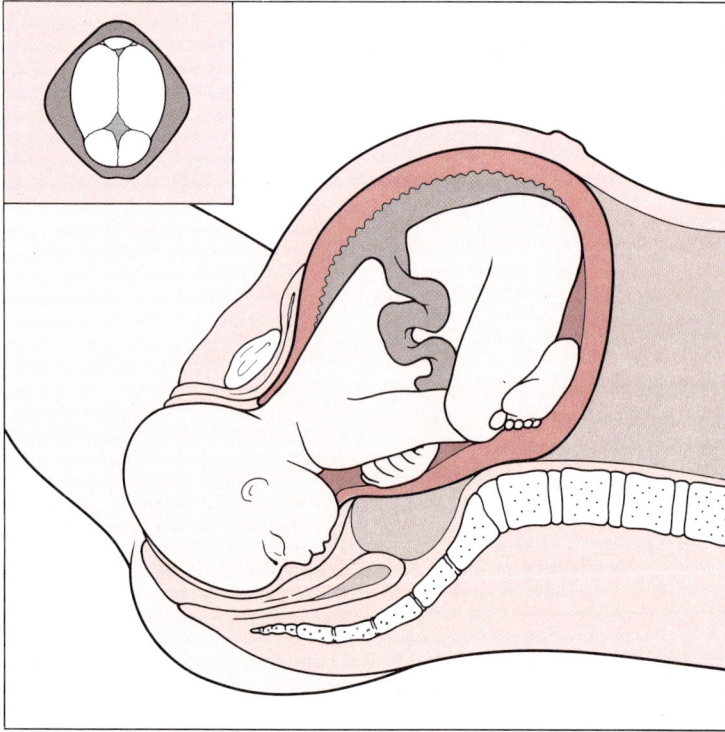

Fig.7.6 The fetal head is at the outlet of the pelvis. Rotation is now complete; the maximum cephalic diameter is aligned with the maximum diameter of the pelvic outlet.

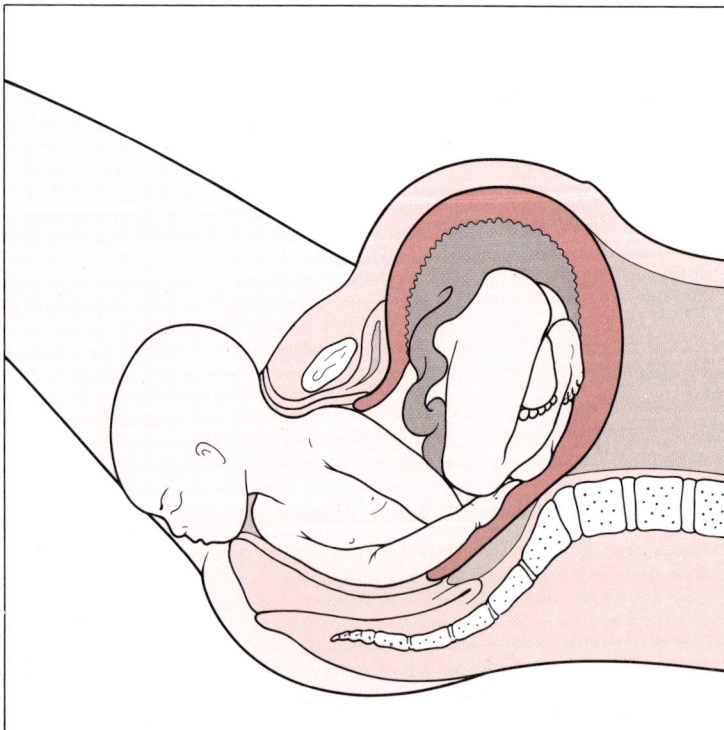

Fig.7.7 Delivery is achieved by extension of the head under the pubic arch.

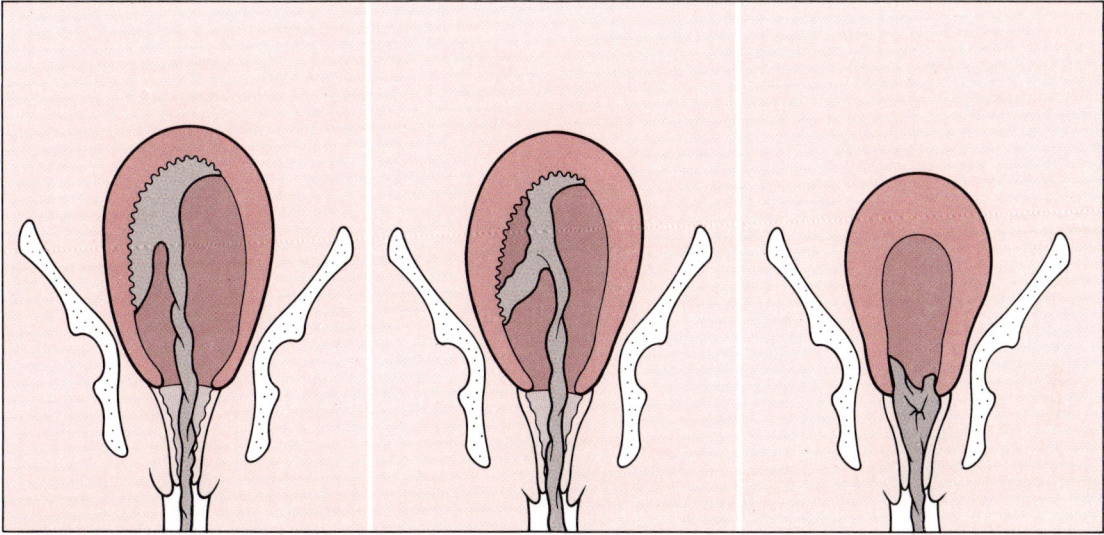

Fig.7.8 Delivery of the placenta. Left: the placental bed and the placenta are about the same size. Centre: further uterine contractions cause the placental bed to decrease in size; the placenta stays the same size and is sheared off.

Right: continued contraction of the uterus causes expulsion of the placenta and membranes through the cervix into the upper vagina.

Third stage

In the third stage of labour, the fibres of the uterine muscle contract and constrict the blood vessels which pass between them. It is this muscular spasm which prevents women from bleeding to death at delivery. The limitation of blood loss from the placental bed does not depend upon clotting in the torn vessels; this process would take too long.

The placenta usually separates from the uterus at the end of the second stage of labour as the baby is being expelled from the body. During pregnancy and most of labour the placental bed and placenta are the same size (Fig.7.8 left), but as the uterus contracts the placental bed becomes much smaller than the placenta. The latter, being almost incompressible since it is filled with blood, is not reduced in surface area and so must shear off (Fig.7.8 centre). It usually follows the fetus down into the lower uterus or the upper vagina (Fig.7.8 right). The uterus rests for a short time after the child is born, but a few moments later contractions may be felt again by placing a hand on the abdomen. This is followed by what used to be referred to as the signs of placental separation. These are actually signs of the placenta passing through the open cervix and down the vagina. The uterus becomes

hard, globular and rises up in the abdomen, feeling like a cricket ball under the examiner's hand. The placenta is being pushed further down the vagina and thence may be guided out by cord traction.

MANAGEMENT OF NORMAL LABOUR

Nearly all women in the United Kingdom (ninety-nine percent) are delivered in a hospital or general practitioner unit. The woman should go there when she thinks labour has started; admission should occur if the membranes rupture, or if regular contractions are coming more frequently than once every twenty minutes.

If antenatal care has been carried out by the same team that attend the woman in labour, full notes will be available at the site of delivery. In some areas, the woman carries her own communication card which contains a summary of these details.

The admitting midwife or doctor should take a short history of the labour, noting when it started and whether the membranes have ruptured. A brief examination should include a check of temperature, blood pressure and urine, and clinical exclusion of anaemia. The abdomen is examined to make sure that

119

the fetus is lying longitudinally and, usually, in a cephalic presentation. If so, engagement of the head should be checked. Vaginal examination is necessary on admission to assess the degree of dilatation and shortening of the cervix and to determine the level of the presenting part in the pelvis.

It is unnecessary to offer the woman an enema on admission. If she has not had her bowels open for several days, suppositories may be helpful, but most women are regular in their bowel habits. There is no need to perform a pubic shave unless a caesarean section is contemplated.

First stage

During the first stage of labour observations, such as blood pressure, pulse rate and temperature, are performed at regular intervals by the attending midwife. The frequency, duration and strength of all uterine contractions should be recorded. This is sometimes done graphically, but descriptions will often suffice. The descent of the fetus is assessed by abdominal examination; the head can be felt leaving the abdomen and entering the pelvis.

The level of the presenting part in relation to the ischial spines of the pelvis is checked vaginally to assess progress. During the same examination, the state of dilatation of the cervix is examined. This should be repeated at intervals of approximately four hours and the results plotted on a partogram (Fig.7.9), which allows a brisk but thorough examination of the woman to be made on the labour ward.

It is important that the bladder does not fill up during labour. As the fetal head moves down into the pelvis, there is often displacement of the bladder from the pelvis into the abdomen, thus stretching the urethra. This may lead to urinary retention. The attendant can often feel the bladder above the pubis and may have to pass a catheter if the woman cannot void urine herself.

Since labour usually lasts for only a few hours, it is probably wise to advise the woman not to eat during this time, but some fluids are allowed. Glucose solutions should be avoided in labour since they can produce a hyperosmolar solution in the stomach, thereby increasing the volume of fluid; this can be a problem if general anaesthesia is required. It is probably not necessary to provide intravenous therapy for most women, but if labour continues for more than twelve hours the woman may need fluid which, to be safe, must be given intravenously; the alimentary route should be avoided.

In the first stage, some women prefer to move around. They feel restless and are happiest walking. Provided the membranes are intact, there is no reason why they should not move around the labour ward or the hospital. Once the membranes rupture, a vaginal examination must be made; if this shows the presenting part to be well engaged, mobility can be allowed. If the presenting part is high, it is wise to stay close to a fetal monitor in case of cord prolapse. If the hospital has long range telemetry (radio) fetal heart rate paging, walking can continue within range of the radio receiver.

During labour, the woman should never be left alone. An attendant, usually a midwife, should always be present, and it is important that the father be allowed to stay in the labour room. Occasionally, in the absence of the father, the woman may wish to be accompanied by a female friend or her mother. The best morale booster is the assurance that everything is normal and going well. Every time an attendant listens to the fetal heart he should tell the mother that all is well, so that she is not unduly concerned by his actions. Analgesia should be administered as appropriate.

Second stage

During the second stage of labour, the woman usually wishes to make expulsive pushing efforts. Indeed, she may want to do this in the latter part of the first stage of labour, and it requires great skill on the attendant's behalf to persuade her to desist. Pushing before the correct time leads to an oedematous cervix, which slows down dilatation.

By this time, the woman may have decided in which position she wishes to deliver. Most women prefer to sit up on a labour ward bed, with pillows or a large rubber wedge supporting the back. This allows the woman to be at an angle of about 30–45° and still be in control of her body. She can, if she wishes, pull up on her own legs and the attendants will then have a clear field in which to assist her.

In a few cases, the woman may prefer to have her baby while lying on her left side in the lateral flexed position, with her body along the edge of the bed. This is particularly useful if a soft bed must be used (the edge is always better supported than the middle) and if only one assistant is present. It is, however, more difficult to perform operative manoeuvres in this position.

Occasionally, women will ask if they can deliver in other positions, for example squatting or in a birth chair. Provided the attendants are familiar with working in this posture, most obstetricians and midwives will agree to such requests.

The worst position in which to have a baby is with the mother lying flat on a bed. The uterus presses down on the aorta and inferior vena cava, causing a reduction of blood flow to the placental bed and thus a diminution of oxygen exchange.

The woman may have been taught beforehand how to push in the second stage. She should hold her breath, tuck her chin onto her chest and, while pulling up the back of her knees, push down into the perineum. Usually, she can hold her breath for fifteen to twenty seconds and so can get in two, three or even four expulsive pushes to each of the uterine contractions, which by this time are lasting for a minute or more. The fetus can be observed moving down the canal by watching the bulge that occurs in the perineum behind the vulva; this leads to a stretching of the anterior wall of the rectum and anal canal, producing a semilunar distension of the anus. In the second stage of labour, inhalation of nitrous oxide and oxygen is probably the best method of analgesia unless an epidural is already being used.

As the fetal head descends to the perineum, the midwife assesses whether the vulva is going to stretch. If there is any doubt, 10ml of local anaesthetic (one percent xylocaine) should be injected into the area in good time to allow an episiotomy to be performed painlessly when required. The head stretches the perineum and crowning is approached. If the perineum starts to tear, an episiotomy is performed in time to prevent a large tear of the tissues. This will allow enlargement of the outlet and the head will crown immediately.

Extension of the fetal head occurs and the baby is delivered by allowing the head to rotate, guiding it towards the mother's anus. This allows the anterior shoulder to escape and the posterior shoulder to be delivered. When the anterior shoulder has been delivered, an intramuscular injection of ergometrine (0.5 mg) or Syntometrine (containing 0.5 mg ergometrine and 5 IU Syntocinon) is given deep into the mother's buttock or thigh muscles to help contraction of the uterus and prevent postpartum haemorrhage.

The baby's nose and mouth may be sucked out before the first breath if excessive mucus is present.

The first inspiration is usually taken within thirty seconds of birth; if this does not occur, the baby should be managed as outlined in Chapter 14.

Once the child is breathing, the cord is usually clamped and divided. This may be done between Spencer Well's forceps or plastic umbilical clips. If the cord is a fat one, as sometimes occurs with large babies, a double tie with silk is probably safer. The baby is wrapped in warm blankets and is given to his mother. Should she wish to put him on her chest for skin-to-skin contact, a warm blanket should be placed over both mother and child.

Third stage

The attendant should put his hand on the woman's abdomen, over a sterile gown, to ensure that the uterus is not rising rapidly and filling up with blood. The first contraction will be felt within a few minutes of expulsion of the baby. This indicates passage of the placenta into the lower segment and delivery can then be attempted. The left hand is placed on the abdomen, with the ball of the thumb over the lower part of the uterus and the palm and fingers embracing the upper part (Fig.7.10). Gentle traction on the umbilical cord guides the placenta down into the vagina. At the same time, the left hand pushes the uterus further up into the abdomen, thus allowing the placenta to pass from the vagina. This is the most efficient way of delivering the placenta and ensures that the uterus is not inverted. The membranes usually follow the placenta in an inverted fashion and are removed by gentle rotation. If they start to split they should be held with ring forceps, which can then be used to rotate the membranes into a loosely twisted rope and make delivery easier. The placenta and membranes should be checked for completeness soon after delivery. An estimate of blood loss should be made and recorded in the notes.

If an episiotomy has been performed or if a tear has occurred, repair should be carried out promptly. This is best learned in the labour ward but the principles are illustrated here (Fig.7.11). The repair is performed in layers under local anaesthesia, using an absorbable material such as catgut throughout.

121

PARTOGRAM

Special Instructions

OBSTETRIC	PAEDIATRIC	ANAESTHETIC
1 previous caesarean section	1 paediatrician present	1 watch if epidural requested
2 not for long labour	if any problem at delivery	

NAME

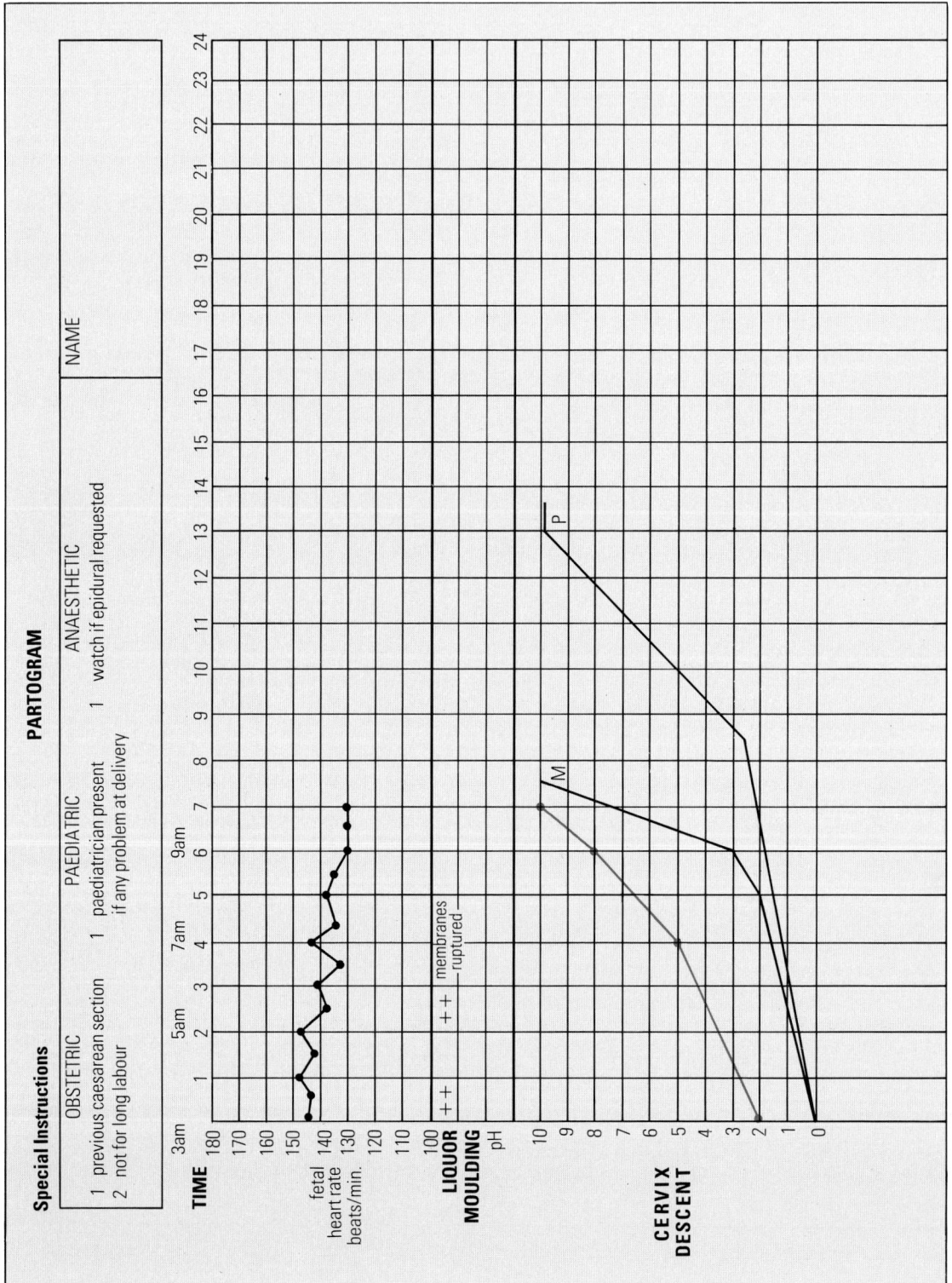

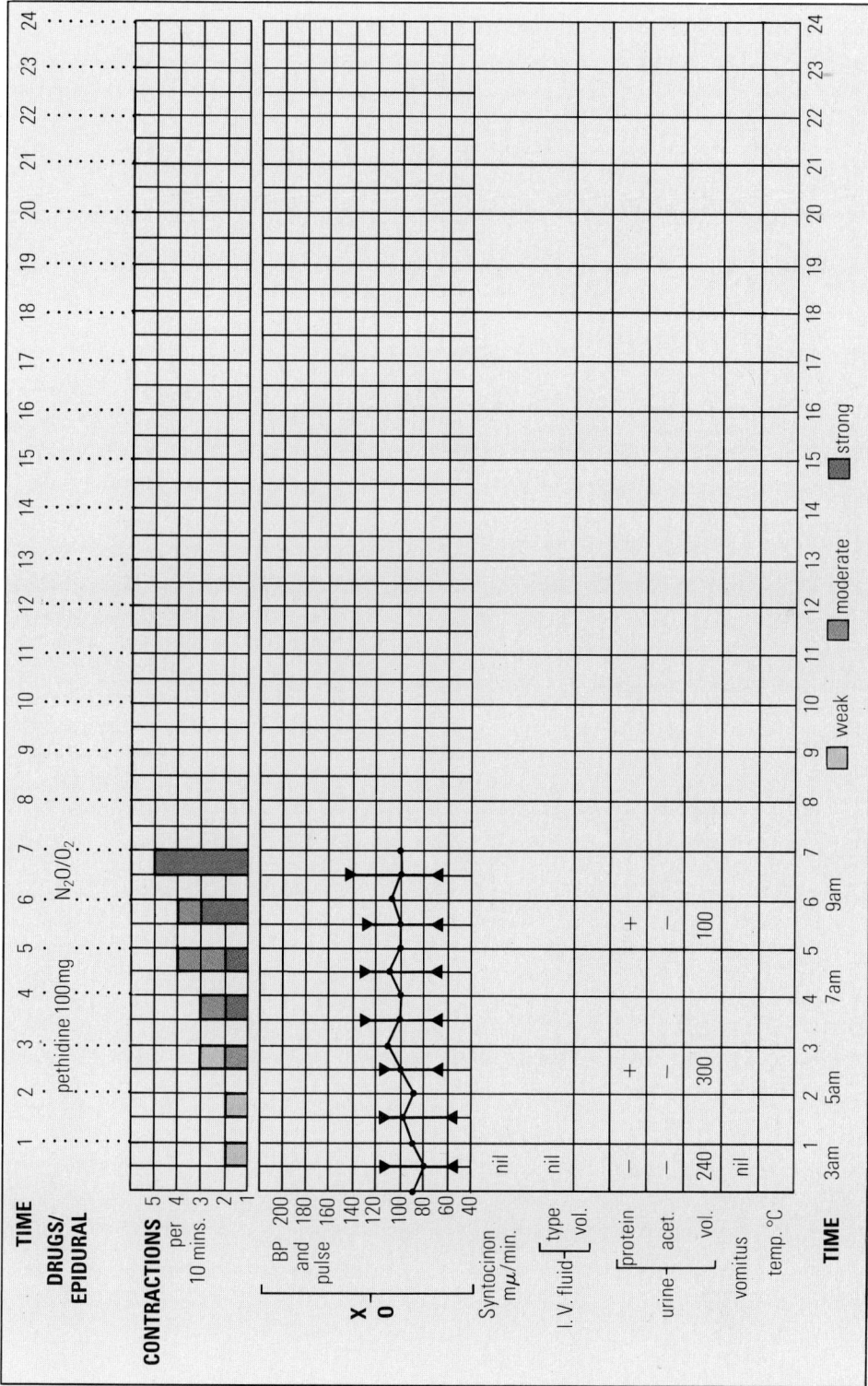

Fig. 7.9 Partogram. In the upper part, the fetal heart rate is recorded and the dilatation of the cervix is plotted. This is compared with two lines, showing the expected dilatation in a multiparous woman (M) and in a primiparous woman (P). If the actual chart of dilatation deviates too far to the right from either of these, the labour has slowed down. Other aspects of observation and management are entered on the lower part of the chart. This chart represents a multiparous woman who started slowly but had a normal labour eventually.

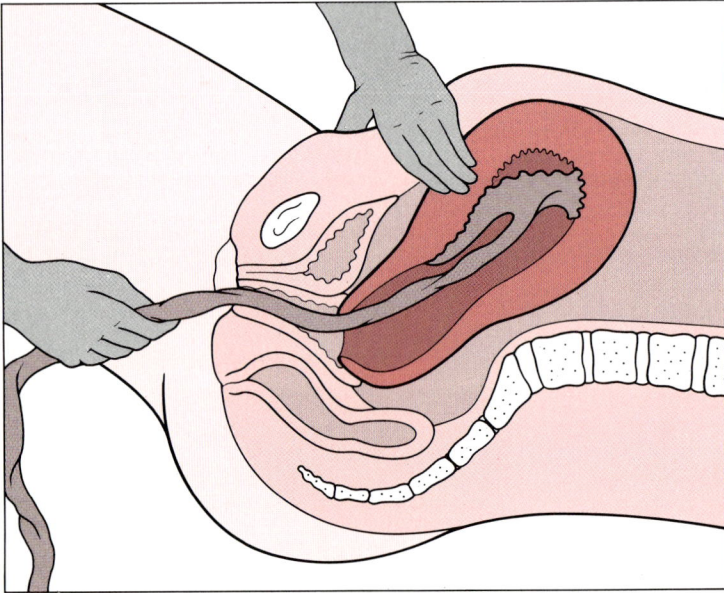

Fig.7.10 Delivery of the placenta. The flat of the deliverer's left hand is placed on the mother's abdomen, the ball of the thumb lying over the lower part of the uterus. The right hand provides gentle traction on the cord which protrudes from the vulva. The left hand moves upwards, putting counter pressure on the uterus as the right hand pulls down.

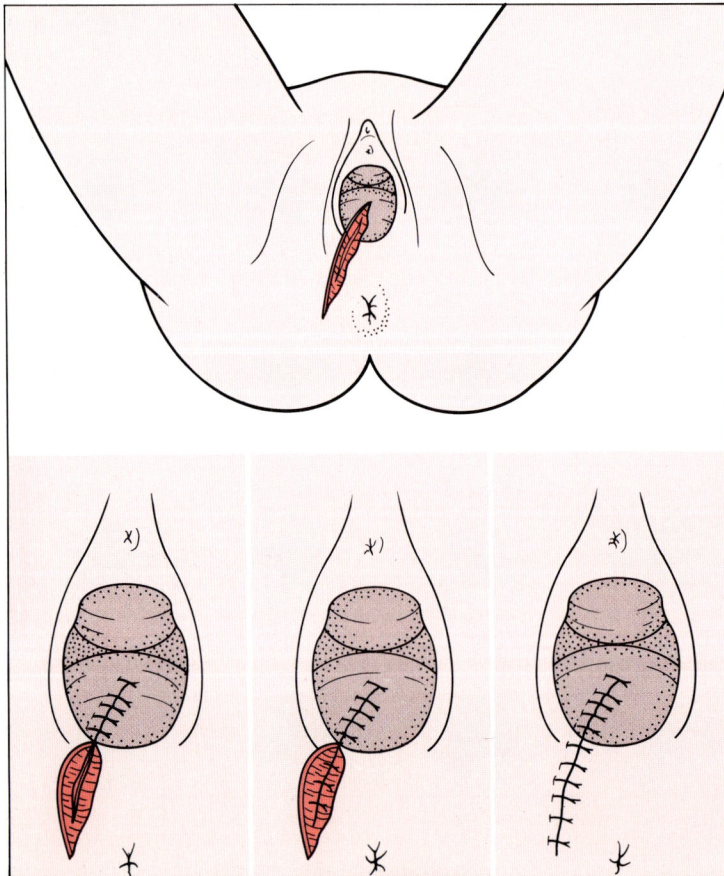

Fig.7.11 Repair of an episiotomy (upper) Lower left: the vaginal epithelium is closed as far as the fourchette. Lower centre: the perineal muscles are brought together with a few interrupted sutures. Lower right: the skin of the perineum is repaired with continuous or interrupted absorbable sutures, particular care being taken in the area of the fourchette.

ANALGESIA AND ANAESTHESIA

Pain relief in labour is a basic function of maternity care. The ideal analgesic should work swiftly, provide adequate pain relief for the mother, and have no side effects on the mother, the fetus, or the newborn baby. Such an agent does not exist. Whilst most anaesthetic drugs are transported rapidly to the fetus, their concentration within fetal tissues is usually low, and generally they have no serious effect. However, some, such as pethidine, which exerts a depressive action on the respiratory centre, may remain in the newborn child for some hours or days after delivery. Balanced against this must be the beneficial psychological effects of analgesia. The influence of anxiety on the uteroplacental circulation may reduce exchange; the removal of stress might improve the fetal state.

In addition to the obstetrician, the anaesthetist, with his more potent methods of analgesia, is now an accepted member of the obstetrical team. It is necessary to differentiate between analgesics, which reduce pain by reducing pain sensitivity, and anaesthetics, which remove consciousness with concomitant depression of the central or peripheral nervous systems. In the former group are nitrous oxide, injectable analgesics and regional analgesics; in the latter are general anaesthetics.

Analgesics

Nitrous oxide

This inhalational analgesic is available in cylinders, premixed with fifty percent oxygen. It is usually self-administered and the mother should be taught how to use the face mask during the antenatal period.

Inhalation of nitrous oxide must commence as soon as the contraction is felt. Ten to twenty seconds will elapse before maximum analgesia is achieved and this will occur when the woman needs it most, at the height of the contraction. Since nitrous oxide is absorbed and expelled across the respiratory membranes, there is a swift rise in concentration in the maternal blood after inhalation and an equally rapid fall when the woman stops inhaling. Hence, nitrous oxide is relatively safe.

Pethidine

This strong analgesic, which has an antispasmodic action on smooth muscle, is probably the most commonly used agent for pain relief in labour in the United Kingdom. It may be given in doses of 50–150mg intramuscularly or, if required urgently, 50–100mg given intravenously over one minute.

Intramuscularly, pethidine takes about twenty minutes to be absorbed and start working, reaching its maximum effect in half an hour; in most people it wears off after two or three hours. It gives good pain relief to most women but a few may experience nausea; it is therefore commonly given with an anti-nausea agent, for example Phenergan.

Pethidine can depress the respiratory centres. At the doses used it does not affect the mother, for she has an established respiratory rhythm, nor does it affect the fetus, since his oxidation depends upon placental exchange. However, if large amounts of pethidine are present in the blood of the newborn, it can depress respiratory action after birth. Consequently, it is conventional to avoid giving pethidine within two hours of birth, although the timing of some deliveries is not precise enough to allow this. Should the baby's respiration be depressed due to pethidine, the action may be reversed by naloxone, which is administered intramuscularly to the newborn child.

Morphine

This opium alkaloid is a stronger analgesic than pethidine. It is administered intravenously as a 10mg dose and is used mostly for prolonged occipito-posterior labours. Morphine depresses the neonatal respiratory centre.

The tranquilizers and sedatives given in labour are not analgesics and are not considered here.

Regional block analgesia

The peripheral nerves are blocked in regional analgesia, thus preventing the passage of pain impulses to the central nervous system.

Spinal analgesia

Lignocaine or bupivacaine may be given into the spinal canal at the level of L3 or L4. This provides good pain relief, but is now less often used in the United Kingdom because it can be associated with a drop in blood pressure. The agent may also track up the central spinal fluid and depress intercostal respiration. This method of analgesia is useful for caesarean section.

Epidural block

Epidural block affords rapid pain relief which lasts for several hours. Lignocaine or bupivacaine is instilled through a catheter into the epidural space. This usually blocks sensory nerve roots T12 to L4. A Touhy needle is passed, under local anaesthetic, through the skin and ligamentum flavum into the epidural space (Fig.7.12). A thin plastic catheter is passed through the needle and because the latter is curved at the end, the tube points downwards into the epidural space. The tube is then pushed a little further into the space and the needle is removed. The analgesic effect may be sustained by topping up the drug via the catheter, which is strapped up over the woman's back to her shoulder.

Epidural block is a good and safe method of analgesia. The introduction and maintenance requires a skilled anaesthetist, although non-anaesthetists, such as midwives and junior obstetricians, may be able to administer the repeated topping-up injections if they are correctly trained. A doctor must be constantly available for cardiorespiratory resuscitation if necessary.

There is usually loss of sensation from the uterus and the anterior abdominal wall; initially the legs may also be involved. This means that the woman does not know when she is having a contraction and so in the second stage of labour, the midwife must inform her whey they do occur; the woman can then coordinate her pushing efforts with the contractions. After an epidural, relaxation of the pelvic floor allows the fetal head to descend much further than usual in the transverse position. Consequently, it does not rotate until later than normal because of the lack of gutter effect at the levator ani muscles. This can often be overcome by waiting for the head to descend before organized pushing is started. Alternatively vacuum extraction, or a manual or forceps rotation can be employed. The incidence of forceps delivery may be higher amongst those with an epidural, particularly if pushing is started too soon.

Epidural block may be associated with a rapid hypotension following anaesthesia of the autonomic nervous system and loss of vasomotor tone. Blood pressure should be checked frequently and an intravenous drip should be running before an epidural is given.

The most serious side effect of epidural block is a

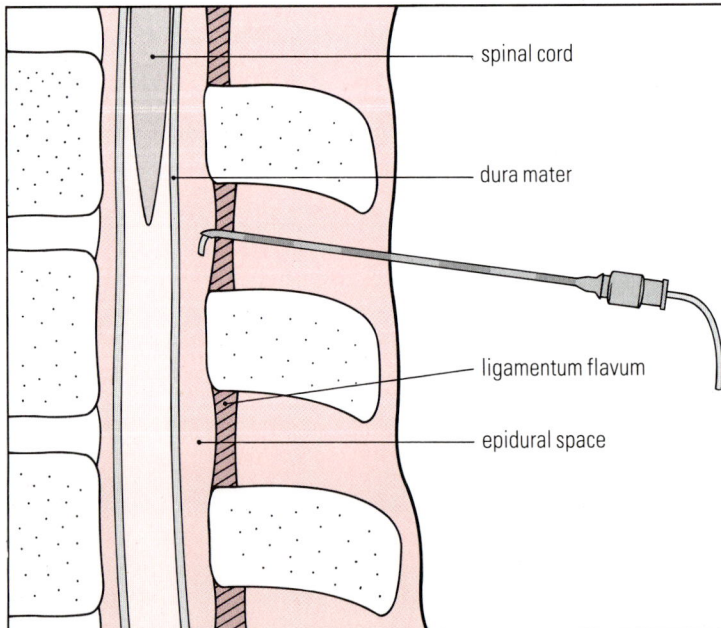

Fig.7.12 Epidural block. A Touhy needle is passed through the skin and ligamentum flavum into the epidural space. A plastic catheter is then passed through the needle, pushed a little further into the epidural space and the needle is removed. Analgesics are administered via the catheter.

spinal cord

dura mater

ligamentum flavum

epidural space

dural tap, which occurs when the dura is accidentally punctured. The woman may then suffer severe headaches for several days. She will require hydration with an intravenous line to supplement her oral fluid intake, and will need a good analgesic, occasionally as strong as morphia, for her headaches.

If the anaesthetist fails to recognize a dural tap and continues with the block, spinal anaesthesia will occur rather than an epidural. This can be very serious, causing arrest of respiration and reduction in blood pressure.

Elective caesarean sections are easily performed under epidural analgesia. The surgeon must be patient and gentle since an epidural may take an hour to have full effect. Under these conditions the woman and her partner can be together and see their child immediately after delivery, compared with the long delays which occur after general anaesthesia.

Paracervical block

Injection of a local anaesthetic agent through each of the lateral fornices of the vagina into the base of the cardinal ligaments leads to blocking of the nerves flowing from the uterus alongside the uterine arteries. Lignocaine (10ml of one percent solution, without adrenaline) can be injected on each side to give good analgesia in the latter part of the first stage of labour. However, it can cause vasoconstriction of the uterine arteries and thus reduce blood flow in the placental bed.

Pudendal block

Lignocaine (one percent) may be injected into the branches of the pudendal nerve where it circumnavigates the ischial spines on each side of the midcavity of the pelvis. It is injected through the upper vaginal wall, 10ml on each side. This can give good analgesia for mid- and lower cavity manipulations, such as forceps deliveries.

Local field block

Infiltration of the vulva and labia with a local anaesthetic agent is often used to relieve pain, particularly to cover an episiotomy. A field block should also be employed when a pudendal block is performed because some areas of the pudenda are not covered by the analgesic effect of blocking the pudendal nerve.

General anaesthesia

General anaesthesia is usually induced by intravenous injection of thiopentone and maintained by inhalation of nitrous oxide. Muscular relaxation is also required to allow laryngeal intubation, and is usually needed for intra-abdominal manoeuvres. This results in an unconscious patient allowing all surgical manoeuvres to be performed. It is essential that anyone having a general anaesthetic is as well prepared as possible. Since no one can predict who is going to need a general anaesthetic in labour, eating is forbidden; thus, a woman requiring anaesthesia will not have a full stomach. Regurgitation of stomach contents with overspill into the trachea can produce an aspiration pneumonia (Mendelson's syndrome). This is a particular risk at the time of intubation, when the acidic contents of the stomach may be regurgitated up the oesophagus, over into the trachea and down to the lungs. In order to prevent this, cricoid pressure is always applied at the time of induction until the cuffed endotracheal tube is in site and has been inflated. If general anaesthesia is to be used in labour, it is essential that it is administered by skilled anaesthetists and not by junior doctors with less experience.

Non-pharmacological analgesia

Between ten and fifteen percent of women delivering in the United Kingdom have no formal analgesia. Whilst some of these are multiparous women who come in late in labour, the others make use of non-pharmacological methods.

Psychoprophylaxis is a method of distracting the woman's thoughts, so that the pain is more manageable. The technique must be learnt carefully in the antenatal period and is best reinforced by a co-operative partner or midwife who also knows the technique. Its use may well postpone formal analgesia, reducing the amount required.

Transdermal nerve stimulation (TNS) is used by some women. A low-grade electrical current is run through the skin of the back or the legs, under the control of the patient. This produces mild counter-irritation and so distracts the mind from the uterine pain.

Hypnosis is used in some centres. Again, the woman

127

needs training in the antenatal period; she and the attendant must be together throughout labour. This is very expensive on the attendant's time and works only for receptive women; it is safe for the fetus.

FETAL MONITORING

The fetal heart rate must be measured and recorded during labour. For many years, a monoauricular stethoscope was used. This enables the obstetrician to listen to the fetal heart through the abdominal wall, providing a coarse guide to the fetal state. Unfortunately, the recordings are intermittent and the heart cannot be heard easily during the time of greatest stress, that is, during uterine contractions. Consequently, if a fetus is considered to be at a higher risk than normal, more intensive monitoring is required.

The signal

The fetal heart rate may be detected by several methods:
- Heart sounds can be picked up by a microphone on the anterior abdominal wall and the rate can then be recorded continuously. Unfortunately, this is not efficient in labour because of noise interference produced by the uterus and by the woman moving around the bed.
- The electrical activity of the fetal heart could be picked up in the same way as is an adult electrocardiograph (ECG). This is not very clear if it is measured through the maternal abdominal wall because of the confounding effects of the stronger electrical activity of the mother's heart, which produces a signal about twenty times stronger than the fetal heart. Direct access to the fetus through the cervix, following rupture of the membranes, allows a much clearer trace to be recorded. This may be achieved using fetal electrodes (Fig.7.13).
- The alterations of flow in the major vessels of the heart can be detected by the reflection of ultrasound waves. The signal is a clean one and can be obtained through the mother's abdominal wall. A transmitter/receiver may be strapped in place, thus obtaining a good continuous fetal heart rate record before the membranes are ruptured.

All of these methods can produce a continuous fetal heart rate trace which may be shown on a screen or printed out on a paper record. Figs.7.14 and 7.15 show normal cardiotocographs during labour. The

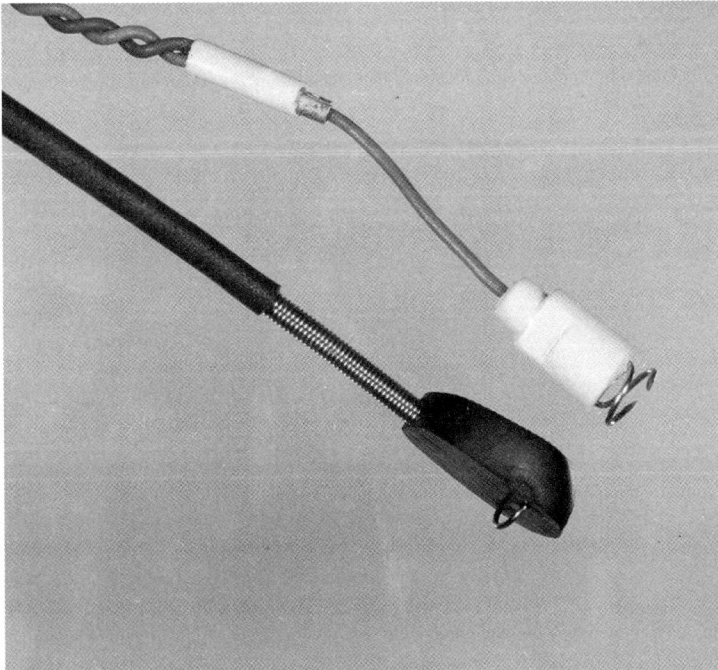

Fig.7.13 Fetal electrodes. The Double Helix (upper) depends upon a screwing action to pierce the fetal skin. In the Copeland (lower) the wire loop can be retracted by rotation of the electrode stem but when released against the fetal scalp, it pierces the skin and provides good electrical contact. Both types are disposable.

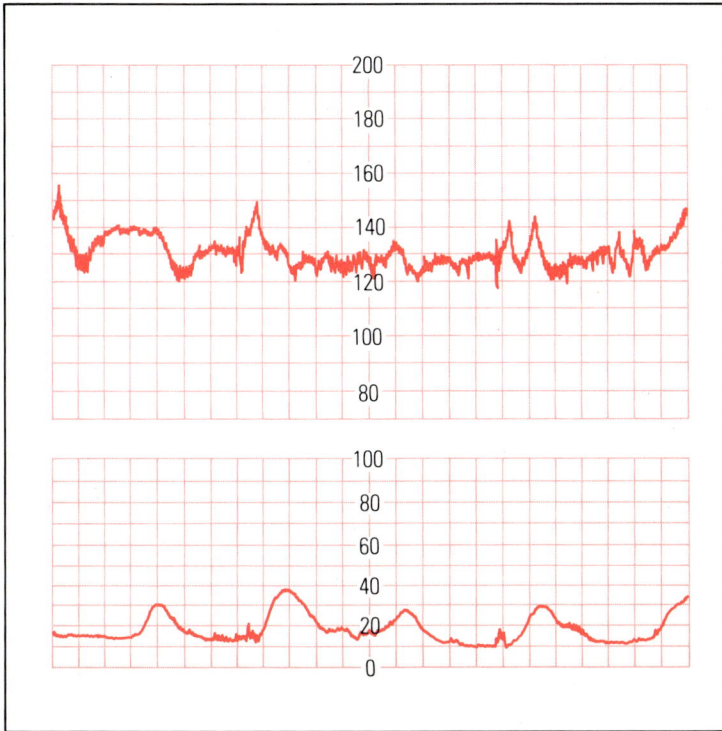

Fig.7.14 Cardiotocograph trace. In this case, labour has only just started and contractions are not very strong or long lasting.

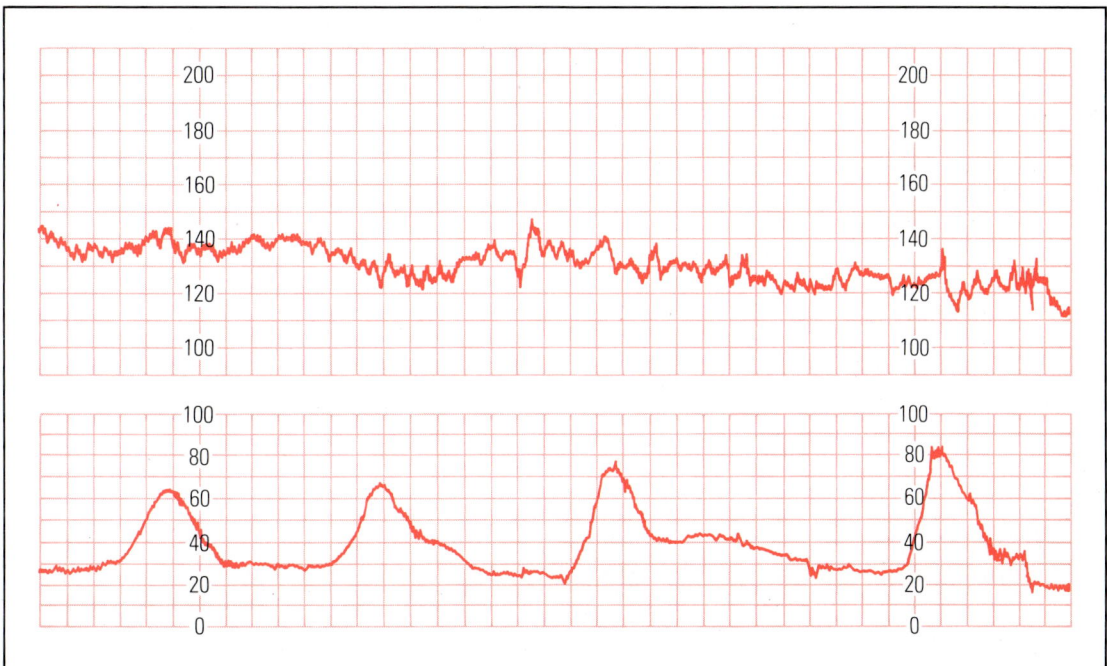

Fig.7.15 Cardiotocograph trace taken at the end of the first stage of labour. Contractions are much stronger and longer lasting than in Fig.7.14; the baseline tone is raised.

129

fetal heart rate is shown on the upper trace of each cardiotocograph; the lower trace indicates the frequency, length and strength of uterine contractions non-quantitatively.

Fetal heart rate variations

Abnormalities in the heart trace are considered in three groups:
• Alterations in heart rate
• Baseline variability
• Periodic heart rate variations

Alterations in heart rate

The fetal heart rate is usually fairly constant at between 140 and 150 beats/min but if hypoxia occurs a tachycardia (Fig.7.16), with a heart rate well above 160 beats/min, may follow.

A more severe change is fetal bradycardia (Fig.7.17), where the fetal heart rate stays persistently below 120 beats/min. This is considered a more dangerous sign of fetal hypoxia than tachycardia.

Baseline variability

The fetal heart responds to a series of nervous, endocrine and biochemical stimuli so that the built-in sinoatrial node impulses are modified by the environment. Consequently no heart rate is absolutely regular, but has a variation of between 5 and 10 beats/min. If the variation is less than 5 beats/min the trace appears flatter (Fig.7.18); the heart is not responding

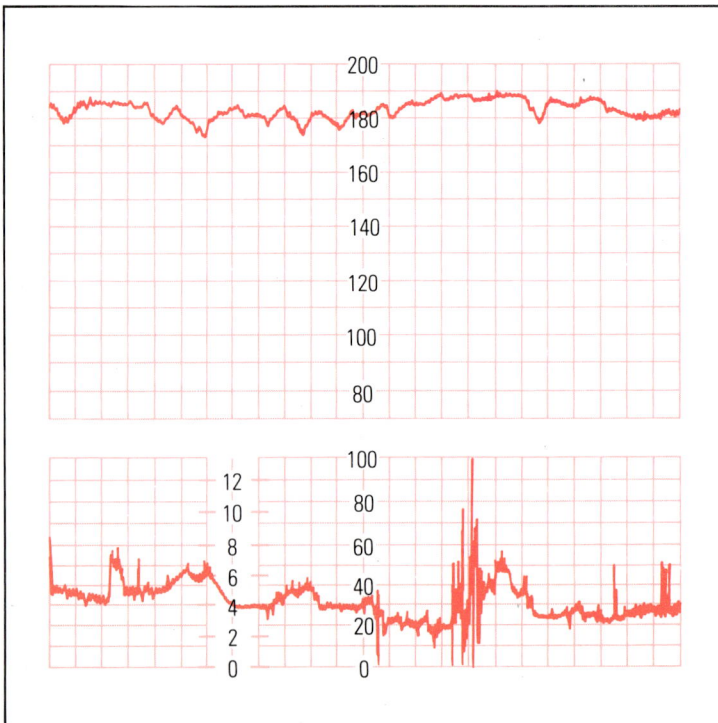

Fig.7.16 Fetal tachycardia. The heart rate is about 180 beats/min; there is some loss of baseline variability.

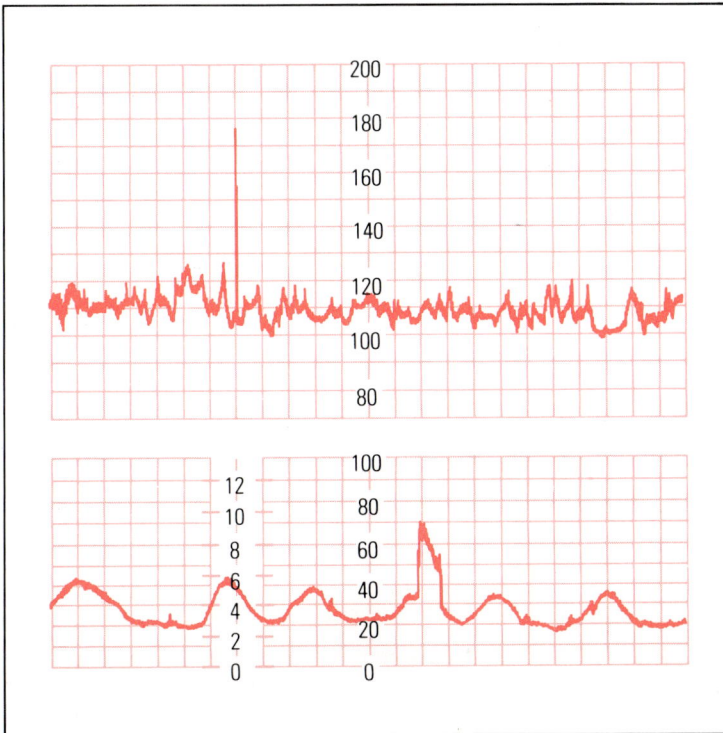

Fig.7.17 Fetal bradycardia. The heart rate is less than 120 beats/min but has maintained a good baseline variability.

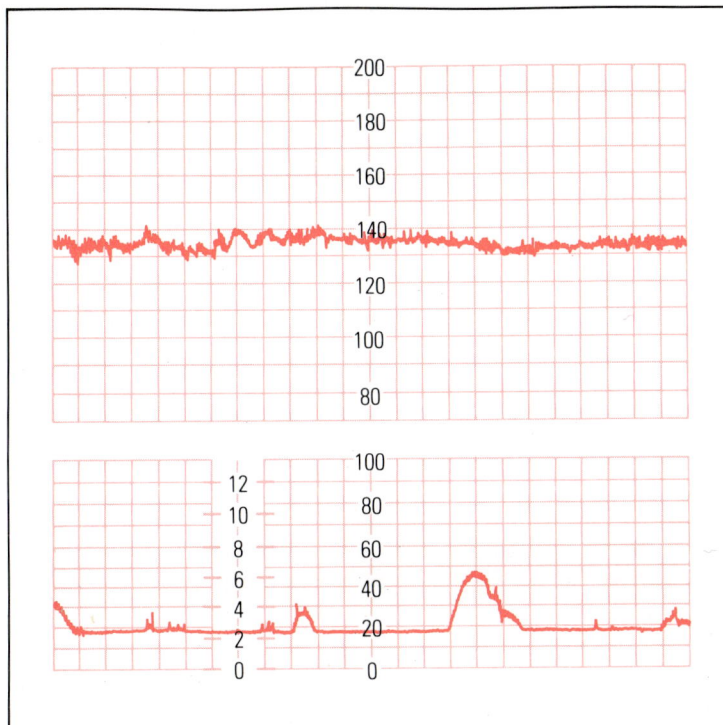

Fig.7.18 Loss of baseline variability. The variability is less than 5 beats/min for most of the trace, indicating a depressed metabolism.

to normal changing environmental stimuli, implying a depressed metabolism. The most common cause for this is hypoxia; the loss of baseline variability is a sign that the fetus is heading into danger.

Periodic heart rate variations

Each time the uterus contracts the placental bed is constricted, so that the blood supply is reduced. The fetus may respond to this, showing a variation in the heart rate which coincides with the uterine contractions. Fig.7.19 shows that during each uterine contraction there is a concomitant acceleration in the fetal heart rate; this is normal and implies that the heart is active. Similarly, brisk decelerations may occur (Fig.7.20), where the heart slows with each contraction. Provided each deceleration occurs soon after the beginning of each uterine contraction, the traces appear to mirror one another so that the apex of the contraction corresponds to the nadir of the deceleration. These are considered to be early decelerations and are not of serious significance.

If the fetal heart is becoming even more hypoxic, it becomes more sluggish in its response. Thus, as uterine contractions occur, the decelerations of the fetal heart rate occur later (Fig.7.21), so that each deceleration follows each uterine contraction. A gap of thirty seconds between the onset of the contraction and the onset of the deceleration of the heart rate indicates a late deceleration.

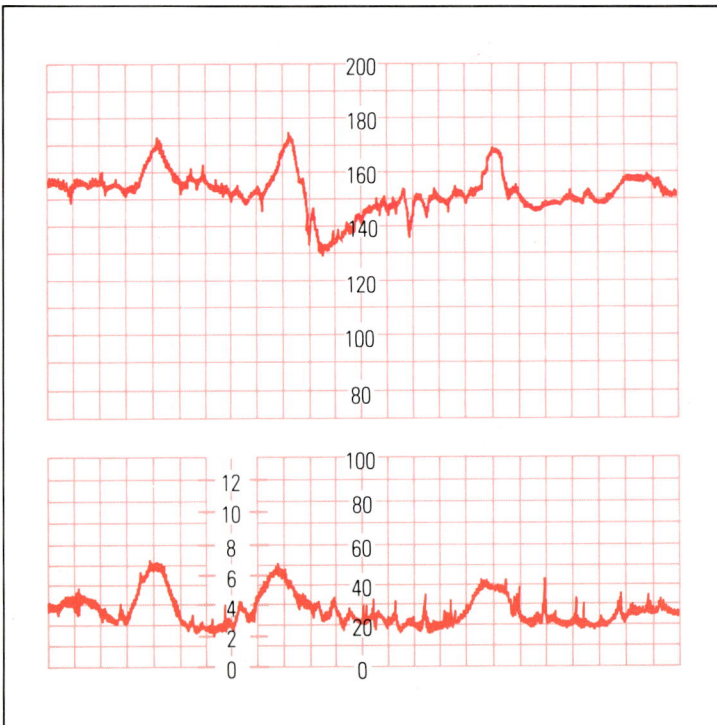

Fig.7.19 Periodic accelerations. The fetal heart rate accelerates with each uterine contraction.

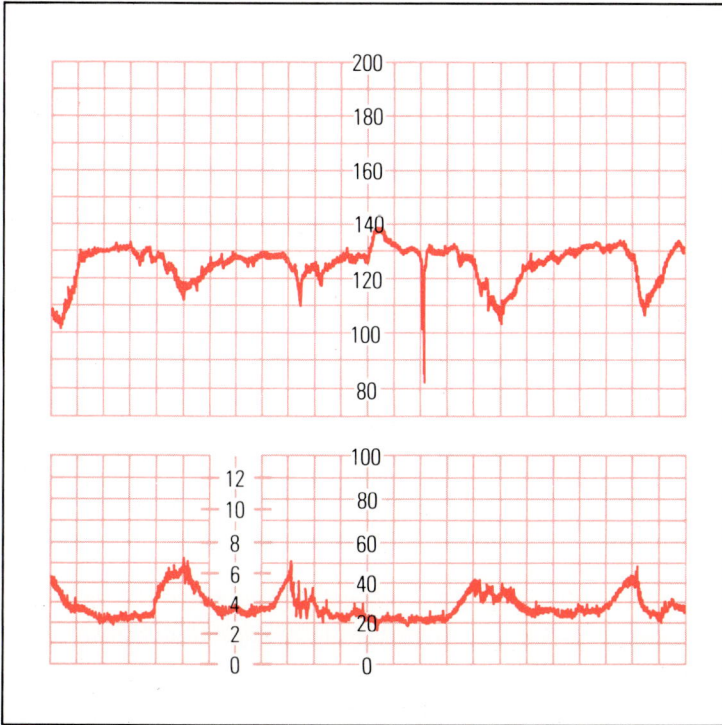

Fig.7.20 Early decelerations. The heart rate decelerates with each uterine contraction. Each deceleration starts close to the beginning of each uterine contraction and the upper trace provides a mirror image of the lower one.

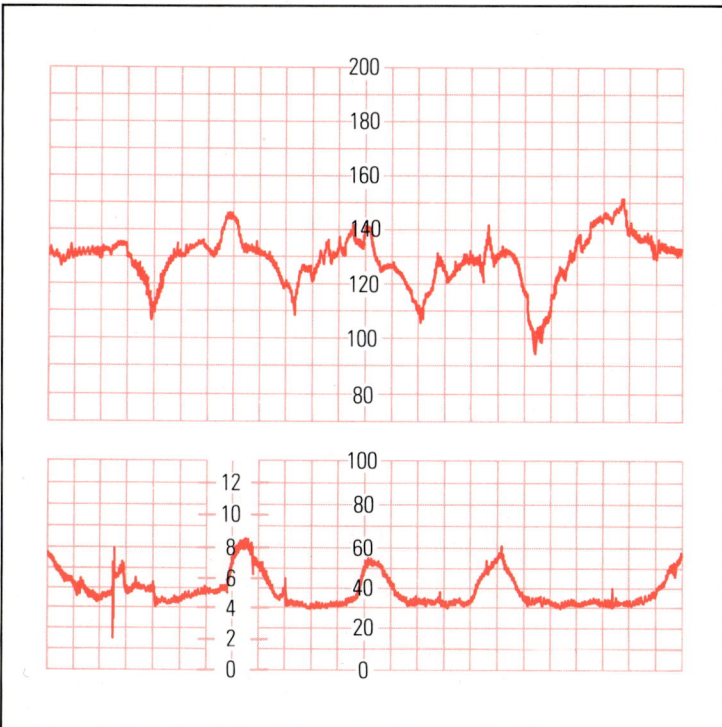

Fig.7.21 Late decelerations. Deceleration following each contraction indicates some sluggishness in the response of the fetal heart.

Often in the labour ward a variable pattern occurs on the trace (Fig.7.22); this is a mixture of early and late decelerations and some which occur with no concomitant uterine contractions. Such a trace is usually considered to be due to intermittent compression of the umbilical cord around a limb or a part of the fetal body; it does not usually have serious implications for the fetus.

Significance of fetal heart rate variations

The fetal heart rate can be monitored continuously in those who are considered to be at higher risk. In early labour, monitoring is usually performed using the ultrasound method through the abdominal wall. Later, once the membranes have ruptured, a scalp clip may be attached to the fetus to obtain direct recordings. Provided the rate stays between 120 and 160 beats/min, the background variability is good and the periodic alterations are either accelerations or early decelerations, the fetus is unlikely to be hypoxic. However, should loss of variability or late or variable decelerations occur, the fetus should be investigated further. In the United Kingdom, this would mean checking the biochemistry of the blood following fetal scalp sampling. In the future, better methods of recording the fetal heart rate may be developed, which may remove the need for fetal blood sampling.

Fetal acid–base balance

Lack of oxygen in the fetus produces an increase in carbon dioxide, while anaerobic respiration produces an increase in metabolites such as lactic and pyruvic acid. Both are associated with a reduction in pH of the tissues and the circulating blood. This can be detected in a very small sample (0.2ml) of fetal blood, which can be obtained from a small prick in the presenting part.

A tapered tube is passed through the cervix once

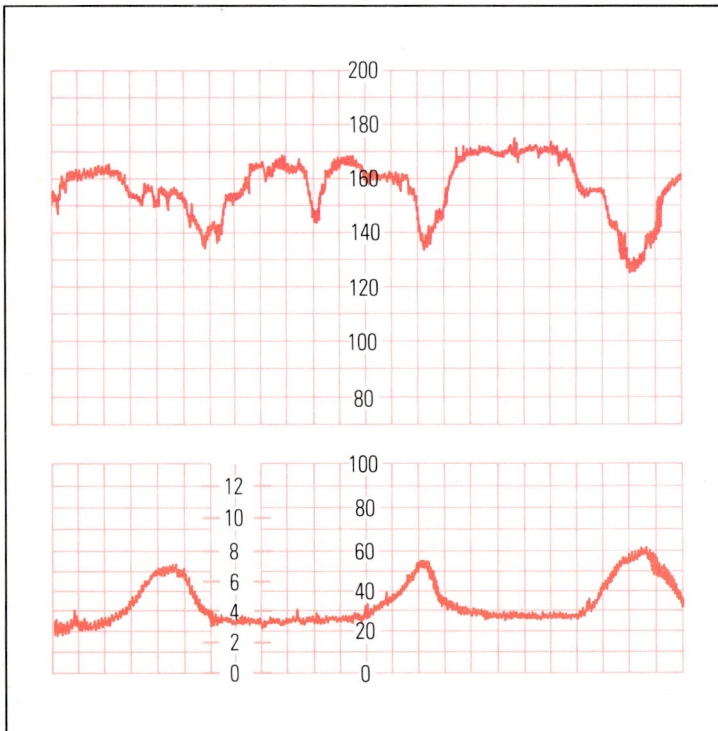

Fig.7.22 Variable decelerations. The fetal heart rate drops, sometimes in relation to a contraction and sometimes independent of it. The relationship between uterine contractions and the heart rate is not constant.

dilatation is more than 2cm. It can be positioned against the fetal head and a small sample of blood drawn into a preheparinized tube. The blood is analysed immediately to give pH level (Fig.7.23) and, if required, base deficit measurements. This is a safe procedure and provides a more accurate account of what is happening in the fetus than the heart rate trace alone. Unfortunately, while fetal continuous heart rate monitors are available for all women in labour in the United Kingdom, only a third of units have equipment to check the acid–base status.

Fetal electrocardiography

The problems of filtering out the fetal electrical heart activity from that of the mother are enormous, but they can be solved; with the proper computer programming a clean fetal ECG trace can be obtained (Fig.7.24). This is interpreted in a similar way to an adult ECG and so early warning of fetal hypoxia can be obtained. This is a new method but will probably become much more widely used in the United Kingdom within the next five years.

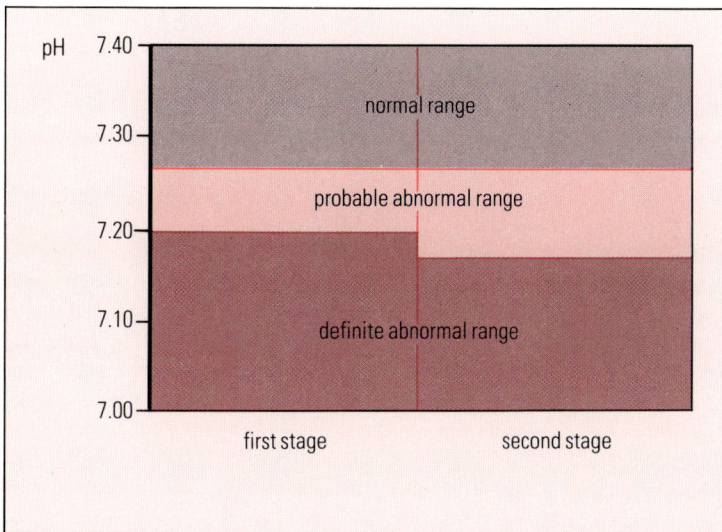

Fig.7.23 Fetal capillary blood pH values in normal labour. The pH usually stays above 7.25; if it is below 7.20 in the first stage or 7.18 in the second stage, immediate delivery is required.

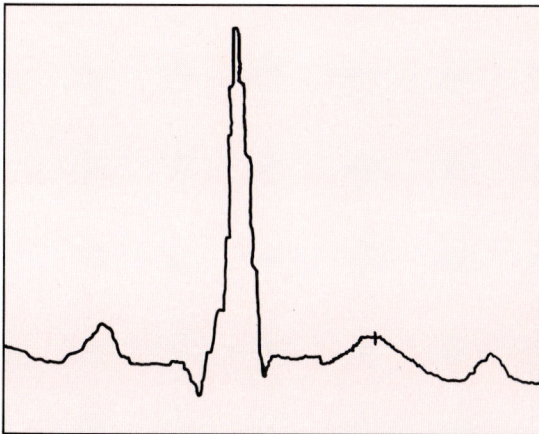

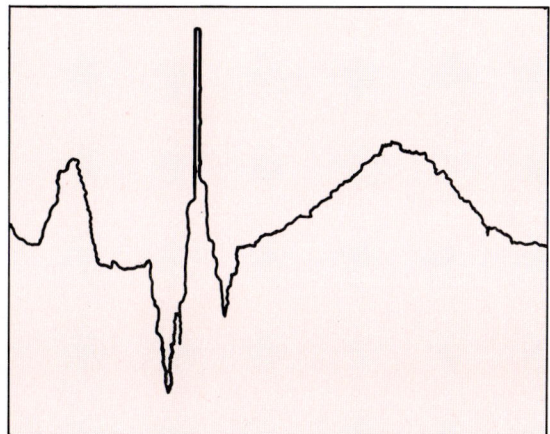

Fig.7.24 Electrocardiography. Left: filtered ECG waveform of a normal fetus. Right: filtered ECG waveform of a hypoxic fetus. The signal is obtained using a fetal scalp electrode and then undergoes computer enhancement to obtain a clear result. Courtesy of Dr. L. Jenkins and Prof. E. Symonds.

EXAMINATION OF THE NEWBORN CHILD

When delivery is complete, the attendant should help the mother and father get used to the newborn child. A good way of doing this is to examine the child on the same bed as the mother, after the parents have been allowed to hold their baby. It is good practice for the person delivering a baby always to exclude congenital abnormalities; such an examination can be done swiftly, but performing it in the presence of the parents reassures them.

After general observations of the breathing pattern and tone of the baby, examination begins at the head. The anterior fontanelle is checked, as are the sutures joining it. The shape and position of the ears and of the eyes are examined, looking for epicanthal folds or extra folds of skin in front of the pinna. The face is checked for features of Down's syndrome and the lip for cleft. Slip a clean little finger into the mouth to check the hard palate for any gaps.

The upper limbs are checked, making sure that the number of fingers is correct and that the palmar creases are normal. The chest is checked for breast enlargement and the heart is listened to. A faint systolic murmur is commonly present, but the heart rate is so fast at this stage that this is often not heard. Should a murmur be present, it should be checked daily until it disappears.

The abdomen is examined, counting the number of vessels in the umbilical cord (two arteries and one vein), and the groins are examined for hernias. The anus should be open and if meconium has not yet been passed, a thermometer slipped into the anus ensures patency and checks the baby's central core temperature at the same time.

The genitalia should be checked. In the female, there is no point in forcing the labia apart, but the clitoral size should be assessed. In the male, the end of the penis should be examined for hypospadias and one should check the scrotum to ensure that two testes are present. It is wise to run a hand down the back to exclude a meningocele, and to make sure there is no mildline hairy patch to suggest a spina bifida occulta. The straightness of the spine can be assessed at this early stage to ensure the absence of congenital kyphoscoliosis.

The lower limbs are examined to count the number of digits on the foot and to check that there is no talipes; the dorsal surface of the foot should be able to touch the anterior tibial surface. Check also for congenital dislocation of the hips, one at a time, by flexing each to 90° with the knee in flexion. The examiner's thumbs are placed, one over each of the hip joints and, if they can be dislocated, a 'clunk' will be felt over the acetabulum when the hip is abducted.

Soon after delivery, the baby should be weighed to the nearest gram or quarter of an ounce. The head circumference and the crown to heel length should be measured. These measures may be set against population derived weight/gestation and length/ gestation charts (see Chapter 13). It must be remembered that these charts are derived by examining fetuses actually born at these various stages of gestation and may not represent the normal range for babies from healthy pregnancies. Cross-sectional measures of natural events like this include a large degree of the pathological along with the normal; this applies particularly to weight and length changes in the late twenty and early thirty weeks of gestation.

8. Induction of Labour

INDICATIONS FOR INDUCTION

The common conditions for which labour may be induced are listed in Fig. 8.1. Hypertensive disease, intrauterine growth retardation and some cases of postmaturity threaten the viability of the fetus due to poor placental bed blood flow, and fetal death may result. If the fetus dies or is abnormal, induction of labour may be necessary to prevent the mother from undue prolongation of the pregnancy with a dead or abnormal child. Rhesus incompatibility is now a rare condition, but a few cases still exist where serious rhesus disease calls for premature induction of labour. If a diabetic condition is not under stringent control there may be an increased tendency for the fetus to die in the last few weeks of pregnancy, and prophylactic early delivery may be necessary.

Many gross fetal abnormalities such as anencephaly and spina bifida are now recognized sufficiently early in pregnancy for therapeutic abortion to be undertaken. If anencephaly presents later in pregnancy, induction of labour is then sometimes indicated.

METHODS OF INDUCTION

Modern methods of induction of labour may be surgical or medical and, in many cases, the two methods are combined.

Surgical methods consist of rupturing the membranes through the cervix, and until comparatively

REASONS FOR INDUCTION OF LABOUR
pre-eclampsia
intrauterine growth retardation
postmaturity
antepartum haemorrhage
maternal disease e.g. diabetes
intrauterine death or severe abnormality diagnosed late
rhesus incompatibility

Fig. 8.1 Indications for induction of labour. The first three conditions constitute 80% of the indications in the United Kingdom.

recently, these have been the most widely used. Once a vaginal examination has been made and a finger introduced through the cervix to establish that there is no contraindication to this method (Fig. 8.2) the membranes are ruptured by either a toothed or a hooked instrument, such as an Amnihook (Fig. 8.3). Women with a low-lying placenta could suffer antepartum haemorrhage and the obstetrician must be careful, when seeking to induce labour, to ensure that there is no placenta lying in the region of the cervical os.

Medical induction of labour used to be by intravenous infusion of oxytocin in gradually increasing amounts until satisfactory uterine contractions were obtained. The rate of infusion must be controlled carefully, since it can overstimulate the uterus. The woman must not be left unattended for at least twenty minutes after starting the induction, to ensure that oversensitivity of the myometrium leading to hypertonic contraction (Fig. 8.4) does not occur. More recently, prostaglandins have been used, either as a gel introduced between the membranes and the cervix or, much more simply, as a pessary containing 3mg of PGE_2 in an inert base. This is inserted high into the vagina and, in most cases, contractions follow within a few hours. If the cervix is long and unripe, a second pessary may be required some time later to induce labour, the first having ripened the cervix.

The choice of method of induction depends on the clinical circumstances and materials available. If the cervix is tightly closed so that a finger can barely be introduced through it, medical means must generally be chosen first; prostaglandin pessaries are useful in such cases. If, however, the cervix is ripe, surgical rupture of the membranes may then be chosen.

COMPLICATIONS

The complications of surgical induction include injury to the cervix by the instrument or, rarely, injury to the fetal head itself if excessive force is used. Whilst injury to the cervix is uncommon, if the umbilical vessels from the cord to the placenta (vasa praevia) run along the membranes over the cervical os, injury to these vessels is almost certain to occur. Furthermore, unless scrupulous asepsis is utilized, infection could be introduced. Because of

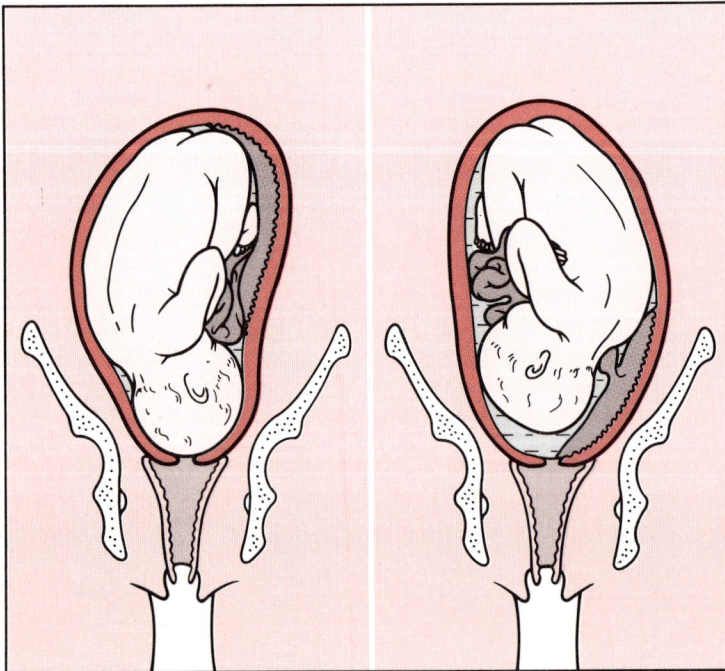

Fig.8.2 Left: placenta in the normal fundal position with the head well down in the pelvis. This fetus is correctly positioned for surgically induced labour. Right: Low-lying placenta with the head high in the pelvis. The obstetrician should not be inducing a woman in this situation.

the risk of infection, a caesarian section may be considered if the patient is not near delivery twenty-four hours after artificial membrane rupture with adequate stimulation of uterine contraction with oxytocin.

The main complication of medical induction of labour is overstimulation of the uterus causing tonic uterine contractions, so reducing the oxygen supply to the fetus. If a prostaglandin gel is inserted through the cervix, there is a small risk of injury to the placenta or the vessels supplying it. Overstimulation of the uterus is more likely in the highly multiparous woman who has already had five or more pregnancies. Oxytocin or prostaglandins must be used cautiously in these circumstances, and it should be remembered that prostaglandin cannot be regulated in the same way as an oxytocin drip if overstimulation should occur.

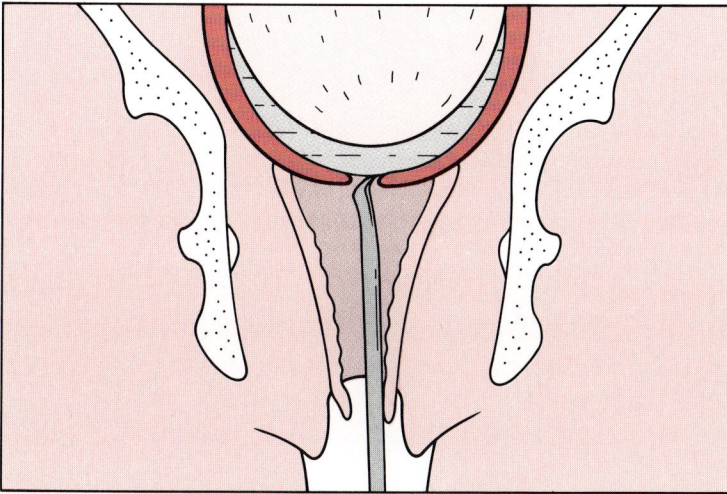

Fig. 8.3 Surgical rupture of the membranes can be achieved by a small plastic hook which snags the membranes.

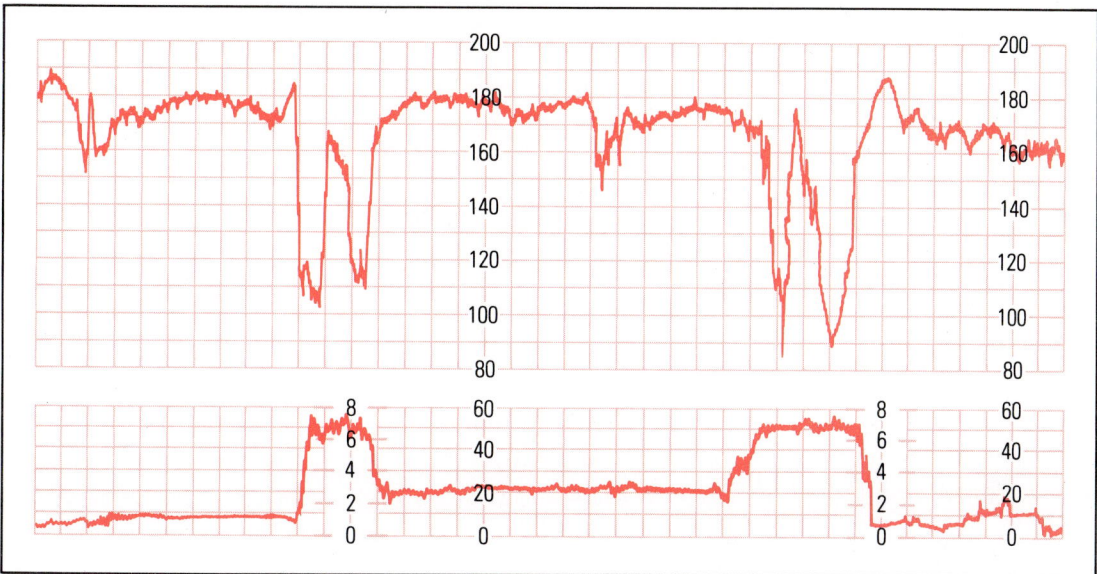

Fig. 8.4 Hypersensitivity to oxytocin. The uterine pressure trace shows the uterus going into spasm; no induction should take place without uterine pressure being monitored.

9. Abnormal Labour

PRETERM LABOUR

A preterm labour is one which occurs before thirty-seven weeks gestation.

Causes

Preterm labour may occur in a variety of circumstances (Fig.9.1). It may be spontaneous, as is often seen in association with twins, polyhydramnios or cervical incompetence, or it may be iatrogenic, when preterm labour is induced for a variety of indications such as intrauterine growth retardation or worsening pre-eclampsia.

Fetal risks

The immature fetus is at risk of cerebral haemorrhage because the fragile cranial bones provide insufficient protection for the brain, the choroid plexuses are more susceptible to hypoxic damage, and there is an increased susceptibility to inefficient clotting mechanisms.

Management

The management of preterm labour involves the following principles:
● Avoid hypoxia.

AETIOLOGY OF SPONTANEOUS PRETERM LABOUR
younger age
poorer socioeconomic class
fatigue and work
smoking
incompetent cervix
multiple pregnancy
abruptio placentae

Fig.9.1 The aetiology of preterm labour.

- Avoid depressing the fetal respiratory centre with excessive analgesic drugs.
- Use epidural analgesia.
- Use caesarean section, particularly in breech presentations.
- Aim to reduce trauma to the fetus, particularly the skull, in vaginal delivery. Forceps may not be necessary, but a wide episiotomy is often required unless the perineum is extremely lax.

It is now recognized that hypoxia, in particular, jeopardizes the survival of the child born prematurely. It is for this reason that careful intrapartum monitoring of the fetal condition should be employed and early recourse to caesarean section available.

Preterm labour may often be prevented by increased rest and it should be suggested that, from mid-pregnancy onwards, the woman lies down in the middle of the day. Should the cervix be incompetent (Fig.9.2), a cervical suture may be inserted close to the level of the internal os (Fig.9.3). Tocolytic agents, such as betasympathomimetic drugs (salbutamol or ritodrine), are often employed and can be valuable in certain circumstances.

Cervical incompetence

Cervical incompetence is usually caused by damage to the internal os. This may happen inadvertently at dilatation and curettage or at vaginal termination of pregnancy. Occasionally, it follows a previous, apparently normal delivery; generally, however, cervical incompetence may be suspected from a previous obstetric history of mid-trimester abortion or early preterm labour. Rupture of the membranes is often the first sign and this is rapidly followed by expulsion of the fetus. In these circumstances, the insertion of a suture close to the internal os is best performed at around fourteen weeks in the subsequent pregnancy.

Tocolytics

Betasympathomimetic drugs have been used to prevent and treat preterm labour. They act on the myometrium and postpone contractions for hours or days but properly conducted, random trials have shown no evidence to indicate that they improve the outlook for the fetus. It may be that the fetus in a spontaneous preterm labour is better off outside the uterus than inside. There has been a reduction in the use of betasympathomimetic tocolytic agents in the developed world. Their main use now is probably to postpone labour temporarily whilst some other line of management can be implemented, for example the *in utero* transfer of the fetus to a tertiary care centre, or the administration, via the mother, of steroids which help to induce maturation of the fetal respiratory system.

In utero transfer

A woman in preterm labour is at risk of producing an immature infant. This will require intensive neonatal

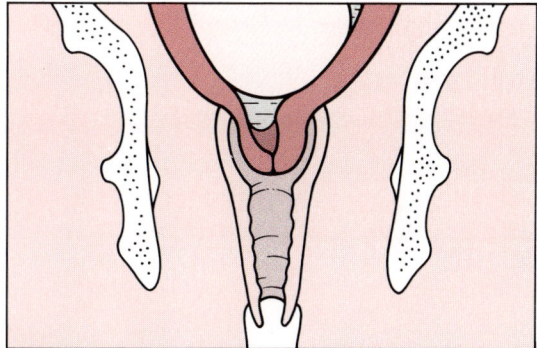

Fig.9.2 Cervical incompetence. This is usually due to previous damage to the cervix which splits the internal os, leaving a defective sphincter (left).

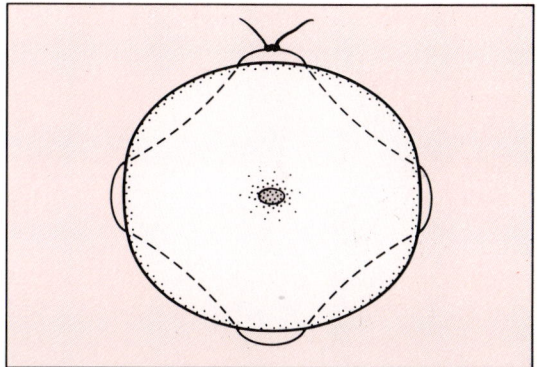

Fig.9.3 Management of cervical incompetence. A suture should be placed around the cervix like a purse string. Here, the suture has four bites into the cervical substance and is tied in front of the cervix. The knot is left with an inch-long end in the vagina and is cut at about 37–38 weeks gestation.

care, particularly if the gestational age is less than thirty weeks. Consequently, the woman should deliver close to the best neonatal unit available, which often means transferring her care in pregnancy to another hospital. Such *in utero* transfer is necessary for women who develop severe raised blood pressure in mid-pregnancy or who have signs of impending preterm labour. The transfer is performed during labour by agreement between the donor and recipient hospitals. The policy of *in utero* transfer is designed to benefit the baby, who can then be delivered straight into the neonatal care in which he may stay for the next few weeks.

MALPRESENTATIONS

A malpresentation is a presentation other than by the vertex; of these, breech presentation is by far the most common.

Breech presentation and labour

Breech presentation may occur in three forms (Fig.9.4):
- Complete breech. Both the hips and knees are flexed.
- Incomplete breech. The legs may be extended, with flexed hips but extended knees. This is the most common type of breech, and may present difficulties because the legs splint the body and interfere with lateral flexion.
- Footling presentation. The hips are much more extended, with the knees flexed and the feet dangling just over, or sometimes through, the cervix. This occurs more commonly in smaller, less mature breech presentations.

Footling presentations are more dangerous than the others because the presenting part does not form such a good fit in the pelvis and cord prolapse may therefore occur. In addition, the feet tend to slip

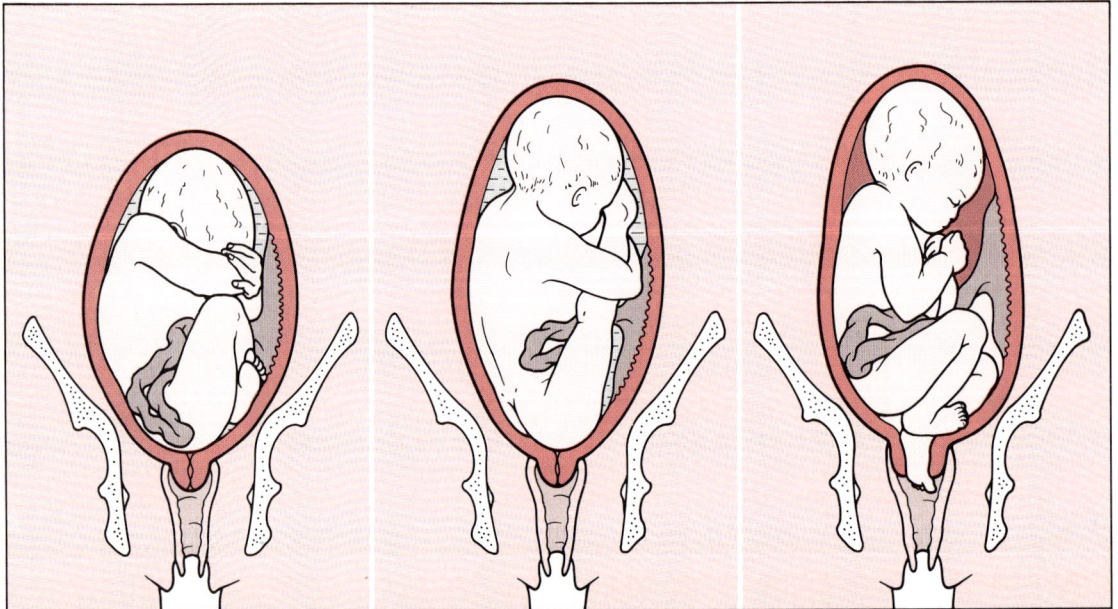

Fig.9.4   Left: complete breech. The thighs are flexed on the body and the legs flexed on the thighs, thus the buttocks are presenting and the feet are low in the pelvis. Middle: incomplete breech. Although the thighs are flexed on the abdomen, the knees are extended so that the legs are alongside the head. Right: footling presentation. The thighs are poorly flexed against the abdominal wall, so that the foot is over the cervix and comes down soon after membrane rupture.

through the undilated cervix, which gives the woman the feeling of wanting to push; this may result in delivery of the child's body, but not the head, through an incompletely dilated cervix, and consequently the child may die.

The incidence of breech presentation at term is approximately three percent, but it is much more common in preterm deliveries; at approximately thirty weeks gestation, twenty-five percent are presenting as a breech.

Not all of the causes of breech presentation are known, but the following are considered possibilities:

- The legs may be extended, thus preventing the fetus from kicking against the bony pelvis to turn itself round from a breech into a vertex presentation.
- The fetus may have additional space in the uterus due to polyhydramnios or multiparity, breech presentation being more common in both of these conditions.
- Engagement of the head may be prevented by the presence of a fibroid or a placenta praevia, and the presentation reverts to breech.

In most cases, however, the cause is unknown.

The use of external version (Fig.9.5) in the management of breech presentation is debatable. Many believe that spontaneous version is so common that it is unnecessary to use external manipulation to convert the fetus to a cephalic presentation. However, some still employ this method, which should be performed on a conscious patient and only if the fetus is not too large and the abdomen not too tense. If the woman is anaesthetized, it will be hard for the operator to judge how much force to employ in trying to turn the baby and injury to the uterus or placenta may result. If the fetus is too large and the abdominal wall tense, the attempted version will be unsuccessful and the patient may be caused considerable discomfort. If, however, the manoeuvre is performed under the appropriate conditions and at the correct time, the fetus should stay in the vertex position.

The risks of external version include preterm labour, placental separation, injury to the uterus itself, and, very rarely, prolapse of the cord (see Fig.9.12). All these complications are more likely to occur if

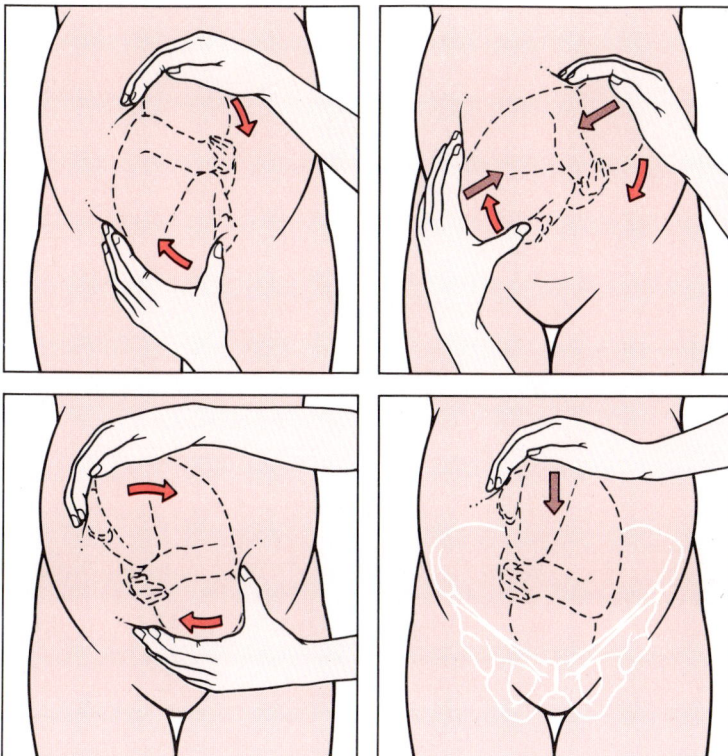

Fig.9.5 External cephalic version. Upper left: the fetal buttocks are displaced from the mother's pelvis and flexion increased by pressing down and forwards on the fetal head. Upper right: the fetal buttocks are disempacted from the pelvis and pushed into the iliac fossa whilst the head is gently brought down the side of the uterus. Lower left: once past the transverse position, the buttocks usually proceed rapidly up towards the fundus and the head moves towards the pelvis. Lower right: the head should now be capable of being pressed down into the pelvis.

the attempted version is carried out under general anaesthesia.

The use of version is now less common because of the possibility of these complications occurring. Furthermore, if vaginal delivery is not to be allowed, there is no point in performing external version; similarly, if the fetus is abnormal or if twins are present, external version is contraindicated.

Breech labour can be allowed under the following circumstances:

- The fetus should not be too large.
- The fetus should not be at higher risk than usual of compromise. Risk of hypoxia, which always occurs during normal delivery, and more so in breech, might be fatal in a fetus which is already compromised (e.g. due to pre-eclampsia).

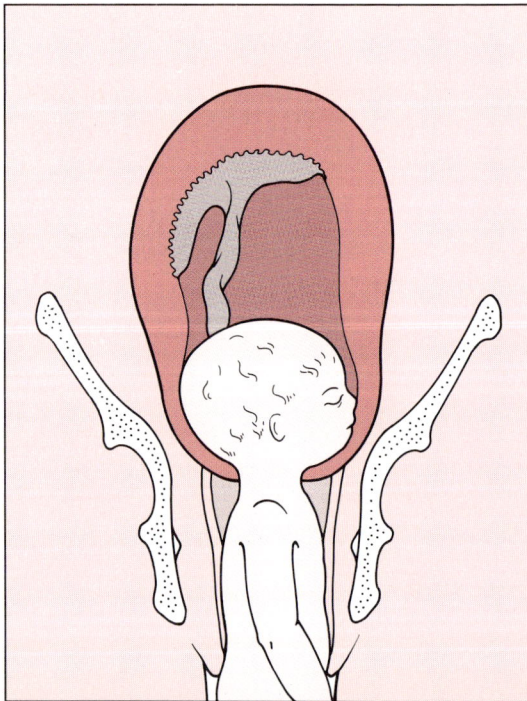

Fig.9.6 The buttocks can pass through an undilated cervix, especially with small babies. They will be rapidly followed by the legs, the body and even the fetal shoulders. The head cannot get through an undilated cervix, even though it is very small.

- The pelvis should not be contracted, hence X-ray pelvimetry should be performed in most cases. Delivery of a baby breech-first through a contracted pelvis is dangerous for the fetus, since, if the head moulds very quickly, cerebral haemorrhage is almost certain to result.
- There should be no other high-risk maternal factor such as elderly primiparity or poor obstetric history.

A proper assessment for breech delivery includes clinical assessment of fetal size, a vaginal examination to assess the bony pelvis and the condition of the cervix and vagina, X-ray pelvimetry to measure the size of the pelvis as precisely as possible, and ultrasonic cephalometry to measure the biparietal diameter of the fetal head and gain a further impression to fetal size. Since the head is the last part of the child to be born, it is not possible to test precisely the cephalopelvic relationship until the last moment of the second stage. Consequently, all available methods must be used to exclude the likelihood of cephalopelvic disproportion. Should such disproportion exist, the operator would have no alternative at this late stage but to continue with delivery by the vaginal route with, almost certainly, serious injury or death to the fetus. If the fetus is unusually large or the pelvis inadequate, complications are more likely to occur and elective caesarean section should be performed. An epidural anaesthetic is usually recommended for analgesia during labour.

During the second stage of labour, the following principles apply:

- Before pushing starts, it is essential to check for full cervical dilatation. Pushing prior to this (Fig.9.6) may result in a dead child.
- It is preferable to monitor the fetus continuously.
- An anaesthetist and a paediatrician should be present in the delivery room during the second stage.

Good technique during the performance of breech delivery can make all the difference between a live, healthy child and one who is brain-damaged, injured or dead. At any stage, complications may arise which a skillful operator should be able to circumvent. One of the most difficult complications is extension of the arms, which may arise due to injudicious pulling on the fetus at an early stage in the delivery; pulling should always be avoided. Once the body of the fetus has been delivered (Fig.9.7), the head, which is still in the uterus, is encouraged to flex on the fetal body, in the vagina, so that a smaller cephalic diameter will present. The fetus may be drawn downwards and backwards to obtain this flexion. Several techniques are available for the delivery of the head (Fig.9.8), but what is most important is that it be brought gently through the pelvis to avoid the risk of cerebral haemorrhage. Once the nose and mouth have been delivered, the baby can breathe freely, so the rest of the delivery can be as slow as is necessary.

Complications

The hazards of breech delivery can affect both the fetus and the mother. The fetus may suffer a cerebral haemorrhage from passing too quickly through the pelvis, or asphyxia from passing through too slowly. Other parts of the body such as the hip or arm may also be injured resulting, for example, in hip dislocation, fractures, or Erb's palsy.

The mother may suffer soft tissue injury and a severe tear due to the manipulations that are sometimes necessary. Those which give rise to soft tissue injury are most likely to be performed if a complication arises in the delivery. Extension of the arms is particularly likely to result in maternal damage.

Owing to these potential dangers in breech delivery, caesarean section is now used in forty percent of all cases of breech presentation in the United Kindgom and in a much higher proportion in the United States.

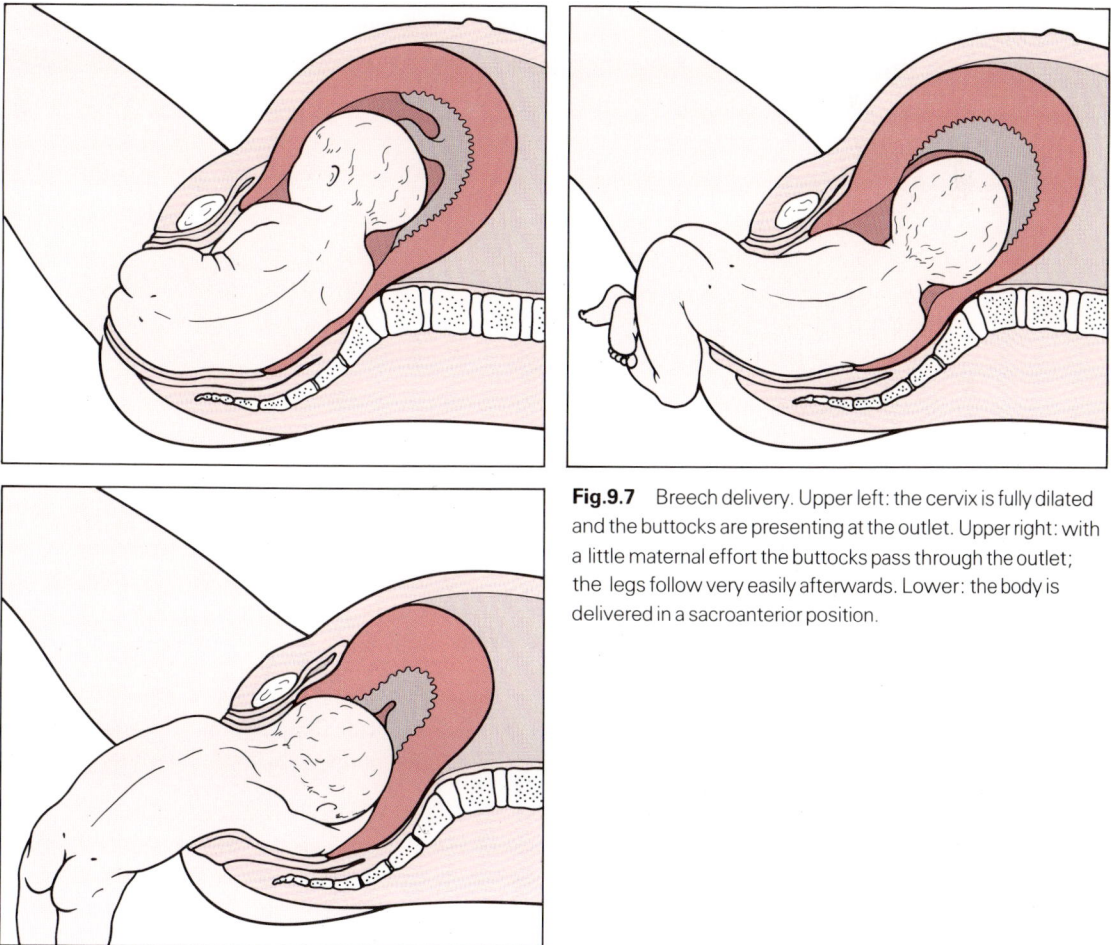

Fig.9.7   Breech delivery. Upper left: the cervix is fully dilated and the buttocks are presenting at the outlet. Upper right: with a little maternal effort the buttocks pass through the outlet; the legs follow very easily afterwards. Lower: the body is delivered in a sacroanterior position.

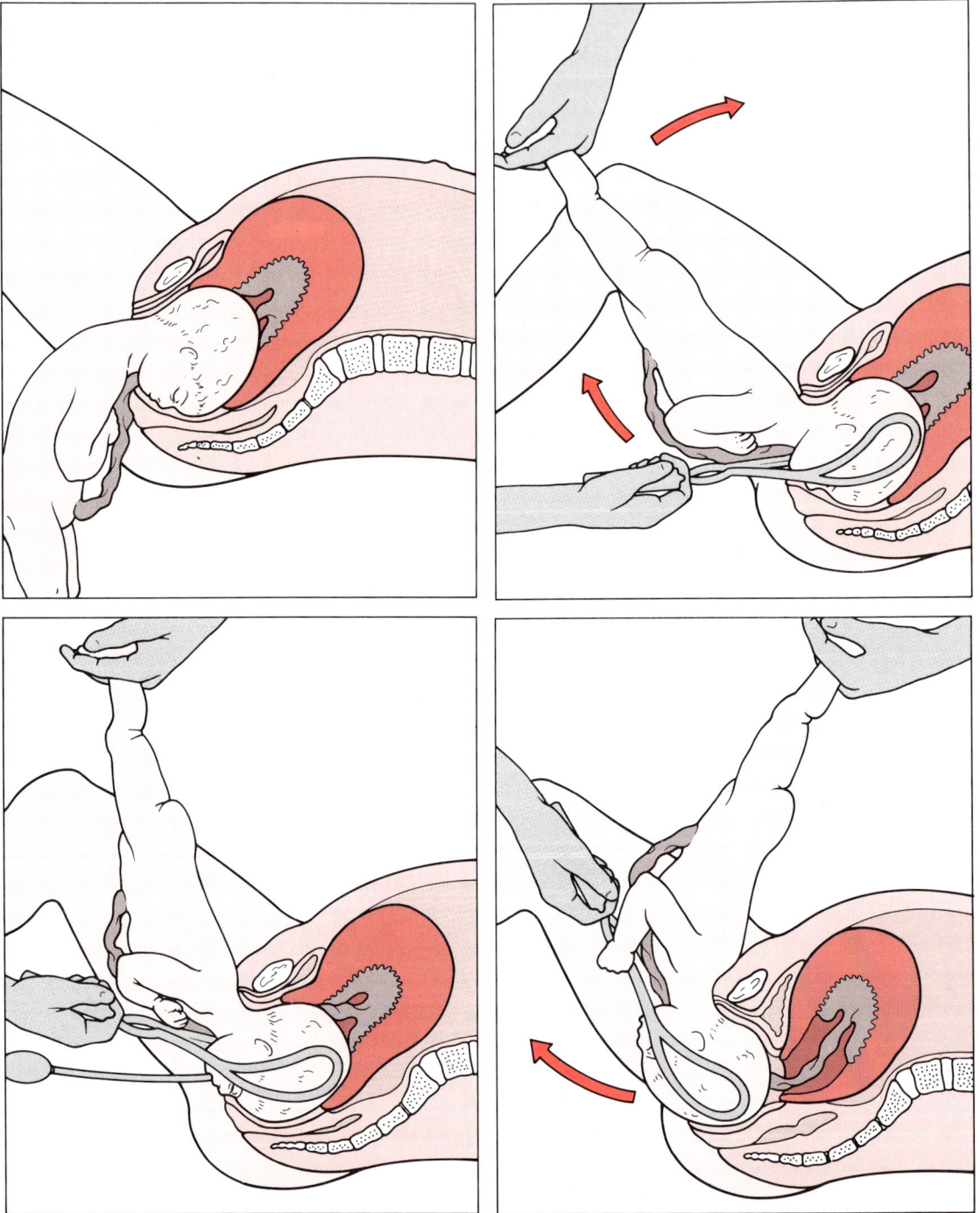

Fig.9.8 Delivery of the head. Upper left: the head has rotated to the occipitoanterior position behind the symphysis pubis. Upper right: a pair of forceps is slipped onto the baby's head to guard it and to control the rate of progress through the pelvis. Lower left: once the nose and mouth are delivered over the perineum, mucus extraction allows the child to breathe freely. Lower right: the rest of the head is delivered.

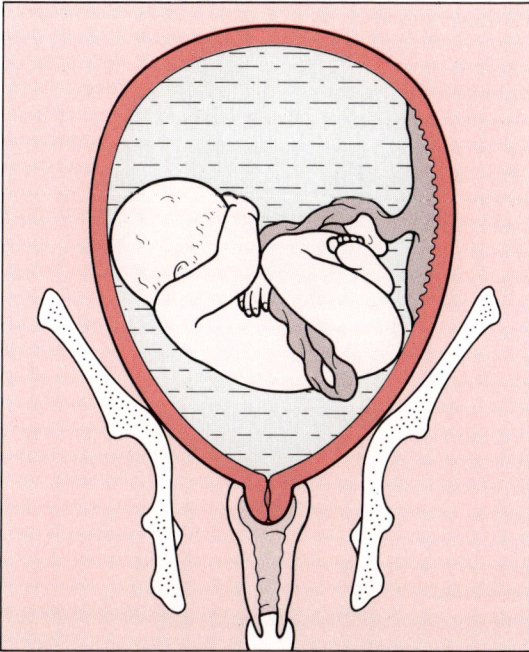

Fig.9.9 A transverse lie is characterized as one where the long axis of the fetus is at right angles with the long axis of the mother. This illustration also shows one of the common causes of the condition, excessive amniotic fluid.

Transverse and oblique lies

The most common cause of transverse (Fig.9.9) and oblique lies of a fetus in late pregnancy is multiparity, because with increasing parity there is increasing laxity of the abdominal wall muscles and the fetus has greater mobility. Other causes include polyhydramnios, the presence of a pelvic tumour (which keeps the presenting part out of the pelvis), or a bicornuate or septate uterus (Fig.9.10), to which the fetus adapts more readily in a transverse or oblique lie.

These possible causes must be considered when the patient is seen in later pregnancy with a transverse or an oblique lie. Polyhydramnios or the presence of a pelvic tumour can be determined by examination, but the possible presence of a bicornuate uterus can be suspected only from a previous history of a similar abnormality, or from an unusual shape of the uterus on palpation; a septate uterus cannot be diagnosed during the pregnant state.

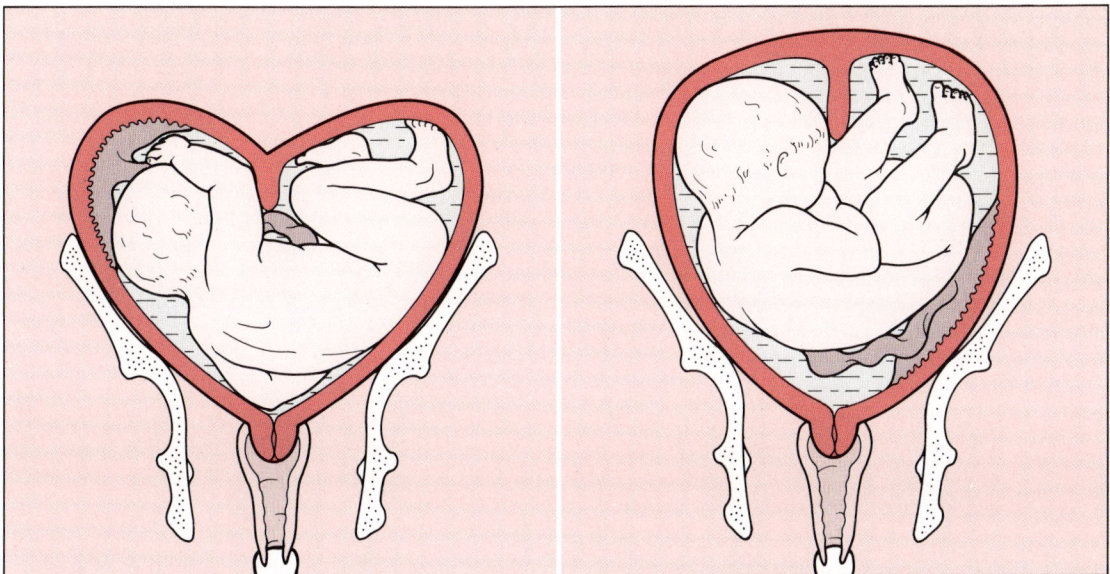

Fig.9.10 Diagnosable causes of a transverse lie. Left: a bicornuate uterus in which the fetus grows in a transverse position from mid-pregnancy. Right: a subseptate uterus, in which the fetus cannot kick himself round because the septum interferes with movement.

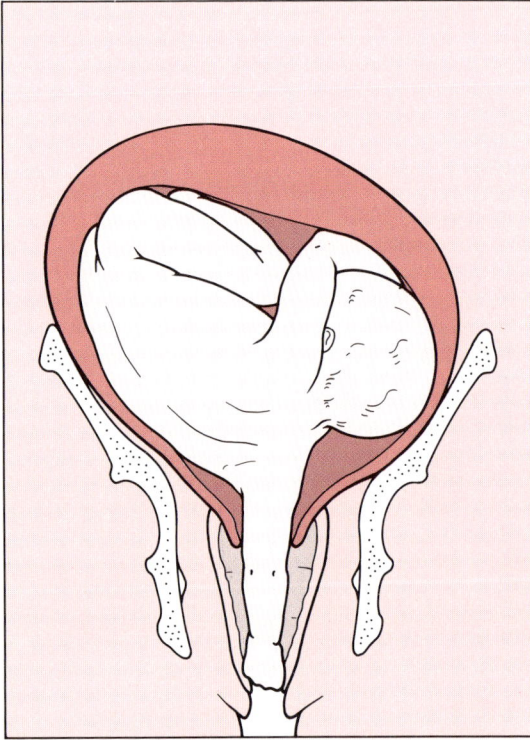

Fig.9.11 Arm prolapse. Labour has started with the fetus in a transverse position. The cervix has dilated to 3–4cm and the membranes have ruptured. An arm has prolapsed into the vagina; this will act as a peg, rooting the baby to this position. Often, by the time an obstetrician sees the woman with an arm prolapse, the baby is dead.

Complications

The complications of transverse and oblique lies include obstructed labour, prolapse of the cord, or uterine rupture if labour starts when the fetus is lying in either of these two positions. Unless a longitudinal lie is achieved during the course of labour, obstruction will occur and serious consequences follow. Very rarely, an arm comes down through the cervix and appears at the vulva (Fig.9.11). A small or a dead child is expelled in a folded-up position, having previously been a transverse or oblique lie. If the fetus is of normal size, the uterus can rupture. Since the fetus cannot be expelled from the birth canal, the upper uterine segment contracts vigorously against resistance, its muscle fibres becoming shorter and

thicker. The fibres of the lower uterine segment become thinner as it is drawn upwards. If the obstetrician should try to introduce his hand to correct the transverse lie, rupture of this thin lower segment is extremely likely; such a rupture will sometimes also occur spontaneously.

If a woman with a transverse or oblique lie is encountered in late pregnancy, the attendant should:
- Exclude a pelvic tumour or placenta praevia.
- Correct the lie if the patient is approaching term and there are no contraindications.
- Possibly induce labour by medical means if correction is unsuccessful.
- Resort to caesarean section at an early stage, since the risk to mother and child is serious.

The difficulty inherent in correction and induction is that, even when the lie is corrected, the fetus may remain in a longitudinal position for only a short time, reverting to a transverse or oblique lie later. For this reason, if labour is to be induced in an attempt to stabilize the presentation, it is usually unwise to rupture the membranes early, since there is then a risk of prolapse of the cord if the lie reverts to oblique.

Cord prolapse (Fig.9.12 left) may arise for a variety of reasons, including association with transverse lie, breech presentation or multiparity. It may be seen in preterm labour, polyhydramnios and twin pregnancy. In general, when the presenting part does not fit the cervix well, the risk of prolapse of the cord is increased. It may also be increased if the cord lies low in the uterine cavity, attached to a placenta praevia. After membrane rupture in a transverse lie, there is nothing to block the internal os and the cord is flushed down in a gush of amniotic fluid.

In the management of a cord prolapse, the attendant should ask himself the following questions:
- Is the prolapsed cord the only abnormality present or is there also, for example, a breech presentation or an oblique lie?
- Is the cord pulsating?
- Is the fetus viable?

If the fetus is alive, the first manoeuvre is to take pressure off the cord either by holding up the presenting part with the hand (Fig.9.12 right), or by putting the patient in the exaggerated lateral position. If pressure on the cord is not relieved, it may go into spasm and prevent proper circulation within the fetus, who is still dependent upon the placental circulation for oxygen. Urgent caesarean section, or forceps or breech extraction may be carried out, depending upon

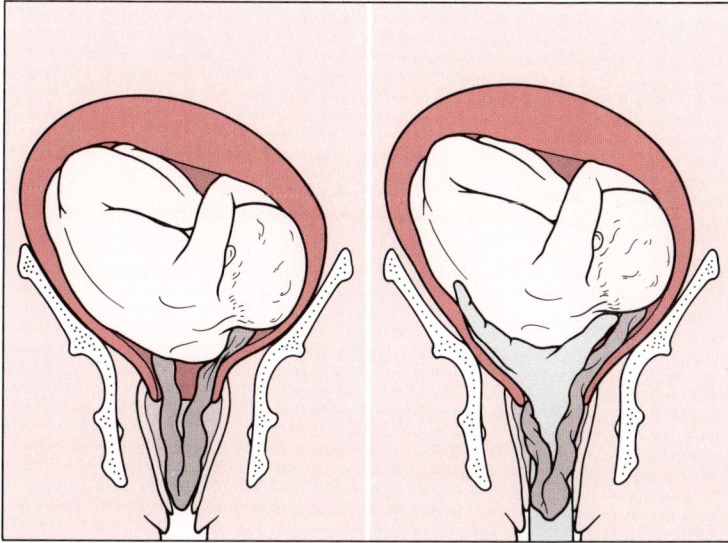

Fig.9.12 Cord prolapse. Left: the cord has prolapsed through the cervix and is appearing at the vulva. Right: the presenting part is held up by the tips of the fingers until a caesarean section can be performed.

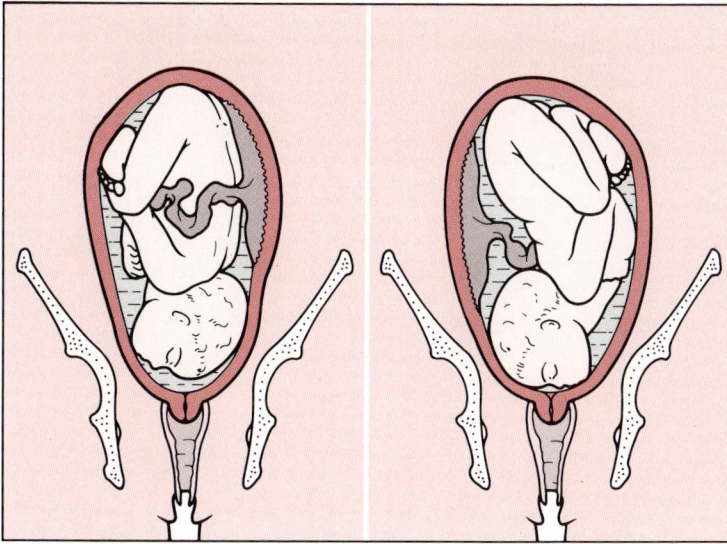

Fig.9.13 Left: brow presentation. The frontal suture is situated over the internal os and the eyebrows are palpable laterally. Right: face presentation. The bridge of the nose is over the internal os. Equidistant on either side of this, the chin and the anterior part of the anterior fontanelle are palpable. The alveolar margins may be palpable within the mouth.

the degree of dilatation of the cervix. Clearly, if the cervix is not fully dilated, caesarean section will be essential: if, however, it is fully dilated, rapid delivery by forceps or breech extraction may be successful.

MALPOSITIONS

Malpositions are defined as any cephalic presentation other than occipitoanterior, for example occipito-posterior, face and brow.

Face and brow presentations

Face and brow presentations (Fig.9.13) are rare, with a prevalence of one in three hundred and one in six hundred labours, respectively. They represent an increased degree of extension rather than flexion of the fetal head. The causes of brow and face presentation include multiparity, polyhydramnios, immaturity, anencephaly (in which only the face of the child is present and the vault of the skull is absent), and pelvic contraction.

149

Face presentation

In face presentation, the 9.5cm submentobregmatic diameter of the fetal head passes through the pelvis, and vaginal delivery is usually possible (Fig.9.14), provided that the chin rotates forward into the mentoanterior position and there is no disproportion. The head descends in full extension and delivers by slight flexion of the head on the body. This is the reverse of the mechanism for a normal vertex delivery, where the head descends with increasing flexion and is delivered over the perineum by extension. For successful delivery of a face presentation, a large episiotomy is usually required, since flexion at the last moment throws the larger submentovertical diameter across the perineum.

Less commonly, the chin rotates posteriorly to the mentoposterior position and labour then becomes completely obstructed (Fig.9.15). As there is no mechanism for delivery in this position, caesarean section must be performed.

The diagnosis of a face presentation can sometimes be made abdominally by noting that the prominence of the head and the back are on the same side. On vaginal examination, it should be possible to recognize a face presentation by palpating the alveolar margins within the mouth. The other facial features are usually too imprecise for recognition because facial oedema during labour often obscures them.

Brow presentation

Vaginal delivery is usually impossible with a persisting brow presentation, since the 13.5cm mentovertical diameter which presents cannot enter the pelvis. Caesarean section is nearly always required. If, however, the head rotates into the occipitoanterior

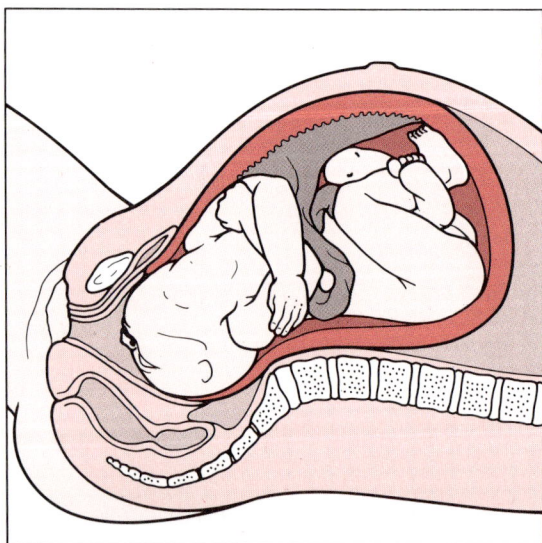

Fig.9.14 Delivery of face presentation. Left: the face has descended and the cervix is widely dilated. The chin is rotating so that it is facing sideways (mentolateral position).

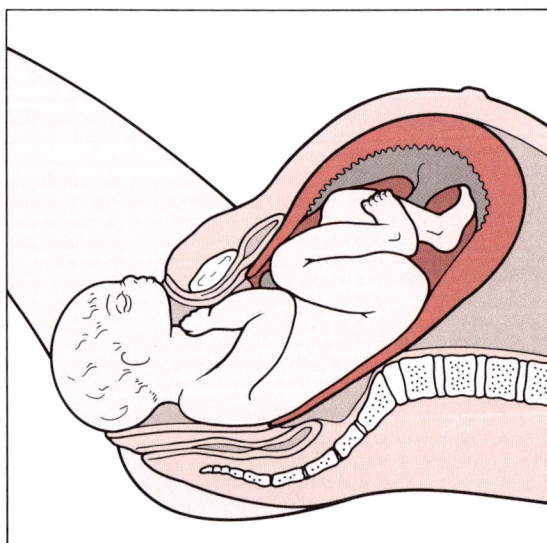

Right: the head descends in full extension, the chin has rotated to the front of the mother's pelvis (mentoanterior position) and is delivering by slight flexion.

position, slight flexion positions the anterior fontanelle immediately over the centre of the os (Fig.9.16). This is one of the better ways in which a brow presentation can proceed, since a slight further flexion would allow engagement in the pelvis and a normal, if long, labour may result in vaginal delivery.

It may be more difficult to recognize a fetus presenting by the brow than one presenting by the face. Diagnosis depends on an unusually prominent anterior fontanelle and on the frontal suture leading to the bridge of the nose when traced with a finger on vaginal examination.

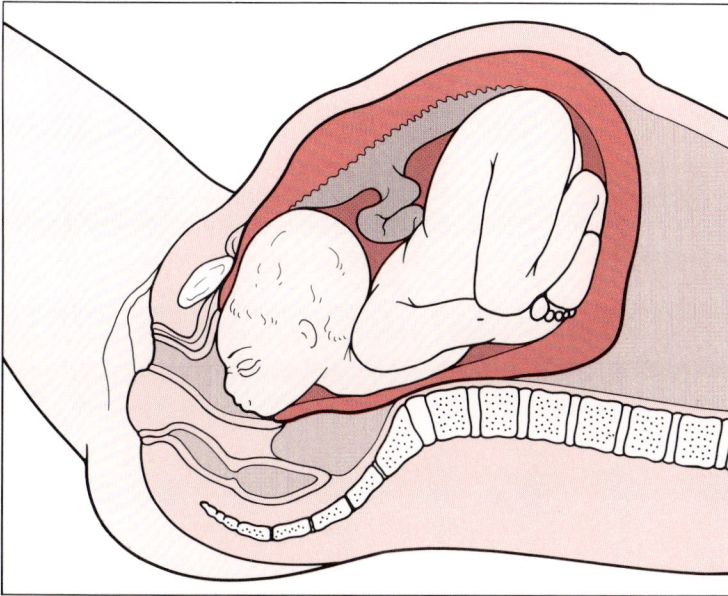

Fig.9.15 Face presentation with a mentoposterior position. The head is jammed in the hollow of the sacrum, as the submentovertical diameter, which is very large, is engaging in the pelvic brim.

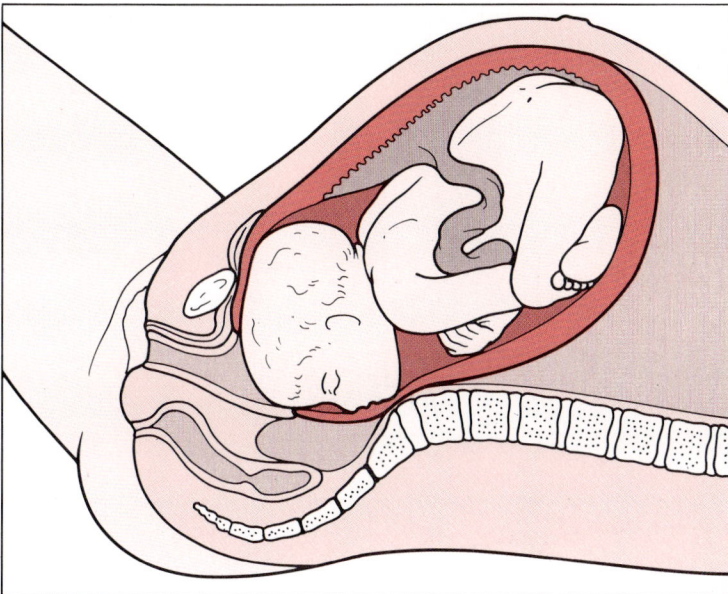

Fig.9.16 Brow presentation. The situation seen in Fig.9.13 (left) has now progressed in labour to about 7cm dilatation. The head has rotated into the occipitoanterior position and has flexed slightly, so that the anterior fontanelle is now immediately over the centre of the os.

151

Occipitoposterior positions

Occipitoposterior positions (Fig.9.17) of the vertex are commonly seen during labour; up to twenty percent of fetuses start labour in this position, with the right occipitoposterior being more common than the left. The head tends to be deflexed, presenting with the 11 cm occipitofrontal diameter engaging. Deflexion may be noticed on abdominal examination, where the palpating fingers on the fetal forehead and occiput will be at the same level through the mother's abdomen instead of the forehead being at a higher level than the occiput, which is the situation in a well flexed head. Unusually prominent limbs are also detectable on abdominal palpation.

On vaginal examination, the occipitoposterior position is recognized by the position of the posterior fontanelle (into which only three sutures are inserted); this will be opposite the right or left sacroiliac joint. The anterior fontanelle (into which four sutures are inserted) is unusually prominent because of deflexion. If there is difficulty in recognizing the position from the fontanelles, palpation of an ear, noting that the pinna points backwards, should identify the position accurately. If the head stays in the occipitoposterior position as it descends in the pelvis, it often becomes less flexed and so presents even larger diameters to the maternal pelvis, producing even further mechanical difficulty.

In delivery of a fetus in the occipitoposterior position, flexion of the head normally increases, allowing the occiput to become the lowest point and to strike the pelvic floor first. The occiput is therefore rotated forwards through 135° (Figs.9.18 & 9.19) to achieve the occipitoanterior position and the delivery is accomplished by extension in the usual manner. Anterior rotation usually occurs late in the first or second stage of labour and this may cause a temporary delay in progress necessitating forceps delivery. Once the head is delivered, the external rotation is variable (45–135°), after which the shoulders are delivered.

If the head remains poorly flexed, however, the sinciput becomes the lowest part, striking the sloping pelvic floor first and rotating forwards; thus the occiput rotates into the hollow of the sacrum producing a direct or persistent occipitoposterior position

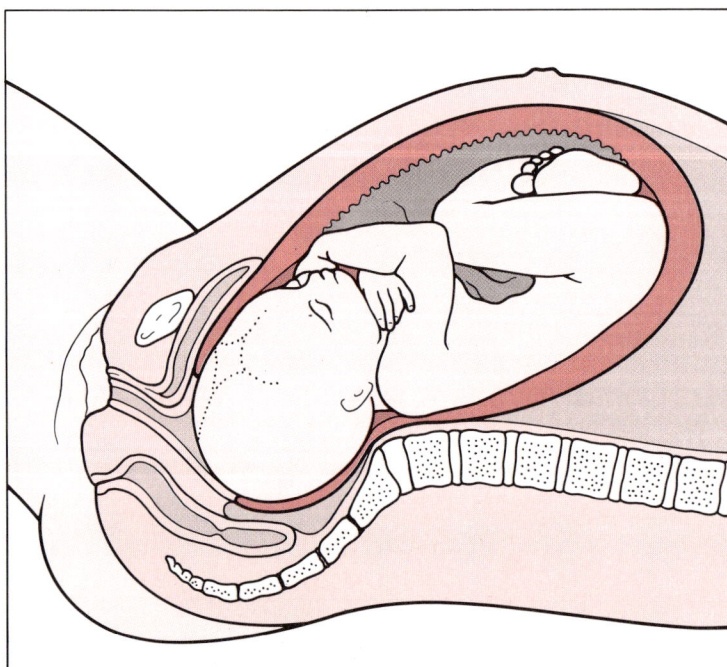

Fig.9.17 Occipitoposterior position. The occiput is in the posterior quadrant of the pelvis and faces the right ala of the sacrum. The head is reasonably flexed in this case, but the anterior fontanelle is in the front of the pelvis and the posterior fontanelle towards the back.

(ten percent of cases). In some cases (fifteen percent), anterior rotation may become arrested at the level of the ischial spines, resulting in deep transverse arrest.

In the management of deep transverse arrest, rotation is imperative to permit vaginal delivery. This may be achieved manually, by Kielland's forceps, or by the use of the vacuum extractor.

If the position is direct occipitoposterior, delivery may be possible face-to-pubis (Fig.9.20), providing the head is reasonably small and the pelvis comparatively large; an episiotomy is almost always required to facilitate delivery and to prevent a large tear. A face-to-pubis delivery is possible in about twenty-five percent of cases. This should not be confused with the face presentation (see Fig.9.14 right), where the face is the leading part. In a face-to-pubis delivery, it is still the vertex of the head that leads, but the occiput is towards the mother's sacrum, and so the baby's face appears from behind the mother's pubis looking upwards.

If there is second stage delay due to a persistent occipitoposterior, forceps delivery may be undertaken provided the head is very low. If the head is at a higher level, however, rotation to an occipitoanterior position is necessary before forceps can be applied. Vacuum extraction may also be used because this allows the fetal head to follow its natural rotation.

DYSFUNCTIONAL UTERINE ACTION

Dysfunctional uterine action may be of three varieties:
- Contractions which are too weak – hypotonic inertia.
- Contractions which are too strong – hypertonic inertia.
- Incoordinate contractions.

Hypotonic inertia

If the contractions are too weak or infrequent, the labour may be augmented by the use of intravenous Syntocinon in a dilute solution to stimulate the uterus. A partogram is essential to follow progress and the observations should ideally be done by just one

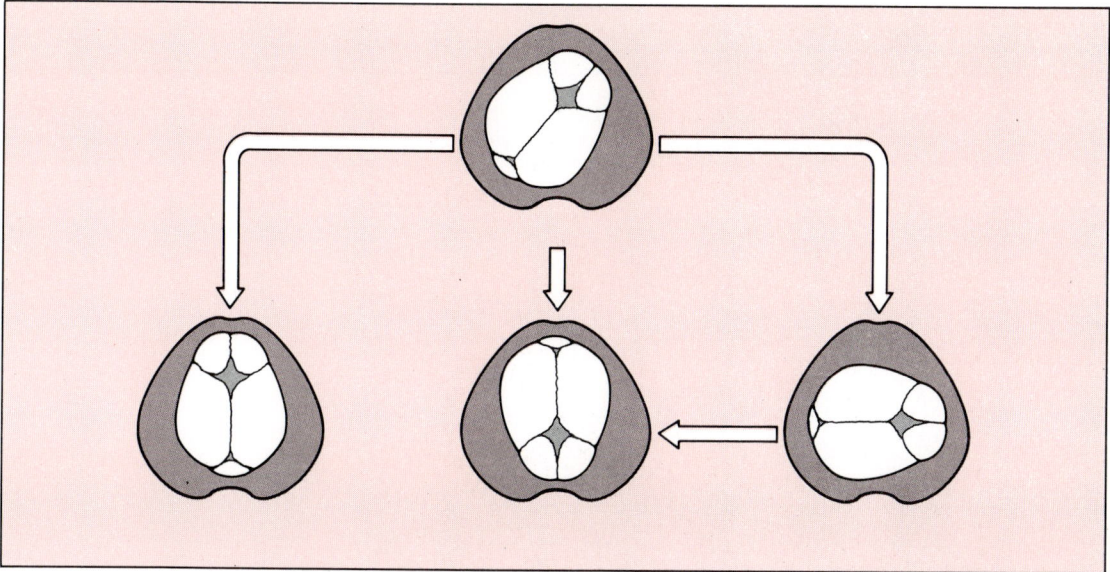

Fig.9.18 Rotation of occipitoposterior positions. The head may rotate through 135° to become occipitoanterior; it may rotate through only a fraction of this (about 45°) laterally and stick in the occipitolateral to produce a deep transverse arrest; or it may rotate directly backwards through about 45° to become a persistent occipitoposterior position.

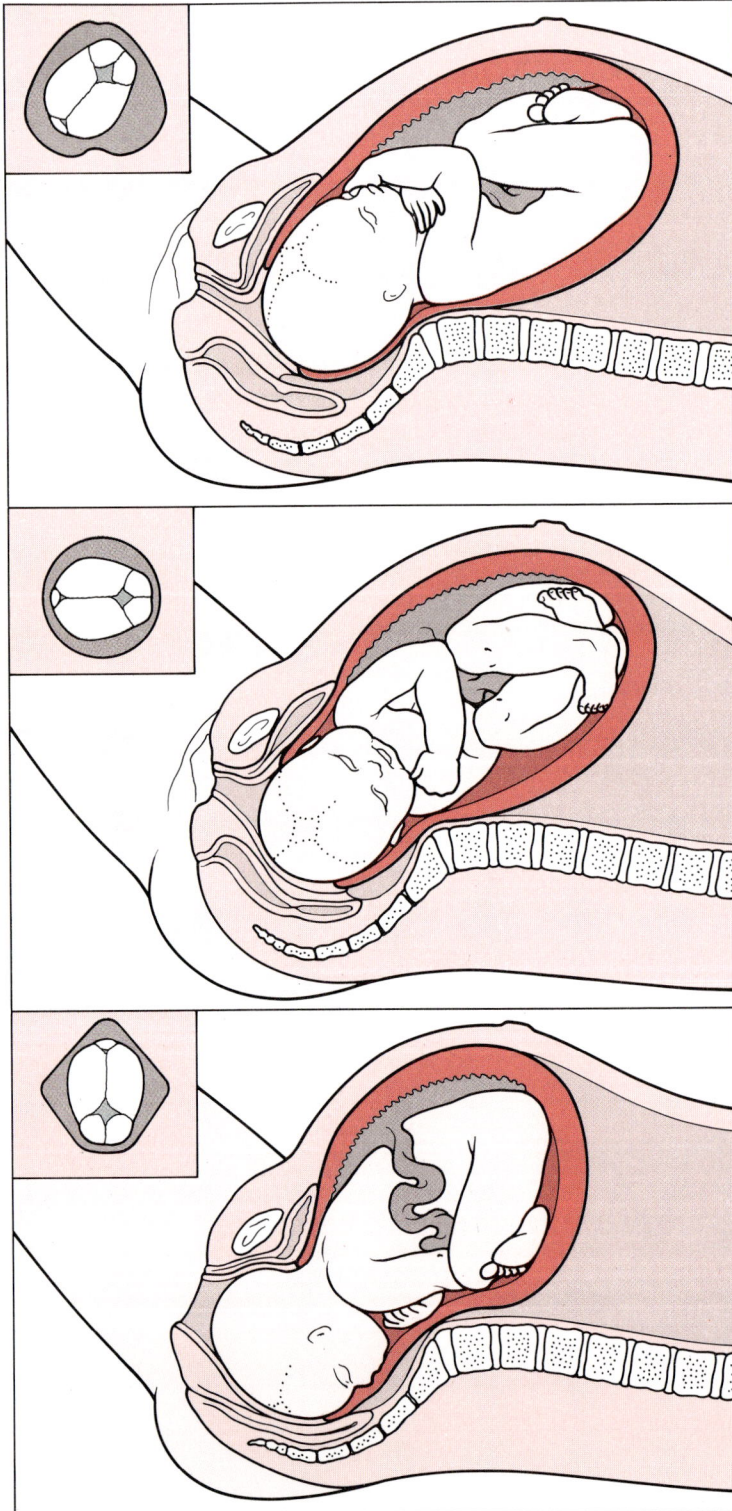

Fig.9.19 Rotation of occipitoposterior to occipitoanterior. Upper: the head is engaged in the occipitoposterior position. Middle: as descent occurs into the pelvis, the head turns first to occipitolateral. This is a long process and could stop in occipitotransverse, leading to deep transverse arrest. Lower: further rotation produces the occipitoanterior position.

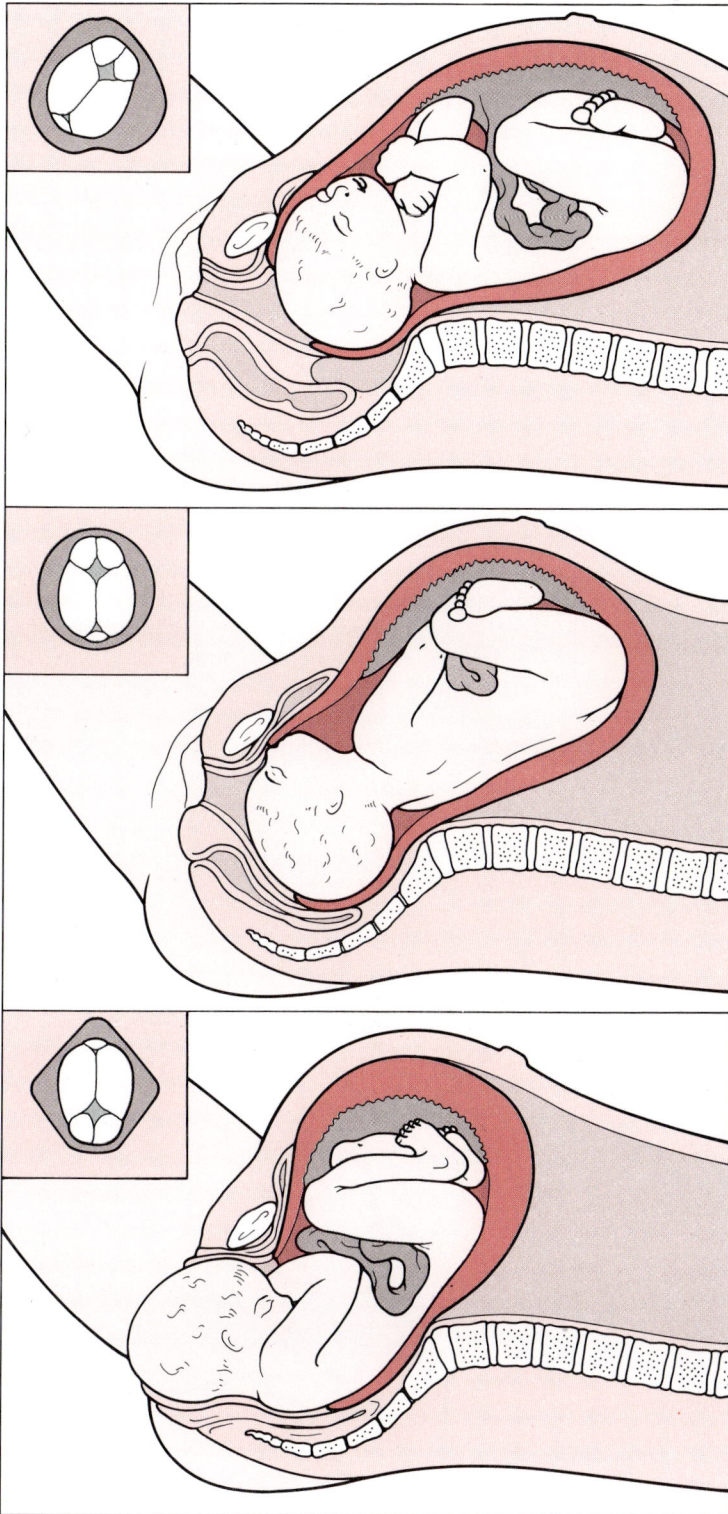

Fig.9.20 Rotation of occipitoposterior to direct occipitoposterior. Upper: the head is engaged in the occipitoposterior position. Middle: the head rotates posteriorly so that the occiput is directly in front of the sacrum. Lower: further progress, by flexion of the head onto the chest allows a face-to-pubis delivery.

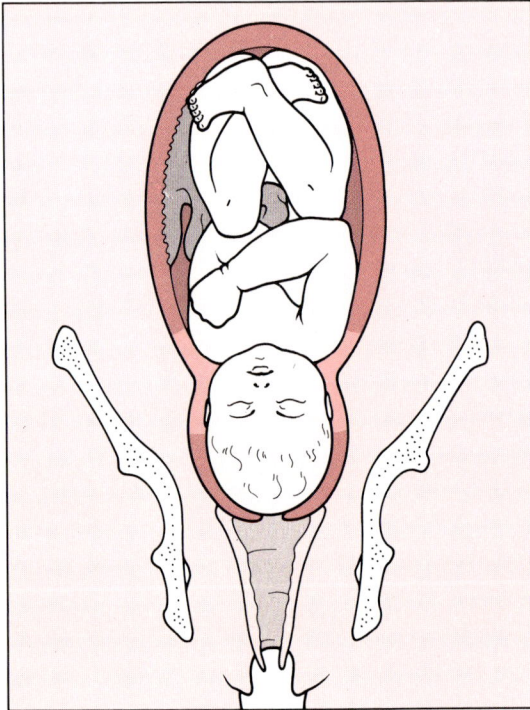

Fig.9.21 Constriction ring. The uterus has moulded itself around the fetus, there is no amniotic fluid, and the chances of this baby delivering are low.

person. If the cervix is soft, taken up and about 2cm dilated, the membranes may also be ruptured to bring the head further down into the lower segment of the uterus. The Syntocinon solution should be run at a drip rate which brings effective uterine contractions every two to three minutes. Alternatively, it may be administered from a well controlled mechanized pump which injects a strictly regulated dose into the intravenous drip fluid. Syntocinon should not be used to drive the uterus into strong contractions because this can cut off the placental bed blood supply and cause fetal hypoxia.

If this management is effective, the uterus will contract at a rate which causes steady dilatation of the cervix and descent of the head. These will be checked on examination and shown on the partogram. The woman may require forceps or vacuum extraction at the second stage of labour for she may be tired after a long labour or the fetal head may not be fully rotated.

If the Syntocinon does not produce coordinated uterine contractions, the head will not descend and the cervix will not dilate. If, after a planned period of Syntocinon progressive stimulation (between four and eight hours) the observations on the partogram still show poor progress, a caesarean section should be considered without waiting any longer.

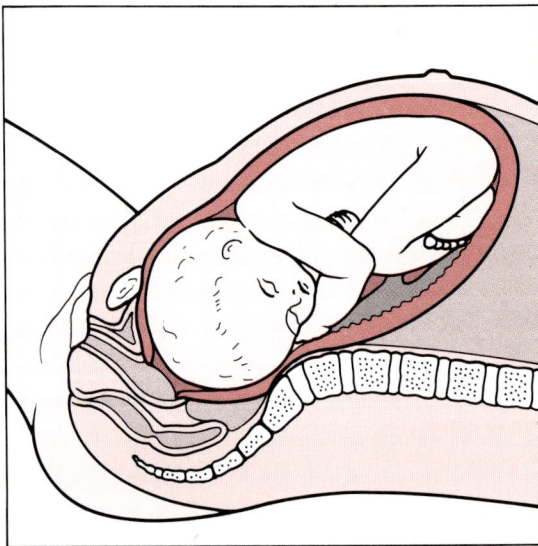

Fig.9.22 Causes of cephalopelvic disproportion. Left: the head is too large because of hydrocephaly. Right: the pelvis is too small for the normal sized baby. Both conditions should be diagnosed in the antenatal period.

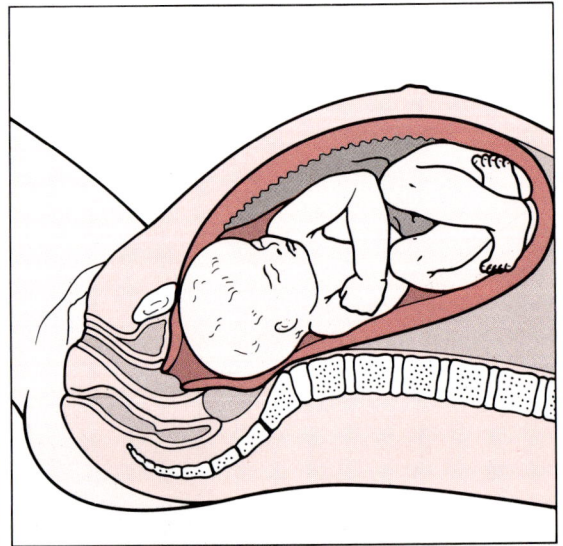

Hypertonic inertia

If the uterine contractions are too strong, they may be reduced by giving an epidural anaesthetic or, if this is unavailable, 150mg of pethidine intravenously. This is not a perfect treatment but it often helps. Should Syntocinon be running, this must of course be reduced, if not stopped, for the uterus might be over-stimulated by the oxytocic drug.

Occasionally, hypertonic uterine contractions lead to a constriction ring (Fig.9.21) which forms around some part of the fetus, for example the neck. If good analgesia does not reduce the contractions, the fetus will not withstand the cut off from the placental bed for long. Continuous fetal heart rate monitoring must be performed and if the fetus shows signs of hypoxia with late decelerations or loss of variability, delivery is by immediate caesarean section.

Incoordinate contractions

Incoordinate uterine action occurs when the contractions on one side of the uterus are not coordinated with those on the other. This produces a rocking effect and is very unusual. It can sometimes be reduced by an epidural anaesthetic, which allows a more normal muscular pattern to take over. If it persists, inco-ordinate inertia will produce a hypoxia similar to that caused by hypertonic uterine contractions, and a caesarian section should be performed.

DISPROPORTION

Disproportion may occur if the head is too big or the pelvis is too small (Fig.9.22). The former may be the result of an abnormality such as hydrocephalus. A very large baby will, of course, have a large head, but perhaps the most common fetal cause of disproportion is deflexion (Fig.9.23), as in the occipitoposterior and brow presentations.

In the occipitoposterior position, the deflexion will result in the occipitofrontal diameter (11cm) being presented to the pelvic brim, and as a result, the head will not enter the brim easily. In a brow presentation, the presenting diameter is the mentovertical (13.5cm), which is much too large to enter the normal pelvis in normal circumstances.

The pelvis may be too small in various circumstances (Fig.9.24):
- The shape may be normally gynaecoid but small in size.
- It may be android, with a heart-shaped brim, prominent ischial spines and a narrow pubic arch.

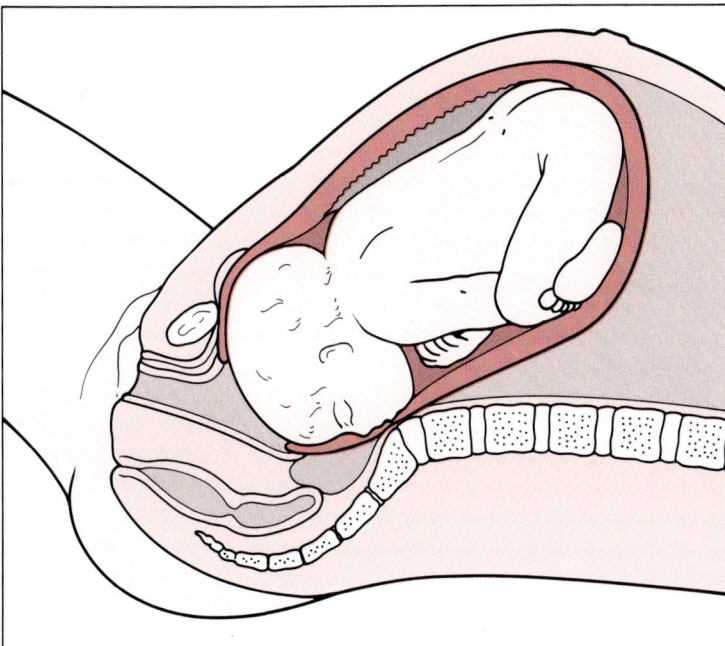

Fig.9.23 A deflexed head. With continued uterine contractions, the head is driven down against the pubis and deflexes further. This may approach a brow presentation.

157

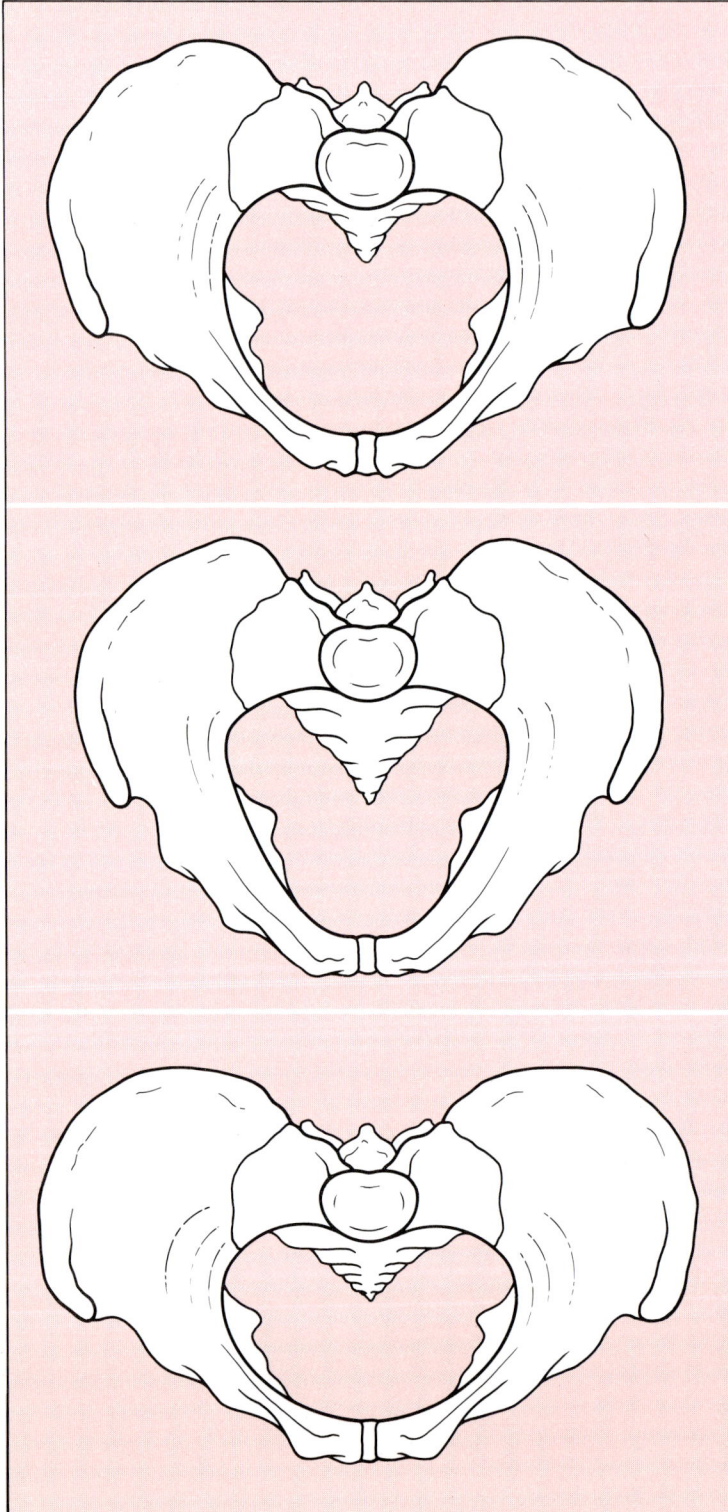

Fig.9.24 Upper: gynaecoid pelvis of normal shape but reduced diameters. The inlet is shaped like a section of a plump apple. Middle: android pelvis. The anteroposterior diameter is long but the front of the pelvis is narrower, allowing less effective room. The sacrum is also rather straight; the inlet is shaped like a plump pear. Lower: platypelloid pelvis. The anteroposterior diameter is reduced but the transverse diameter is increased. The inlet is shaped like a squashed tomato.

It may be platypelloid, being flat with a wide transverse diameter and a narrow anteroposterior diameter.

The pelvis may also be contracted as a result of chronic disease earlier in life, often in childhood. Such conditions include kyphoscoliosis and shortening of the leg (which may follow poliomyelitis or hip disease) or, more rarely, rickets or road traffic accidents.

It must be emphasized that pelvic contraction *per se* is not important, but rather the size and shape of the pelvis in relation to the size and position of the fetus. A mildly contracted pelvis may prevent the passage of a normal sized fetus, but may allow the passage of a much smaller one.

Disproportion may be suspected if a high head is found in the last weeks of pregnancy in a primigravid patient (Fig.9.25). The finding of overlap, when it is possible to palpate the head anterior to the symphysis pubis, should also raise a suspicion of disproportion. If the patient is of short stature or has had one of the previously mentioned disorders, disproportion is again a possibility.

On vaginal examination, disproportion may be suspected if the head remains high despite good contractions. In a normal labour, the fetal head descends and the skull bones overlap to allow moulding (Fig.9.26). If there is a gross degree of disproportion, such moulding may be exaggerated and a large pad of oedema (the caput) is formed over the presenting part. It may deceive the unwary into thinking that labour is progressing because the caput bulges down through the cervix and into the vagina. There is, in fact, no progress, merely more oedema of the fetal head, the bones of which are gripped by the bones of the mother's pelvis.

The management of disproportion may be summarized as follows:
- If the degree of disproportion suspected is minor, a trial of labour may be employed provided there are no unfavourable signs.
- If it is likely that there is major disproportion, a caesarean section should be performed.

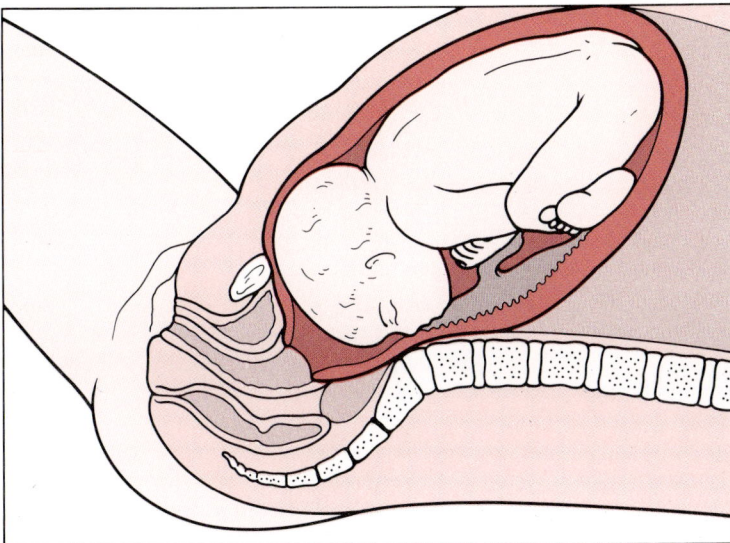

Fig.9.25 Disproportion. The head is too high above the brim and will not engage. The overlap in this case is slightly exaggerated to give the impression of what can be felt on examination.

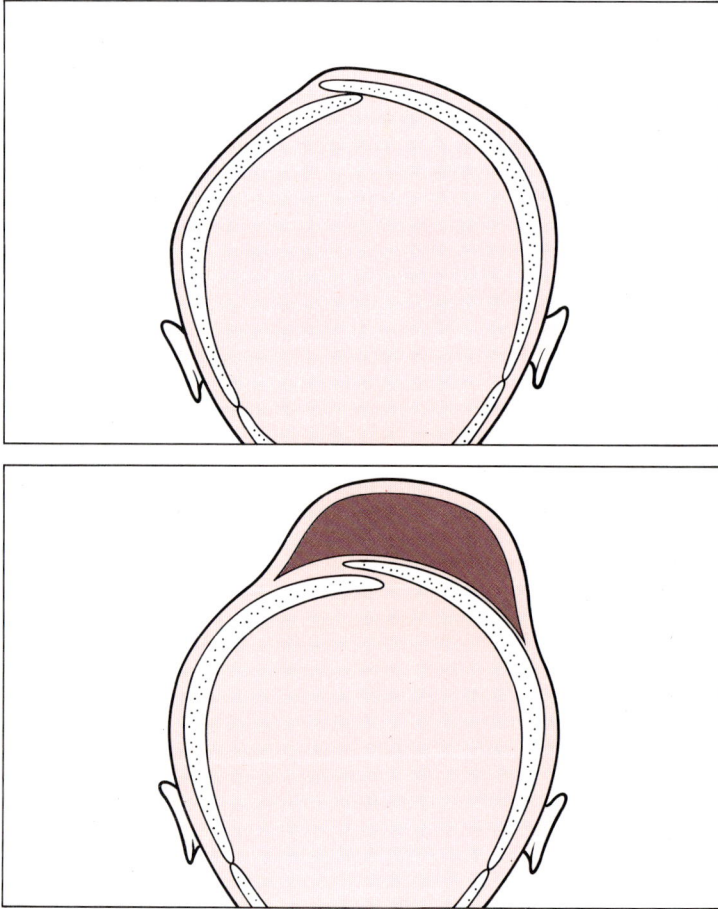

Fig.9.26 Upper: moulding of the fetal head in normal labour.
Lower: exaggerated moulding and a large pad of oedema (the
the presenting part occurs with gross cephalopelvic disproportion.

RUPTURE OF THE UTERUS

Rupture of the uterus is a very serious complication of labour, but rarely occurs nowadays. It is most commonly seen in a patient who has previously had a caesarean section (especially of the classical variety) but may also be seen in patients in whom previous curettage has resulted in perforation of the uterine fundus. Spontaneous uterine rupture may follow an obstructed labour from whatever cause.

Uterine rupture must be suspected if shock becomes evident at any time during labour or if there is sudden loss of the fetal heart. The fetus is commonly expelled through the tear into the abdomen (Fig.9.27) and uterine contractions cease. If the bladder has been involved haematuria may also be present. It may be unusually easy to feel the fetus beneath the abdominal wall after its expulsion from the uterus. Bleeding from the vagina may not be marked, depending upon the extent of internal bleeding.

The first step in treatment is immediate resuscitation by infusion of a plasma expander followed by blood transfusion as soon as this blood is cross-matched. The woman must be given a general anaesthetic and the abdomen opened. Management will depend upon the extent of the tear and upon the patient's previous obstetric history. If the tear is extensive and the patient is multiparous, hysterectomy may be the wisest form of management. It is sometimes possible to repair the tear, however, and the patient may safely carry a later pregnancy but delivery will probably be by elective caesarian section.

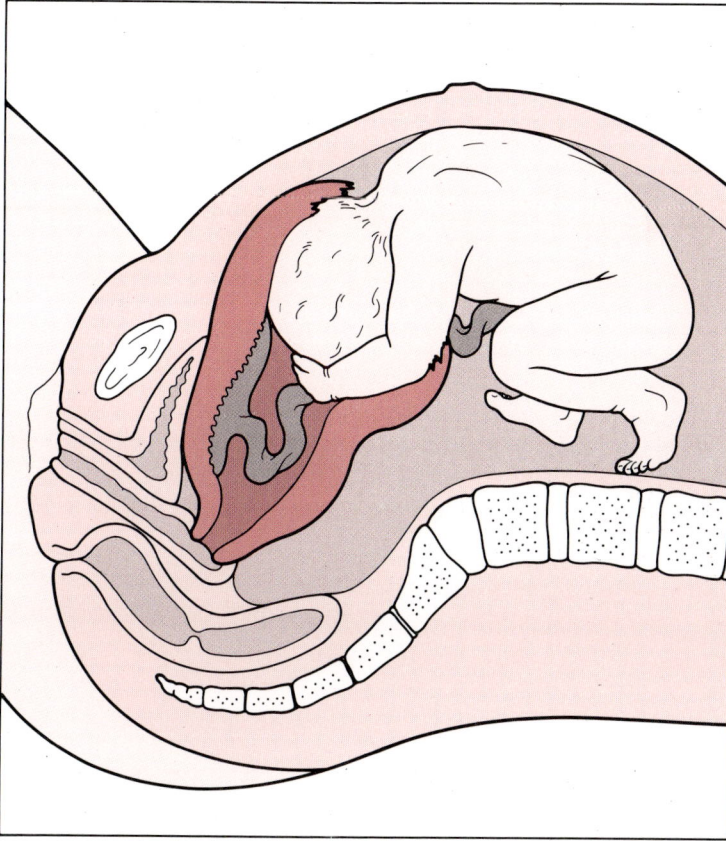

Fig.9.27 Uterine rupture. The uterus has ruptured at the fundus and allowed the fetus to escape into the peritoneal cavity. The fetus will probably be dead and the mother very shocked.

10. Operative Delivery

FORCEPS DELIVERY

A forceps delivery may be indicated if there is fetal distress, delay in the second stage of labour or maternal distress. Certain criteria must exist (Fig. 10.1) before a forceps delivery can be undertaken. The cervix must be fully dilated and the fetal head engaged in the pelvis, there should be no obstruction beneath the head, the bladder should be empty and the membranes ruptured. The presentation should be by the vertex or the face in a suitable occipitoanterior position.

When forceps delivery is undertaken with the largest diameter of the head below the ischial spines, it is a low forceps extraction (Fig.10.2). A mid-forceps extraction (Fig.10.3) occurs when the largest diameter of the head is above the spines, but below the pelvic brim. This can be more difficult than a low forceps

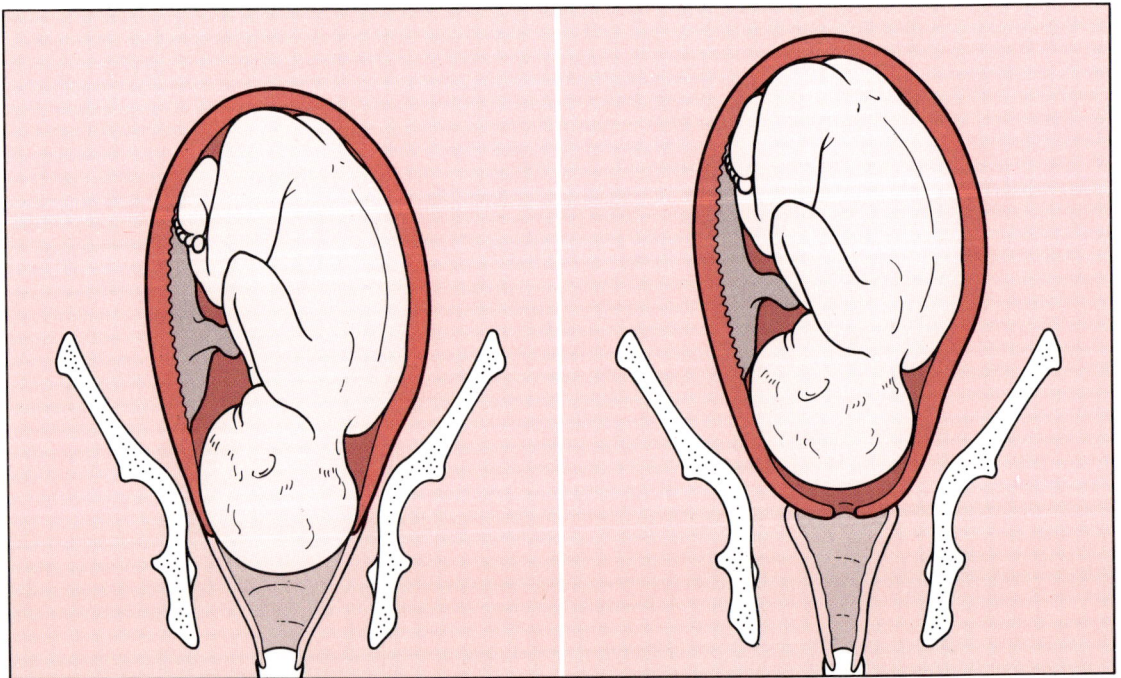

Fig.10.1 Indications for forceps delivery. Left: the cervix is dilated and the head is in the pelvis. Forceps delivery is possible. Right: the cervix is undilated and the head is high. Forceps delivery should not be atttempted.

delivery and requires more skill. If the head is at a higher level than this (Fig.10.4), forceps should not be employed.

Some obstetricians used to use forceps if the second stage of labour continued beyond two hours in a nulliparous woman or one hour in a multipara, but this has changed with the wider use of epidural anaesthesia. If a woman is not pushing actively, the second stage may be allowed to continue for longer, provided any detrimental effects on the fetus are excluded once maternal pushing has started, since this affects oxygen transfer across the placenta. Hence

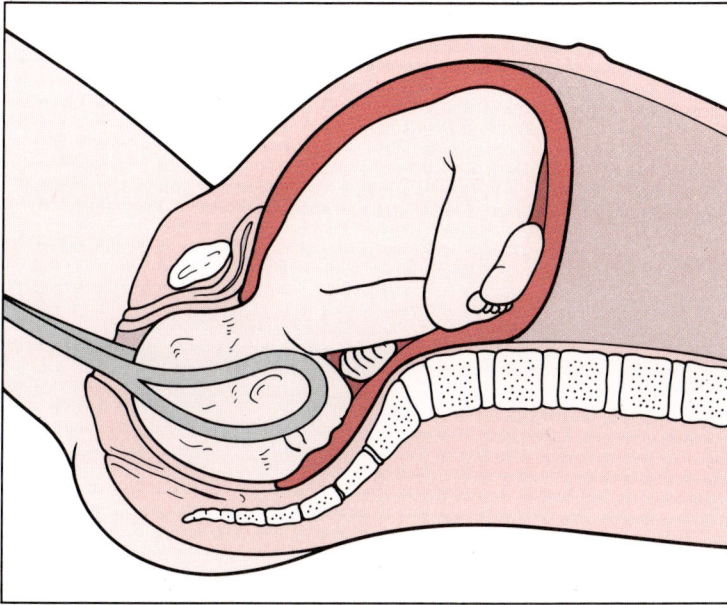

Fig.10.2 The head is in the midcavity and is easily accessible to the operator. A low forceps delivery, a relatively easy procedure, is about to take place.

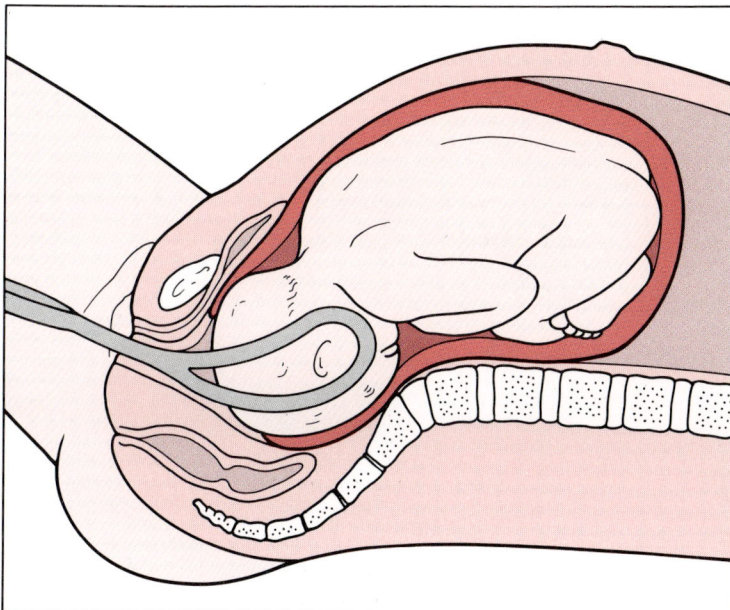

Fig.10.3 The head is rather high in the upper midcavity, although it is engaged. A midcavity forceps delivery is about to be performed. In this illustration the long axis of the fetal head is not quite in the anteroposterior diameter of the mother's pelvis, and a little rotation may be necessary.

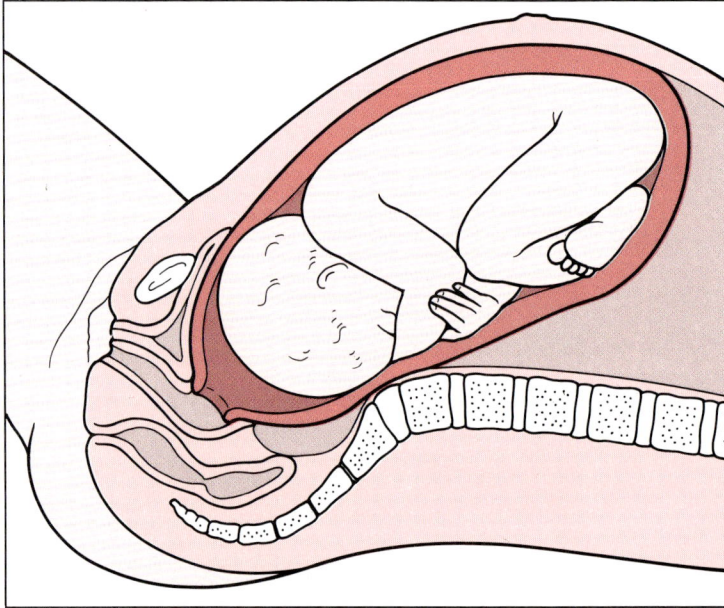

Fig.10.4 The head is not engaged and should not be delivered by forceps. This would involve a high forceps delivery, which is now very rarely performed. Vacuum extraction or, more probably, caesarean section is preferable.

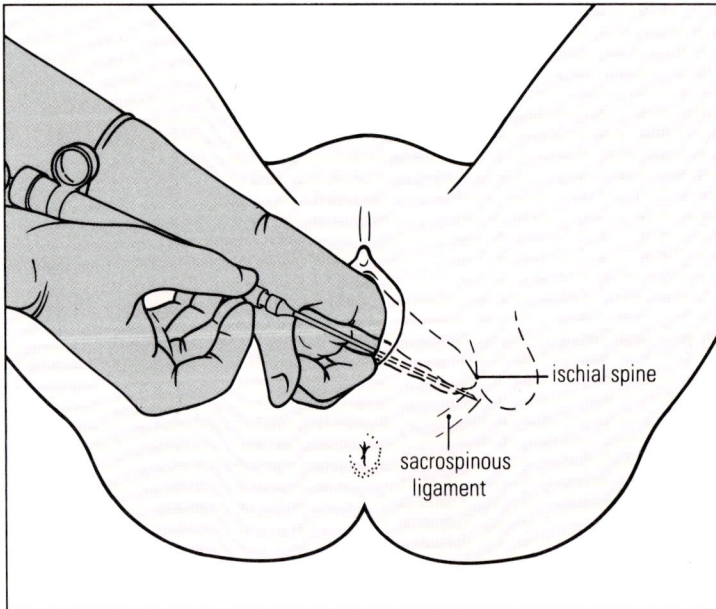

Fig.10.5 Pudendal block. A gloved finger is introduced into the vagina and the ischial spine is palpated. A long needle is then run to this area and 10ml of 1% lignocaine injected around the spine.

continuous cardiotocography, with a good trace of the fetal heart and uterine contractions, should always be employed. Should there be no progress with active pushing, forceps may be needed. It must be emphasized that the delivery of a live, healthy fetus may be incompatible with an undue degree of force during the process of forceps extraction. The obstetrician should ensure that attempted forceps delivery is halted before this stage is reached and a caesarean section performed, even if labour has reached the second stage.

Anaesthesia for forceps delivery may be general

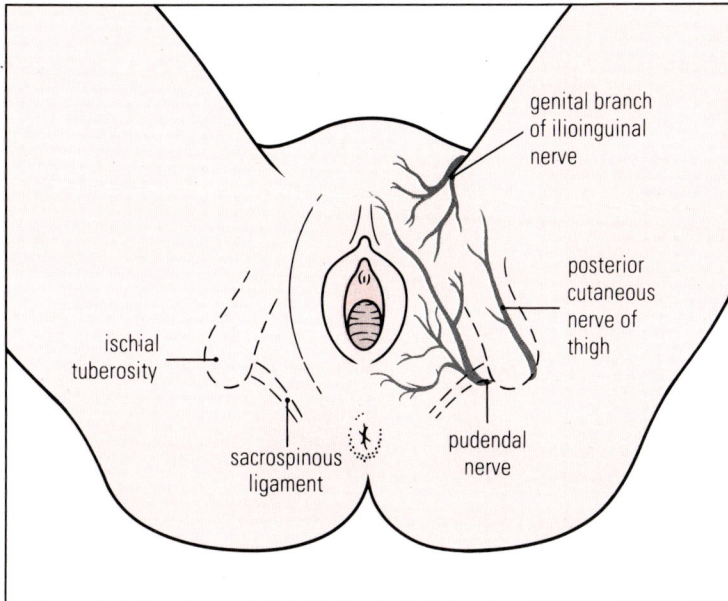

Fig.10.6 Additional nerve supply to the perineum. The areas supplied by these nerves must all be infiltrated to achieve successful anaesthesia.

(which is now usually unnecessary), by epidural or by caudal block if facilities are available. The most commonly employed method is a pudendal block. The first stage is infiltration at the point of the ischial spines where the pudendal nerve passes briefly out of the pelvis (Fig.10.5). In most cases, the pudendal nerve runs around the outside of the ischial spine; in a few, some part of it travels inside. Hence, the wary operator will inject local anaesthetic solution all round the spine. This must be followed by local perineal infiltration to ensure that all the additional nerve supply to the perineum (Fig.10.6) is blocked. This consists of a branch of the ilioinguinal nerve anteriorly, the posterior cutaneous nerve of the thigh posteriorly, and a branch which comes directly from the sacral plexus. If the woman receives only a pudendal block and these other nerves are ignored, the anaesthesia obtained will be imperfect.

Once the perineum has been anaesthetized, the forceps are applied. The left-hand blade is held almost vertically and run along the palm and surface of the operator's fingers, which should cup the fetal parietal eminence . The blade follows the natural curve of the parietal eminence and the vaginal wall is protected by the operator's fingers (Fig.10.7 upper left). It slides easily into position so that the spoon of the blade cups the side of the fetal head. The second blade is introduced (Fig.10.7 middle left) in a similar way, with the operator's fingers guarding the vaginal wall and guiding the blade around the fetal head. If the blades are properly applied, they will meet easily and lock at the same level in the midline (Fig.10.7 middle right). The fetal head is now protected between the blades of the forceps. An episiotomy is then performed and gentle traction exerted in a downwards direction (Fig.10.7 lower left) to achieve delivery of the fetal head.

165

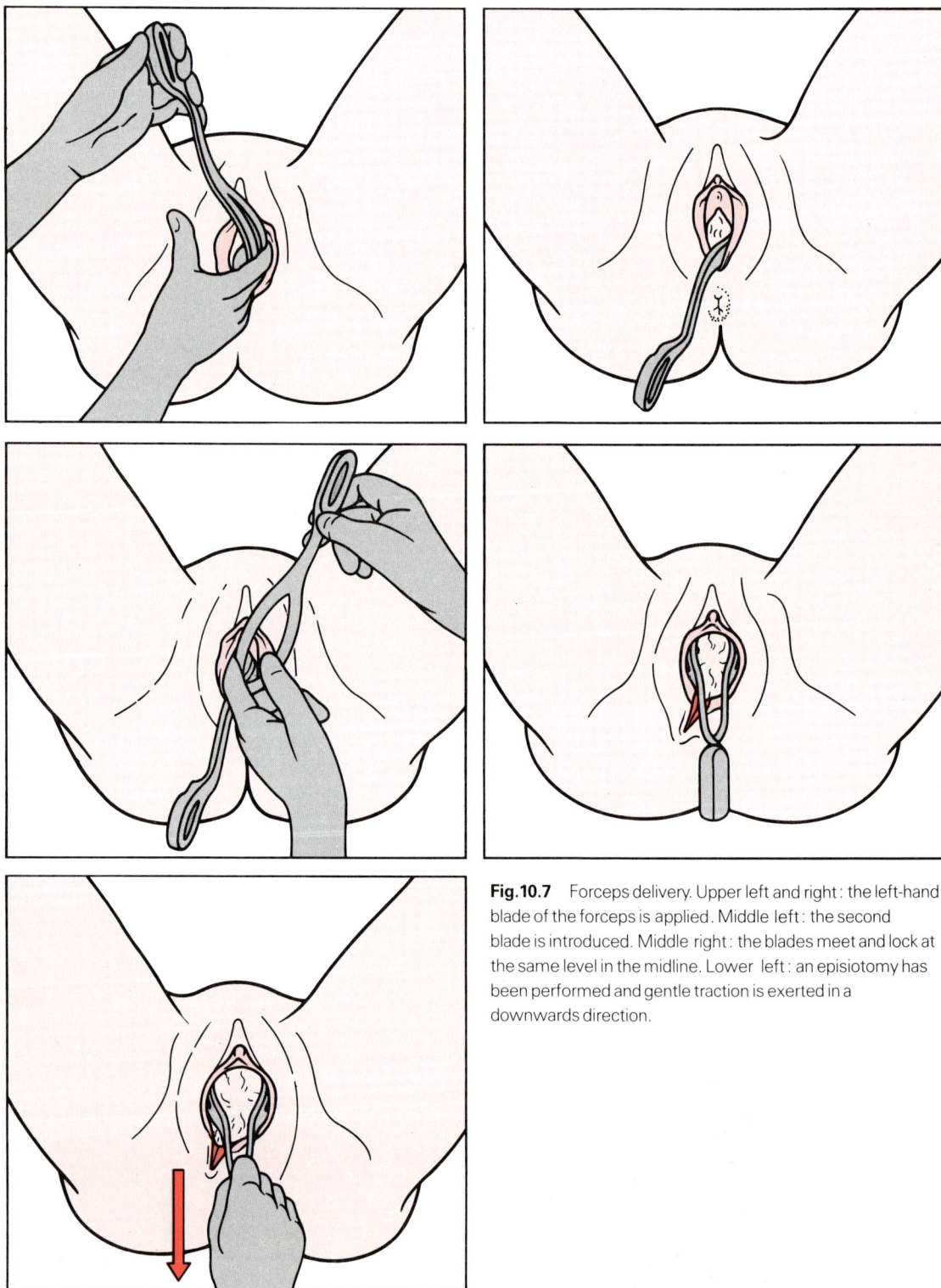

Fig.10.7 Forceps delivery. Upper left and right: the left-hand blade of the forceps is applied. Middle left: the second blade is introduced. Middle right: the blades meet and lock at the same level in the midline. Lower left: an episiotomy has been performed and gentle traction is exerted in a downwards direction.

Rotation to an occipitoanterior position may be required before forceps delivery if the head is in an occipitolateral or occipitoposterior position. This may be accomplished by Kielland's forceps (Fig. 10.8), by the ventouse or, less commonly, by manual rotation.

Various complications may be seen in association with forceps extraction. A perineal tear is likely to occur and therefore an episiotomy is usually performed during the procedure. Vaginal or cervical tears may occasionally be seen, especially if forceps rotation has been used or if the head has been brought down from too high a level in the pelvis. There may be marked haemorrhage from any of these tears and injury to the fetal head. Failed forceps delivery is now a rare event. The most common reasons for failure are use of the forceps before the cervix is fully dilated and failure to recognize that the position is not occipitoanterior. Disproportion is a possible cause of failed forceps, but a rare one.

VACUUM EXTRACTION

The vacuum extractor, or ventouse, (Fig.10.9 left) is now frequently used in Africa and Europe (but not in the United Kingdom and America) as an alternative to low or even mid-forceps extraction. The suction cap of the instrument can be fixed firmly to the scalp of the fetal head (Fig.10.9 right) and the suction employed

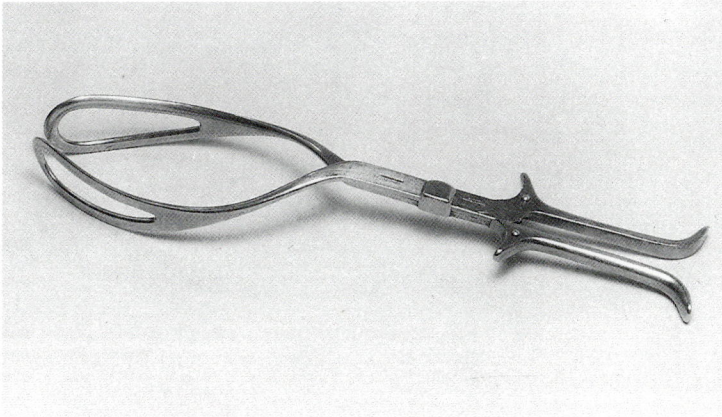

Fig.10.8 Keilland's forceps are straight with no pelvic curve. They allow rotation to occur in the pelvis with less risk of trauma to the soft tissues (such as the bladder base) outside the vagina.

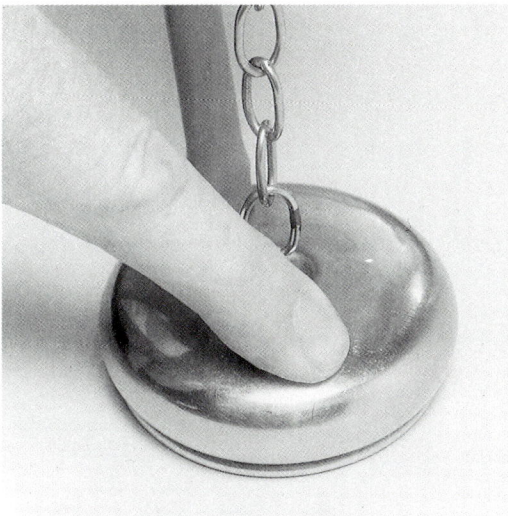

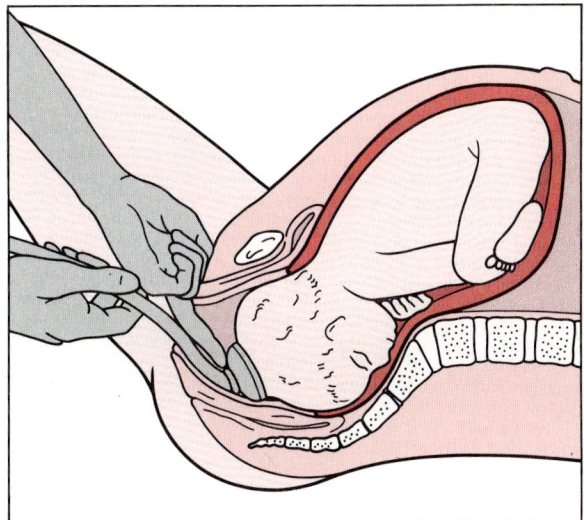

Fig.10.9 Left: vacuum extractor. Right: application of the vacuum extractor.

produces a raised area of chignon within the cap. Extraction of the head (Fig.10.10) may be carried out with little danger of damage to mother or child.

The indications for vacuum extraction are the same as those for forceps delivery and the instrument may be applied when the position is occipitoposterior to effect rotation. In addition, a vacuum extractor cap can be slipped through an incompletely dilated (8–9cm) cervix and used to bring the fetal head down against the cervix with contraction. In this manner, full dilatation can be induced in a few minutes. This is of great use if there is fetal distress at 8cm dilatation in a multiparous woman, since it can be performed much more swiftly than a caesarean section.

BREECH EXTRACTION

This operation is now less frequently performed in the developed world, where it is being replaced by caesarean section. The procedure consists of accelerating the delivery of a breech presentation in the second stage. Indications include:
• Fetal distress
• Maternal distress
• Lack of advance in second stage

These are the same indications as those for forceps delivery in a cephalic presentation, but it must be remembered that with a breech presentation a caesarean section may be preferable in any of the above situations.

Breech extraction can be performed under pudendal block reinforced with intravenous pethidine. However, if time allows, an epidural or caudal anaesthetic is more acceptable to the woman.

At a breech extraction, the operator must provide traction to deliver the baby. The buttocks should be at midcavity or below before the operator hooks a finger into the fold between the thigh and the abdomen of the fetus (Fig.10.11), behind the mother's pubis, and applies traction on his hooked finger. When the breech is low enough he can insert his other index finger into the posterior groin and thereby work on both sides of the fetus.

As the buttocks descend, a generous episiotomy is performed. When both buttocks have been delivered over the perineum, a leg should be brought down, delivery being achieved by flexing the knee laterally (Fig.10.12). Normally, the anterior knee is easier to bring down than the posterior, but in practice, the operator attempts to deliver the leg of the buttock which is lower. After the buttocks have delivered, one

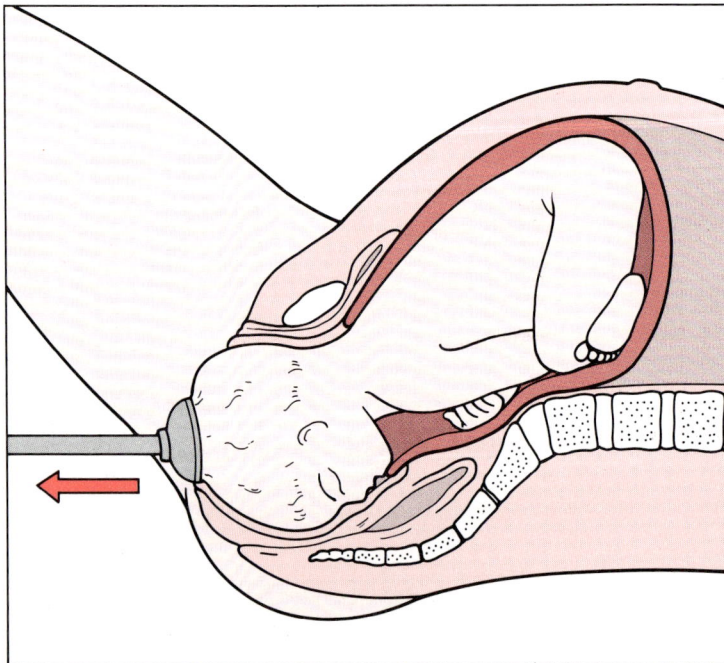

Fig.10.10 The vacuum extractor provides a linear pull only. This must always be in the line of the curve of the pelvis. As the head reaches the outlet, the pull can be elevated so that it is lifting the head over the perineum.

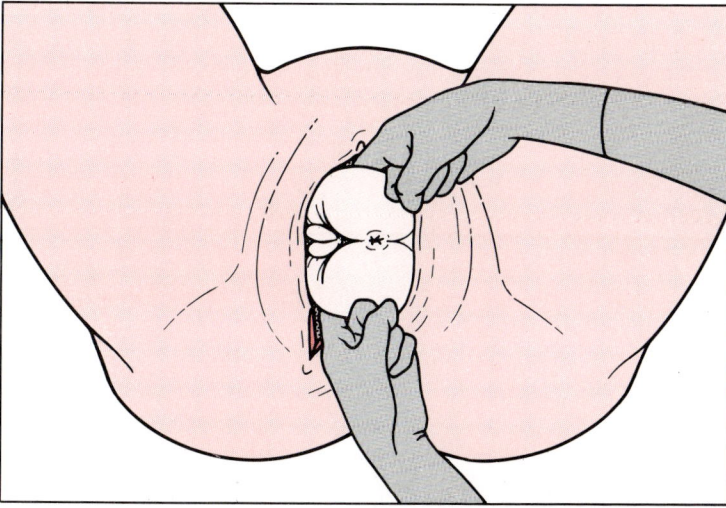

Fig.10.11   Breech extraction. The operator inserts his index fingers into the angle between the fetal thighs and the abdominal wall. A good episiotomy must be made.

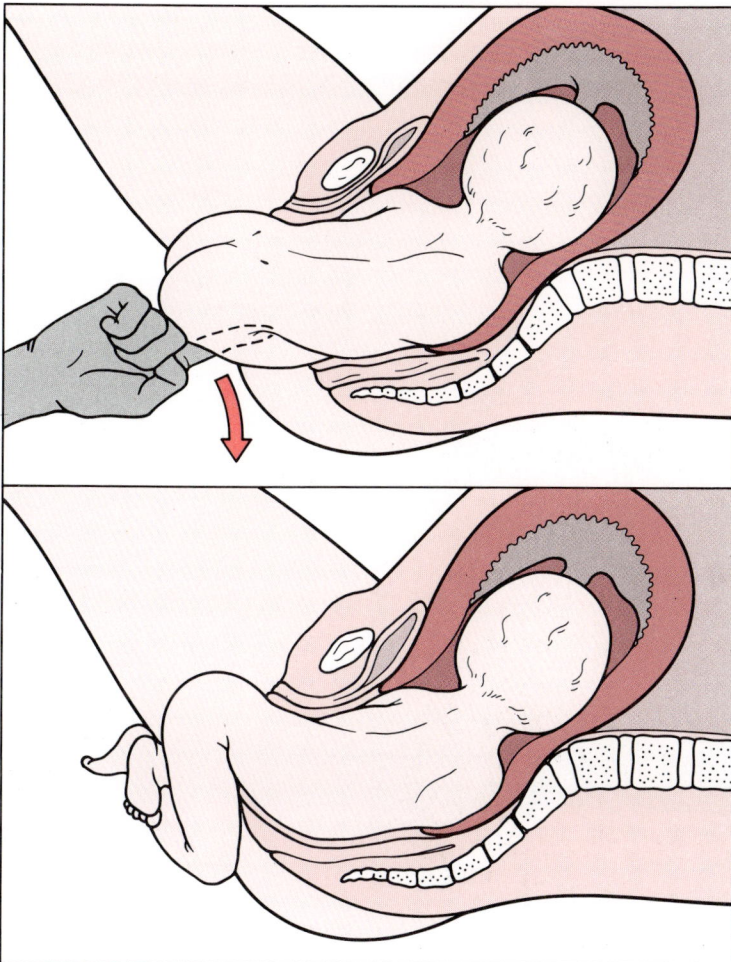

Fig.10.12   Delivery of the legs. Upper: a leg is brought down by passing a finger up to the extended knee and pressing into the popliteal fossa. This allows the knee to flex and usually the operator is then able to bring a leg down. Lower: the buttocks have both delivered and the legs curl up, showing healthy fetal tone.

should ensure that the fetal sacrum rotates anteriorly (Fig.10.13). Extraction is continued by traction on the thighs but not on the fetal abdomen because this could cause damage to the abdominal organs.

The shoulders are delivered by rotation. The fetal posterior shoulder is often lower than the anterior one, but the anterior wall of the maternal pelvis is often shorter than the posterior. Hence, rotation brings the lower shoulder under the shorter wall and the arm is delivered (Fig.10.14). The body is then rotated through 180° in the opposite direction to allow the other shoulder to pass under the symphysis pubis and the second arm is delivered.

Forceps are applied to the aftercoming head (see Fig.9.8) to ease the delivery of the nose and mouth over the perineum. These are used not to speed delivery, but rather to slow the process down and give the operator full control. Once the nose and mouth are outside, the air passages are aspirated and delivery of the head takes place slowly. Once the nose is in the open air it does not matter where the top of the head is.

The perinatal mortality rate with breech extraction is many times higher than with cephalic or breech delivery. This is due to intracranial damage caused by subdural or intracranial haemorrhage or to hypoxia during delivery. Trauma may also affect the femora, intra-abdominal organs (liver, spleen or adrenals), the trunk, or the arms and the brachial plexus at the time of delivery. Maternal morbidity is higher with breech extraction because of the extensive operative procedure involving much manoeuvring of the pelvis.

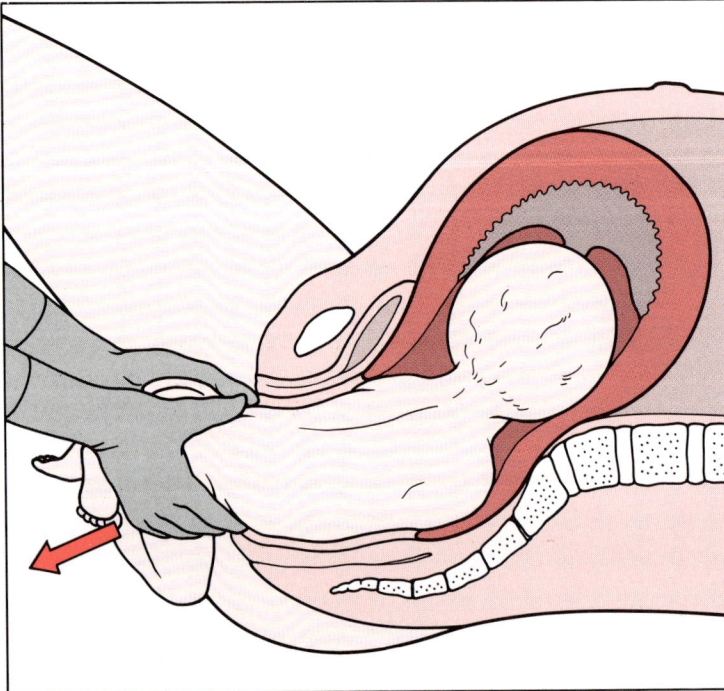

Fig.10.13 The operator grasps the upper thighs in his hands, putting his thumbs over the buttocks, thereby rotating the sacrum anteriorly. Traction is applied and the body usually delivers fairly readily.

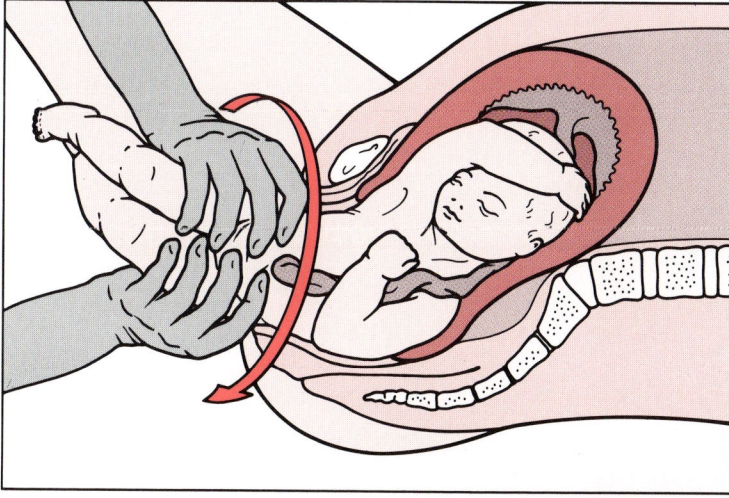

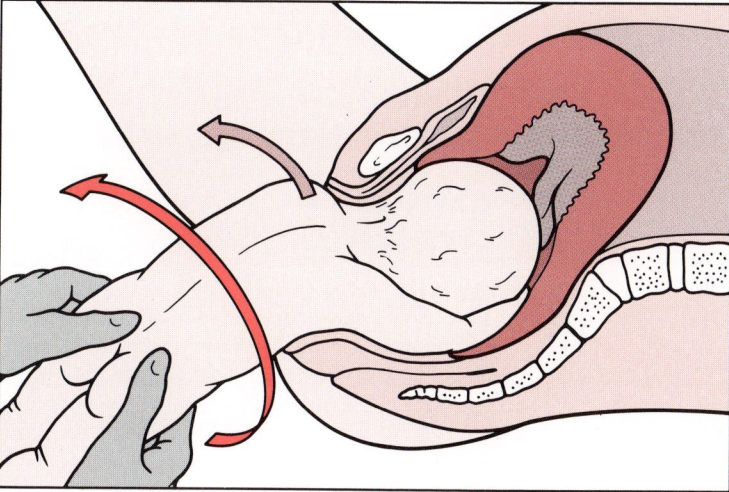

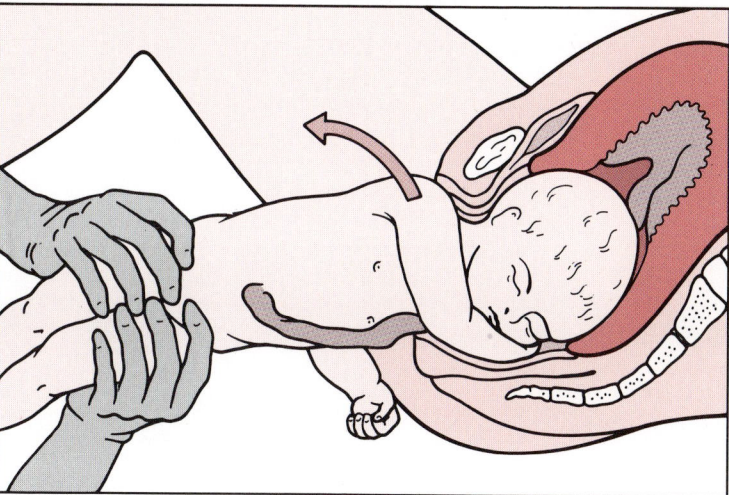

Fig. 10.14 Delivery of the shoulders. Upper: the fetus is rotated through 180° to bring the posterior shoulder under the symphysis pubis. Middle: the first shoulder is delivered. Rotation through 180° in the other direction brings the second shoulder into the anterior position. Lower: the anterior shoulder can now be delivered.

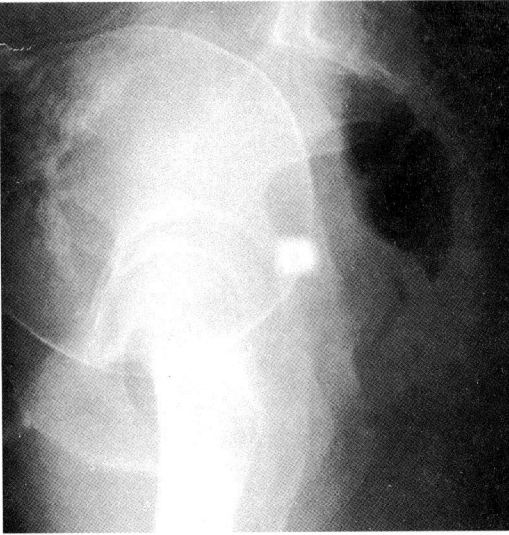

Fig.10.15 Standing lateral X-ray of the pelvis. The fetal head is not engaged for the maximum diameter has not yet entered the pelvic inlet (A–B). There is no sign of disproportion in this case, and the head will progress to the curve (B–D), finally delivering through the outlet (C–D).

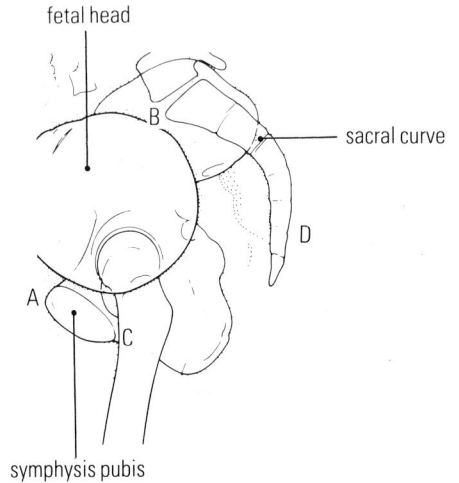

If the obstetrician thinks a vaginal delivery will be hazardous with a breech, a caesarean section should be performed. Indications for this might be:
- Mild pelvic contraction. All women with a breech presentation considered for a vaginal delivery should undergo X-ray pelvimetry. This need not be done if the woman has previously had a large baby (>3.5kg) delivered vaginally. Standing lateral X-ray pelvimetry should ideally show (Fig.10.15):
  - (a) an adequate inlet (anteroposterior diameter >11.5cm);
  - (b) a good curve to the sacrum to allow rotation;
  - (c) an adequate outlet (anteroposterior diameter >12.5cm).
- Large fetus (>3.5kg) with a large biparietal diameter (>10cm).
- Unfavourable fetal position, e.g. extension of the head.
- Accompanying complications, e.g. pre-eclampsia or diabetes.
- Immature fetus.

It is wise to deliver a fetus in a breech presentation between twenty-six and thirty-four weeks by caesarean section. At this stage, about a quarter of all presentations are by the breech. A lower segment operation can be very difficult and sometimes a low classical operation or a transverse incision in the lower part of the upper segment must be performed, placing the woman's future obstetrical career at risk. This should be considered very carefully before embarking on the procedure.

There is no place for trial of labour in breech presentation. Occasionally, however, if the pelvis is adequate, labour may be allowed to start in a breech presentation even when there are minimal doubts about the woman's power to deliver the baby vaginally. Unless the buttocks descend well early in the first stage of labour, the operator should not proceed into the later first stage of labour, but should perform a caesarean section. If breech delivery inadvertently proceeds in a case where there is cephalopelvic disproportion, the body will deliver but the head will not. One is left with the choice of perforating the aftercoming head to remove cerebrospinal fluid and thus decompress the head, or performing a caesarean section, for which the body of the baby must be passed back up through the birth canal. The first procedure is always fatal and the second usually so. The moral is to ensure in the antenatal period that cephalopelvic disproportion does not exist.

CAESAREAN SECTION

Caesarean section may be of the classical variety

172

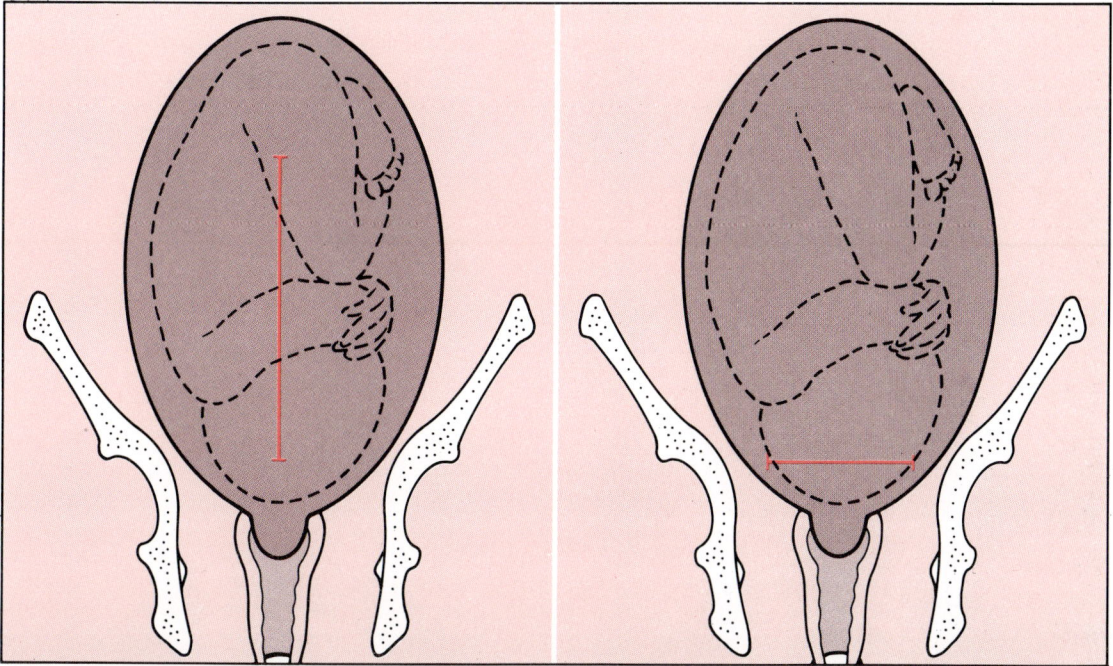

Fig.10.16 Incisions for caesarean section. Left: in the classical variety, the incision is longitudinal in the thicker muscle of the upper segment. This heals badly. Right: in the lower segment variety, a curved incision is made in thinner tissue; this heals better after delivery since it is parallel with the fibres of the myometrium.

(Fig.10.16 left), in which the incision is made in the uterine body, or of the lower segment variety (Fig.10.16 right), in which the thin lower segment of the uterus is incised, usually transversely. Classical caesarean section is rarely employed now, the risk of scar rupture being greater than with the lower segment procedure.

Common indications for caesarean section include placenta praevia, disproportion, obstructed labour from other causes, prolapse of the cord, fetal distress and maternal distress. It is more frequently employed in preterm labour and in breech presentation.

A number of complications may be encountered during or after the procedure of caesarean section. There may be haemorrhage (if the placenta is situated in front of the fetal head), infection, or injury to nearby organs such as the bladder. There are also several possible complications related to the use of anaesthesia, such as inhalation of vomit if a general anaesthetic is employed, or hypotension or a spinal tap if an epidural is employed.

The technique of lower segment caesarean section is briefly illustrated in Fig.10.17. A transverse lower abdominal incision is usually employed, the parietal peritoneum opened, and the loose visceral peritoneum over the lower uterine segment incised. This allows the bladder to be displaced downwards and a retractor to be inserted. A transverse incision in the thin lower uterine segment can then be employed and the head extracted, usually without difficulty. Occasionally, a longitudinal incision is made through the lower segment, but this will often extend upwards into the thicker upper segment and is not favoured by most obstetricians.

Indications for classical caesarean section include fibroids in and adhesions obscuring the lower uterine segment. A transverse lie is difficult to deliver though a lower segment approach to the uterus. After opening the abdomen, the operator should try to convert the fetal lie to longitudinal directly through the intact uterine wall. If this succeeds, a lower segment incision allows delivery of the baby by breech or head first. If, however, he cannot convert the lie, a vertical classical incision is safer.

If the woman has died and the child is still alive, or if there is a desperate emergency threatening the child's life, the quickest caesarian section possible should be performed, which for most obstetricians these days will be through the lower segment.

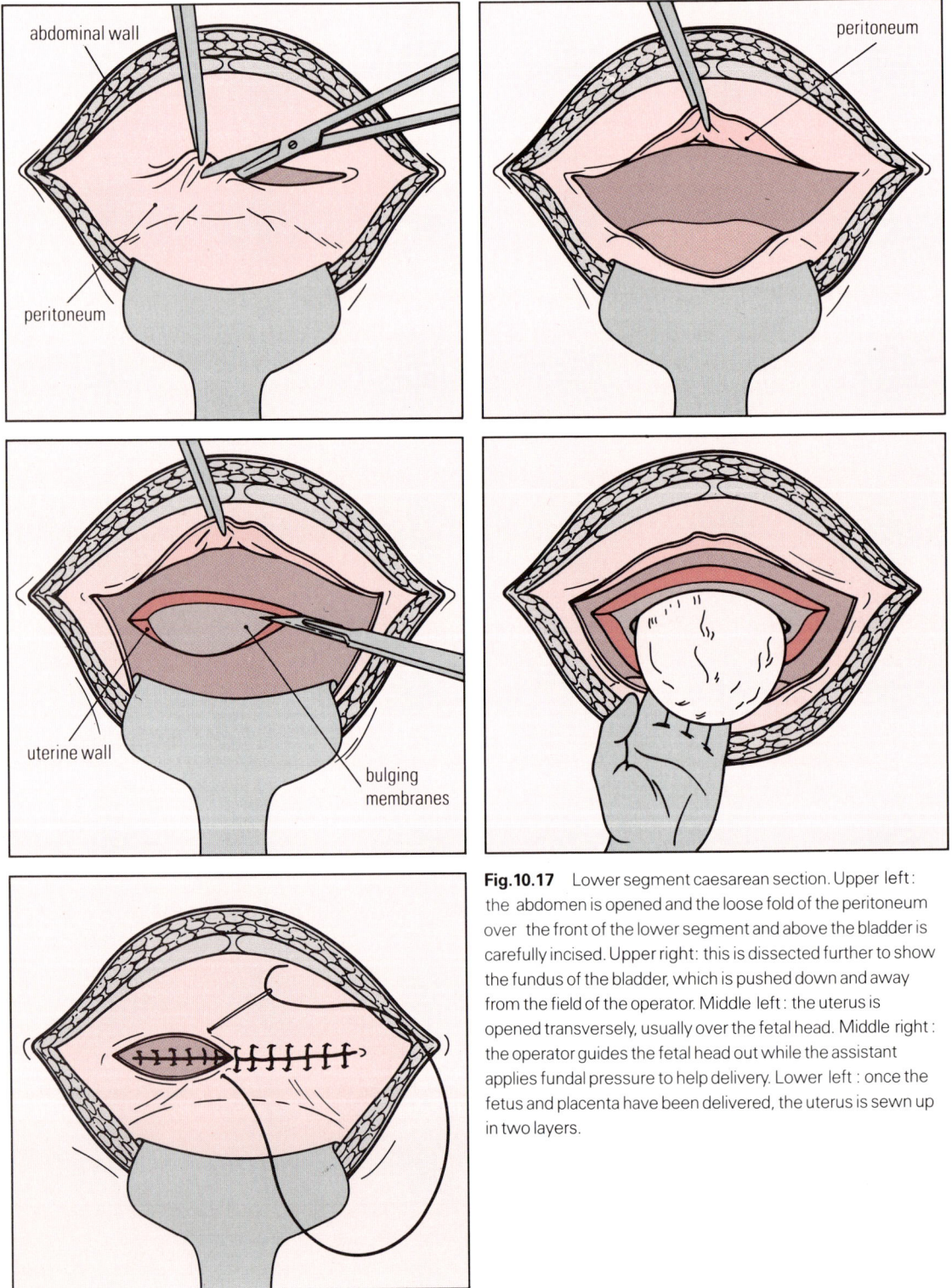

Fig.10.17 Lower segment caesarean section. Upper left: the abdomen is opened and the loose fold of the peritoneum over the front of the lower segment and above the bladder is carefully incised. Upper right: this is dissected further to show the fundus of the bladder, which is pushed down and away from the field of the operator. Middle left: the uterus is opened transversely, usually over the fetal head. Middle right: the operator guides the fetal head out while the assistant applies fundal pressure to help delivery. Lower left: once the fetus and placenta have been delivered, the uterus is sewn up in two layers.

11. Multiple Pregnancy and Delivery

PREGNANCY

A twin pregnancy is seen in the United Kingdom about once in every one hundred deliveries, but in some other countries it is much more frequent, for example occurring once in every thirty deliveries in Nigeria.

Twins may be uniovular or binovular (Fig.11.1). In the former instance, a single oocyte is fertilized in the usual way but, at about the time of implantation, the embryonic cells separate and develop independently as separate fetuses. In binovular twins, two oocytes are fertilized separately by two separate sperms; they develop independently, sharing the same uterus. Uniovular twins have an identical genetic structure, whilst binovular twins are genetically different.

Triplet and quadruplet pregnancies also occur spontaneously but are very infrequent. If ovulation is induced, particularly by gonadotrophins, multiple oocytes are more likely to be produced and triplets, quadruplets or even larger numbers of fetuses may result.

A twin pregnancy usually puts the mother under an increased strain and all the problems of pregnancy are exaggerated. A number of complications are more likely to arise:

- Anaemia. This is principally an iron deficiency anaemia due to the larger drain than usual on the mother's iron reserves. It is also probable that folic acid deficiency will develop because of the increased demand produced by more than one fetus. The fetuses take as much as they require of nutrients such as folate, and since most women do not have much folate in their diet, maternal anaemia is much more likely to develop in a twin than in a singleton pregnancy unless the dietary intake is increased.

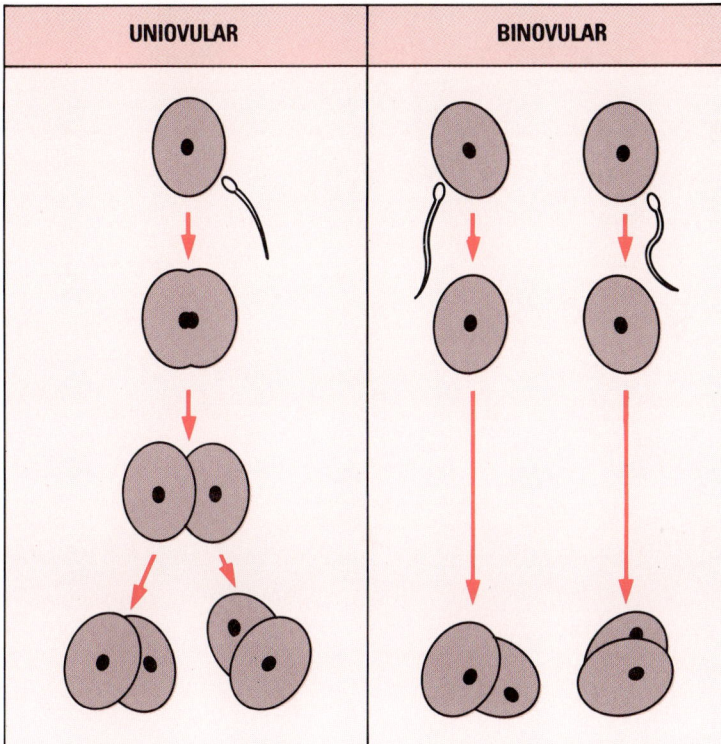

Fig.11.1 Fertilization and early development of twins. Left: in uniovular twins, one sperm fertilizes one oocyte; the zygote separates around the time of implantation to produce genetically identical twins. Right: in binovular twins, two oocytes are fertilized separately by two different sperms to produce genetically different twins.

175

- Pre-eclamptic toxaemia. This is a more common complication of twin pregnancy, occurring in up to one third of cases. The obstetrician should watch carefully for signs of this condition (raised blood pressure and proteinuria) in the antenatal period.
- Polyhydramnios. One or both of the fetal sacs may be complicated by excess amniotic fluid (Fig.11.2).

Both pre-eclampsia and polyhydramnios are important causes of preterm labour, which is itself probably the most important reason for fetal loss in twin pregnancy.

In addition to these complications, the discomforts of pregnancy are aggravated by twins or triplets. Women complain of abdominal discomfort, dyspnoea, swelling of the feet and increasing tiredness in carrying around the large mass of the pregnant uterus. Sleep is more difficult at night and complications such as heartburn may be troublesome.

DIAGNOSIS

In the United Kingdom, the diagnosis of twins is now frequently made by ultrasound (Fig.11.3), with which two fetal sacs can be detected from as early as seven weeks gestation. It is commonplace for patients to have an ultrasound scan to identify a pregnancy in its early stages, and a twin pregnancy may be diagnosed before it could possibly be recognized clinically. Occasionally, when two fetal sacs have been seen on a very early scan, one may diminish and then disappear at a later stage, probably because one embryo has died. Such resorption of a twin may be somewhat more common than was previously supposed, occurring in up to twenty-five percent of cases.

The clinical diagnosis of twins is first made at about twenty-six to thirty weeks by recognizing a uterus

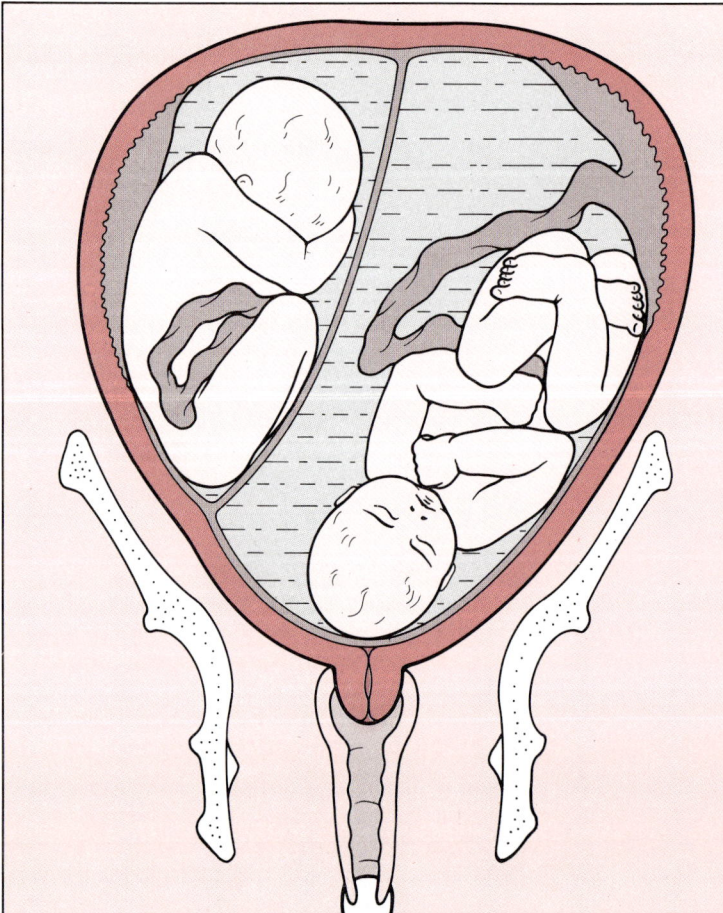

Fig.11.2 Polyhydramnios. This condition is common in twins, occurring in one or both sacs.

larger than would be expected for the period of amenorrhoea. Alternatively, at about thirty to thirty-two weeks, one may find that too many fetal parts can be identified. There are, however, several other causes for a uterus which is larger than expected:

- Wrong dates.
- Polyhydramnios.
- A uterus containing fibroids or the presence of an ovarian cyst in the abdomen (Fig.11.4).
- In later pregnancy, a very large baby.

Abdominal palpation is more difficult in twin pregnancy, but it is usually possible to identify two heads and perhaps a third pole, which will strengthen the clinical diagnosis of the condition. Hearing two fetal heart sounds is a less convincing sign and would only suggest twins if the two rates were significantly different: a single fetal heart may be clearly heard in two different parts of the abdomen. If diagnosed clinically, multiple pregnancy should always be confirmed by ultrasound or an X-ray. Only then can the actual number of fetuses be determined.

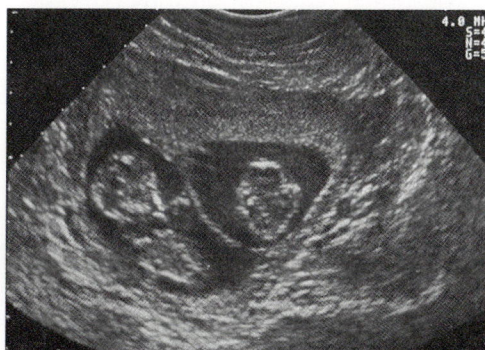

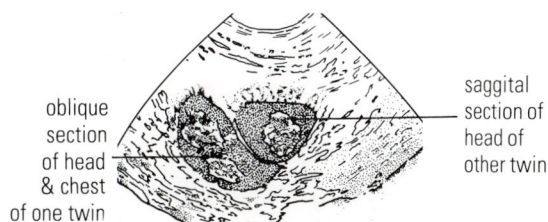

oblique section of head & chest of one twin

saggital section of head of other twin

Fig.11.3 An ultrasound scan taken at twelve weeks gestation showing two sacs with embryonic tissue in each. Courtesy of Dr. R. Patel.

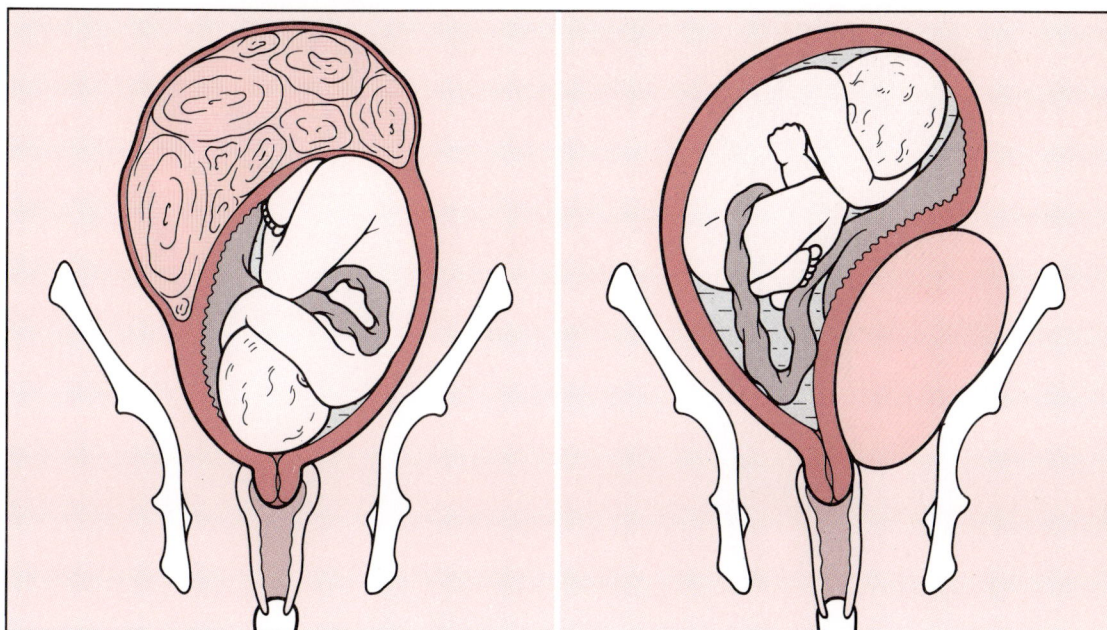

Fig.11.4 Misdiagnosis of twins can be made if a single fetus is accompanied by fibroids (left) or an ovarian cyst (right).

LABOUR

Multiple pregnancy predisposes to many complic-ations of labour. It is often preterm, either spontan-eous, or induced because of pre-eclampsia. Prolapse of the cord is more frequent if the presenting part is not occupying the pelvis when the membranes rupture (Fig.11.5); in these circumstances a loop of cord may easily be washed down. This should be treated as is a prolapsed cord in a singleton pregnancy.

Various presentations may be found in multiple pregnancy (Fig.11.6):
- Both fetuses in a cephalic presentation (40% of cases).
- A cephalic presentation accompanied by a breech (40% of cases).
- Two breeches (15% of cases).
- A longitudinal lie accompanied by a transverse lie (2% of cases). Transverse lie of the first fetus is uncommon, but the second twin is often found in this position after the birth of the first.

- A breech presentation accompanied by a transverse lie (about 2% of cases).
- Both fetuses in transverse lie (about 1% of cases). This is most unusual and is found only in very preterm deliveries.

Labour is generally said to be more prolonged than usual but it is doubtful if this is an important aspect of twin labour.

During the second stage, intervention may be required because of abnormalities of lie and presenta-tion, however, complications of the third stage are more common. In a multiple pregnancy the placental site is large, and the number of sinuses from which bleeding must be controlled is far greater than in a single pregnancy. For this reason alone, postpartum haemorrhage is more likely. Sometimes during twin delivery, one placenta will separate after the first baby is born, putting the mother at risk from bleeding, and representing a serious risk of hypoxia to the second twin if it is this placenta which has separated.

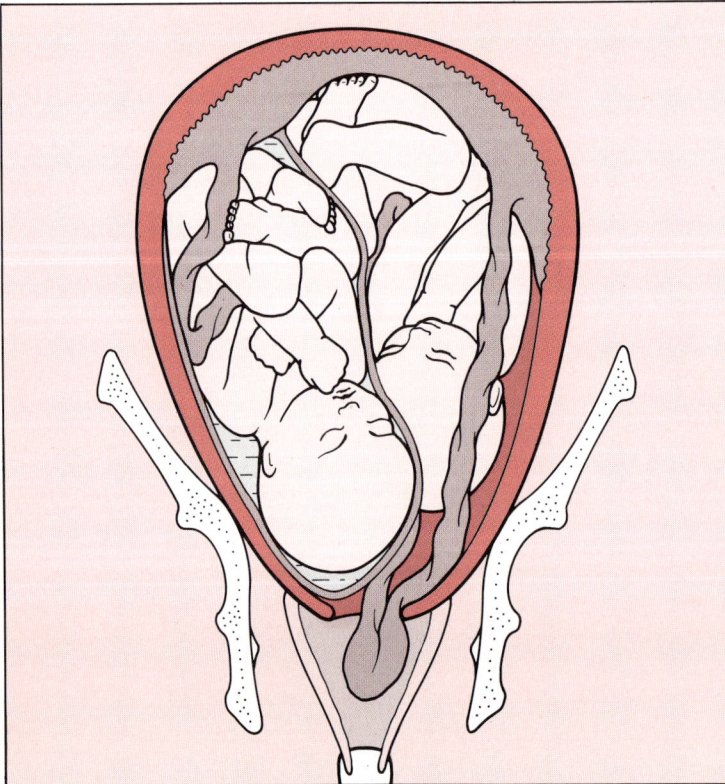

Fig.11.5 Cord prolapse. The membranes of the sac of the second twin have ruptured first and, since the presenting part of that twin is very high, cord prolapse has occurred.

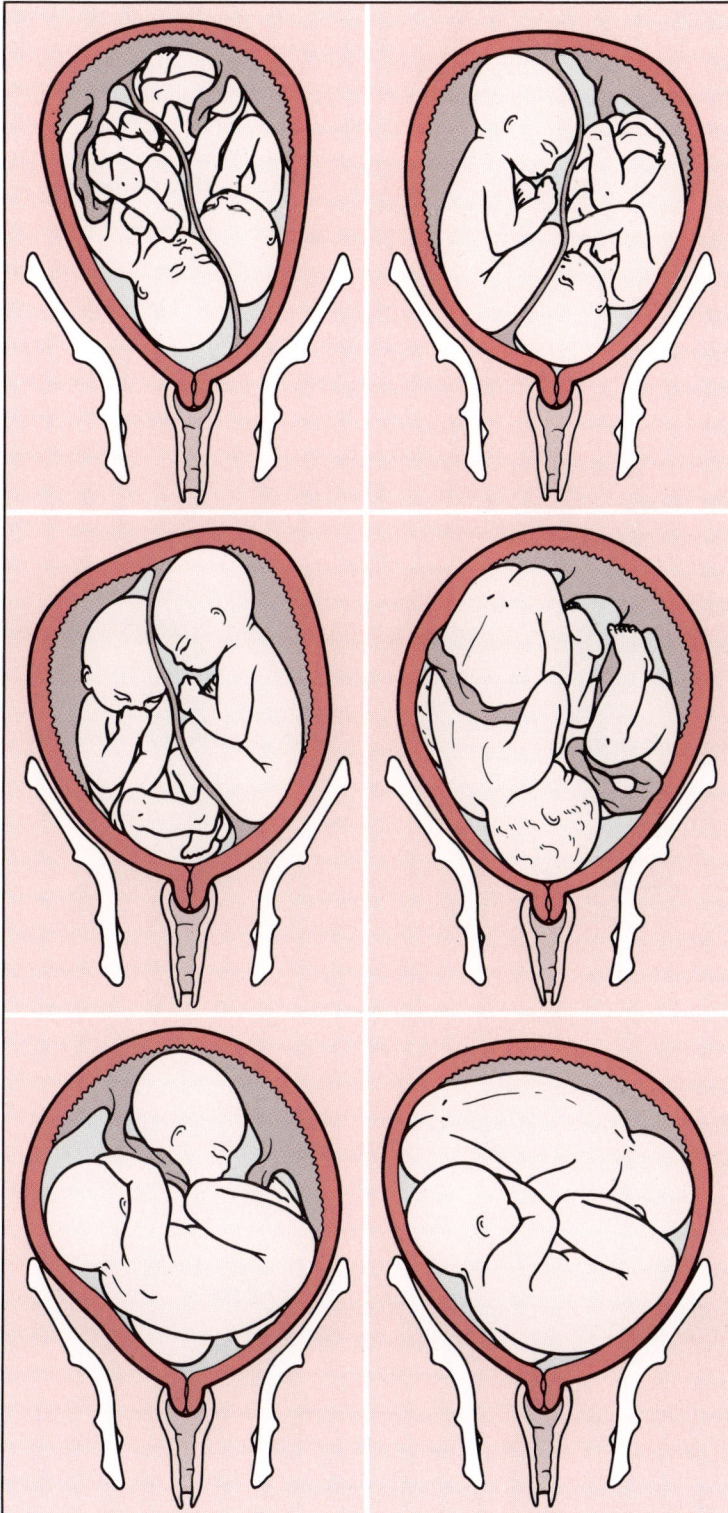

Fig.11.6 Presentation of twins. Upper left: both fetuses in cephalic presentation. Upper right: cephalic presentation accompanied by breech presentation. Middle left: two breeches. Middle right: longitudinal lie (cephalic presentation) accompanied by transverse lie. Lower left: breech presentation accompanied by transverse lie. Lower right: both fetuses in transverse lie.

MANAGEMENT OF LABOUR

Since twin labour often begins early with premature rupture of the membranes, vaginal examination should be made at that point to exclude prolapse of the cord. The management of the first stage is usually along the lines of a singleton labour but it is important to prepare for the second stage. An intravenous line should be set up; epidural analgesia is helpful in case sudden intervention is necessary in the second stage. Two sets of cord clamps will be needed, and forceps and a vacuum extractor should be ready in case they are required. A paediatrician should be present for the delivery, as should an anaesthetist.

Once the first child is born, it is important to clamp the cord in two places and then divide it between the clamps. The abdomen should be palpated immediately to ensure that the second child is lying longitudinally. If this is not the case (Fig.11.7), a prompt external cephalic or internal podalic version should be performed. If this cannot be done, a caesarean section must be carried out immediately. If the second fetus remains in a transverse lie and the membranes rupture, there may be an obstructed labour with the fetus wedged in the pelvis.

If, after the birth of the first twin, the lie of the second is longitudinal, there is little to be gained by waiting. If contractions do not resume after a few minutes, the woman should be given a low dose of oxytocin in the drip. It is best to ensure that the presenting part is in contact with the cervix, after which the membranes may be ruptured and the second twin born. It is most important that great care be taken to prevent postpartum haemorrhage. This may be achieved by administering intravenous Syntometrine with the delivery of the second twin.

Examination of the placenta and membranes after delivery (Fig.11.8) may show whether the twins are uniovular or binovular, although this is not always easy to determine. Even if the placentas were separated originally, they may have become fused into a single mass. One should determine whether, in the septum between the two sacs, there are two amnions and two chorions, which in most cases indicates a binovular pregnancy. This can be tested by stripping the membranes back to the underlying placental substance – the chorion stops at the edge, whereas the amnion runs over the entire surface.

Uniovular twins have several possible configurations of the membranes, depending on the stage of development reached by the embryo before separation into two individuals. Separation of the mor-

ula would result in two placentas and two chorions, whereas separation at the implanting stage (the most common time) would produce one chorion and two amniotic sacs. However, if separation is delayed until after formation of the amniotic cavity (after eight days), the twins will share the same amniotic cavity and so the placenta will have one amnion and one chorion only.

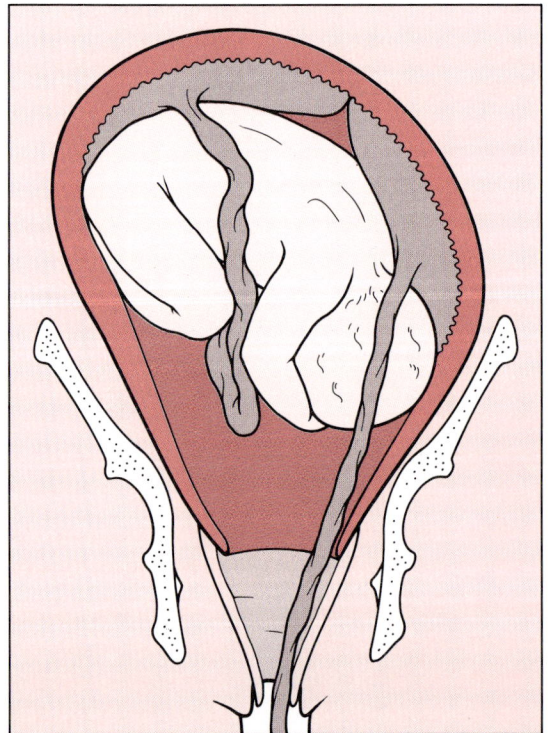

Fig.11.7 The first twin has been delivered but the second is lying obliquely and must be converted into longitudinal lie before safe delivery can occur.

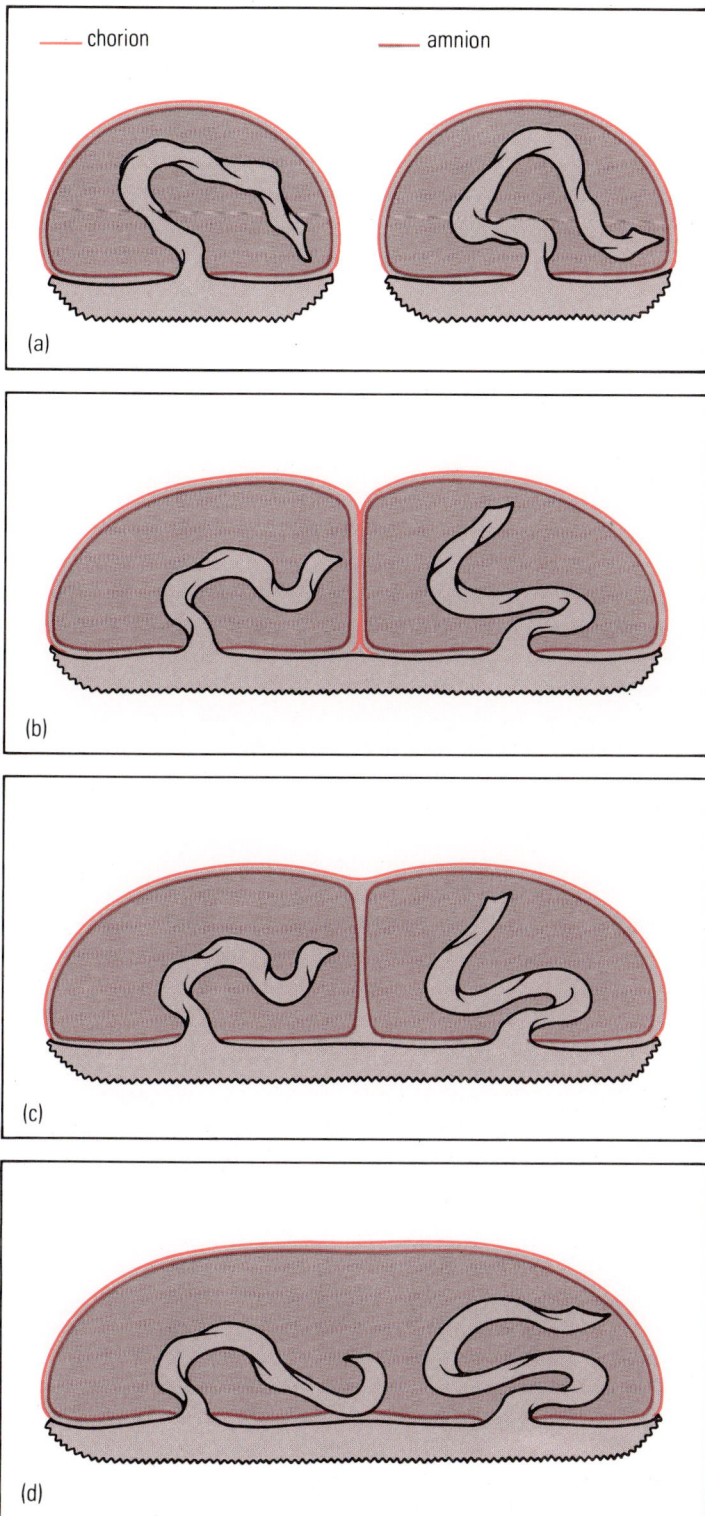

Fig.11.8 Examination of twin placentas: (a) the placentas are completely separate and obviously belong to binovular twins; (b) the placentas appear to have a common substance but the sacs are separate. The septum contains both chorion and amnion – these are probably binovular twins; (c) the placentas are separate but the septum contains only amnion – these are probably uniovular twins; (d) there is no septum between the two sacs – these are uniovular twins.

12. The Puerperium

The puerperium is defined as the period during which the reproductive organs return to their normal condition following labour. It begins with the delivery of the placenta and ends approximately six weeks later.

THE POSTNATAL VISIT

Women make a postnatal visit approximately six weeks after confinement to ensure that they and their pelvic organs have returned to normal. This also provides an opportunity to discuss any paediatric problems which may have arisen, and to consider which family planning method should be employed.

The mother's health is estimated by her appearance, her behaviour and by vital signs such as blood pressure, pulse rate and absence of anaemia. Careful bimanual examination of the pelvic organs is also indicated. One should note whether the episiotomy scar is satisfactorily healed and whether it is tender.

The state of the vaginal walls and cervix (Fig.12.1) is noted on inspection and palpation. Some cervical splitting is commonplace during labour and delivery, so that a slit-like external os is often seen, rather than the circular os of the nulliparous patient. The bimanual examination should determine whether uterine involution is complete; the uterus will be larger than in the nulliparous state but it should be firm. The uterine position should also be noted. Formerly, great attention was paid to anteverting a retroverted uterus (Fig.12.2), but nowadays it is realized that many normal women have a uterus which is tilted backwards.

If the woman brings her baby with her, the child should be examined to ensure that he or she is entirely normal and is thriving. Feeding should be discussed and advice given to the mother as necessary. If she is no longer breast feeding, an enquiry should be made about the comfort of the breasts.

POSTPARTUM HAEMORRHAGE

Primary postpartum haemorrhage

Primary postpartum haemorrhage is defined as bleeding of more than 500ml from the genital tract in the first twenty-four hours after delivery. It usually occurs during or immediately after the third stage of labour. The bleeding may occur with the placenta retained, or after its expulsion from the uterus. Most women can withstand a blood loss of 500ml without any serious effect on their general condition, but a heavier loss, of one litre or more, leads to shock.

If such a haemorrhage occurs and the placenta is retained within the uterus, the following should be the course of action:

- Rub up a contraction by manual pressure on the uterine fundus (Fig.12.3).
- Attempt removal of the placenta by controlled cord traction as soon as a contraction is felt.
- Give one ampule of Syntometrine if the placenta is satisfactorily removed.
- If the placenta cannot be expelled in this fashion, manual removal under anaesthesia should be employed (Fig.12.4).

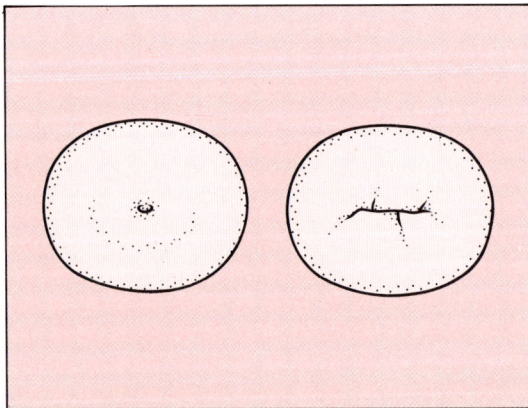

Fig.12.1 Appearance of the cervix. Left: in a nulliparous woman, the cervix is a rounded, small opening not more than 2mm in diameter. Right: in the multiparous, the os has been stretched at the time of delivery and is often linear; however, the canal higher up will not be much wider than in the primiparous.

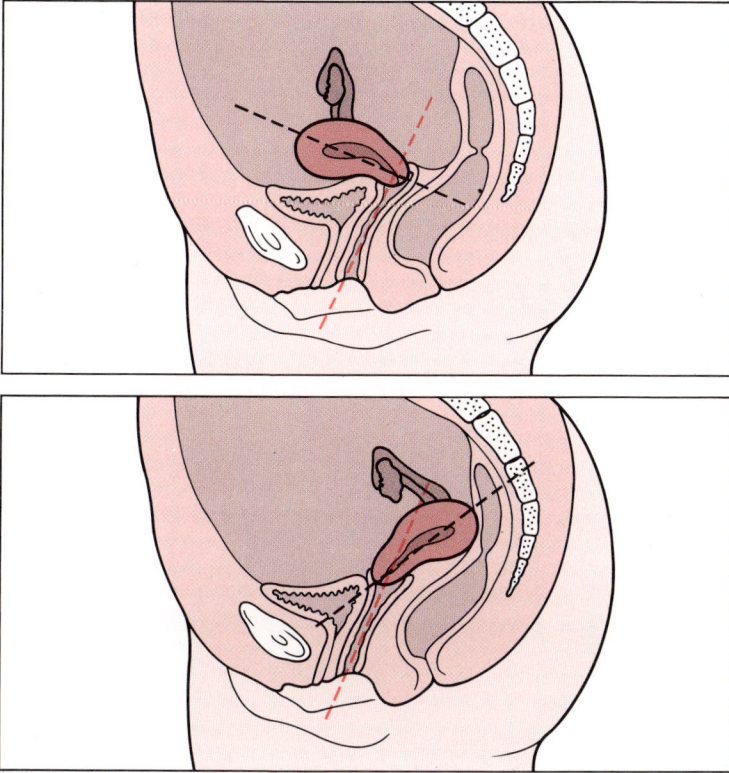

Fig.12.2 Uterine position. Upper: anteverted uterus, with its long axis bent forwards upon that of the vagina. Lower: retroverted uterus, with its long axis bent backwards upon that of the vagina.

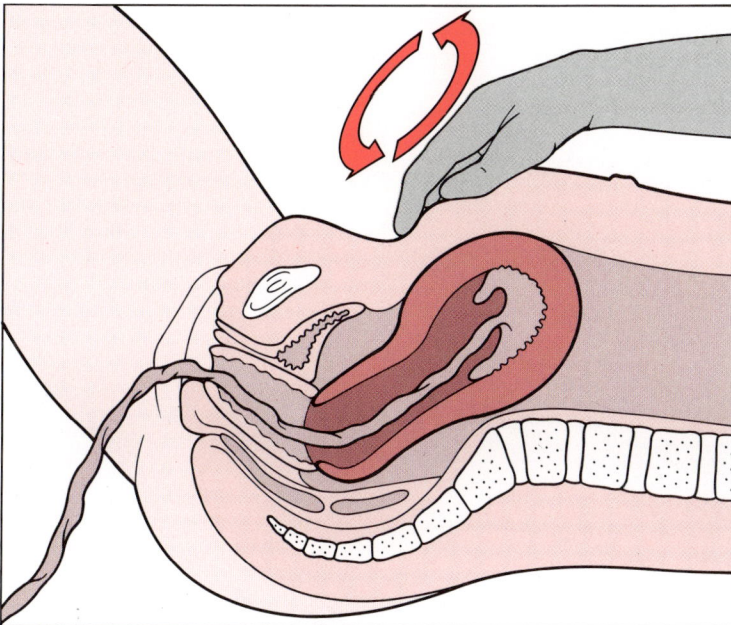

Fig.12.3 Management of primary postpartum haemorrhage. The uterus still contains the placenta, which is attached to its bed at the fundus. A circular massaging action will often stimulate the myometrium to go into spasm.

If the facilities for manual removal under anaesthesia are not immediately available, it is wise to maintain uterine contractions by controlling the fundus digitally and infusing oxytocin at a fast rate.

If the placenta has been expelled and the woman is still bleeding, one should check whether the uterus is contracted or relaxed. If relaxed, the blood is almost certainly coming from the placental site (Fig.12.5). However, if the uterus is firmly contracted and bleeding is still in progress, this is likely to be from a tear in the cervix (Fig.12.6) or vagina.

If the uterus is found to be relaxed, the fundus should immediately be rubbed up with the fingers and one ampule of Syntometrine should be administered. If the woman suffers a heavy blood loss whilst waiting for a uterine contraction to occur, bimanual compression (Fig.12.7) may be necessary, although such a course of action is rare.

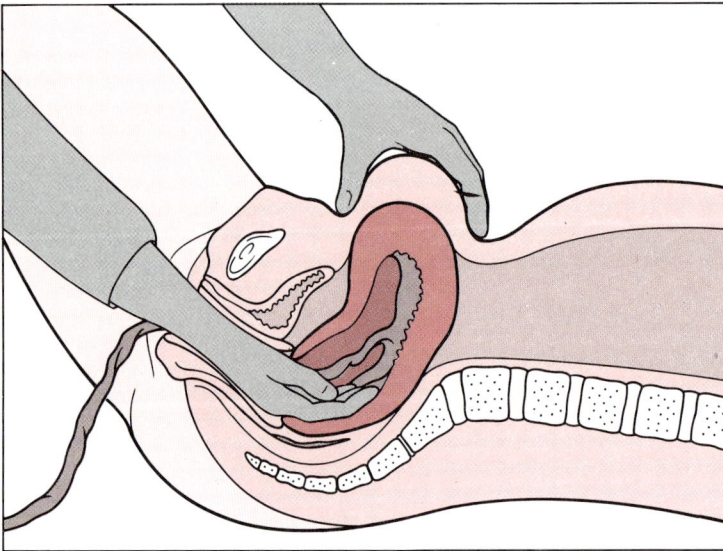

Fig.12.4 Manual removal of a non-detached placenta. The operator's right hand is passed through the cervix, which is quite lax after delivery. It finds a plane of cleavage and starts to separate off the placental bed by gentle side-to-side sweeping movements. Meanwhile, the left hand steadies the uterus and holds it through the lax abdominal wall.

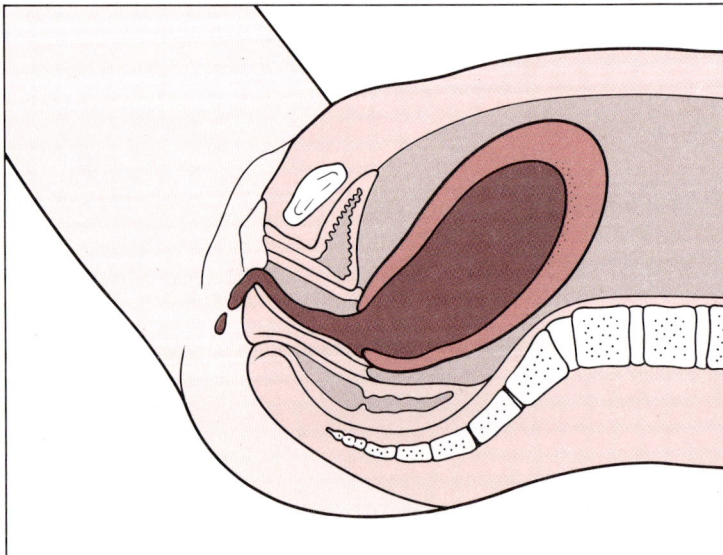

Fig.12.5 Primary postpartum haemorrhage from the placental bed. The uterus is filled with blood clot and cannot contract down; a small trickle of blood continues to be lost.

If the uterus is contracted and it seems likely that the bleeding is from a tear in the lower part of the genital tract, the bleeding area must be identifed as soon as possible. The lower vagina should be examined first and if this is free from trauma, the cervix should be inspected with good analgesia and adequate lighting.

This is best done by placing a pair of sponge-holding forceps on the anterior and posterior cervical lips and gently drawing them down to the vulva so that the cervix can be inspected directly. If a tear is found, it must be sutured effectively; the bleeding will be controlled by a series of through-and-through sutures

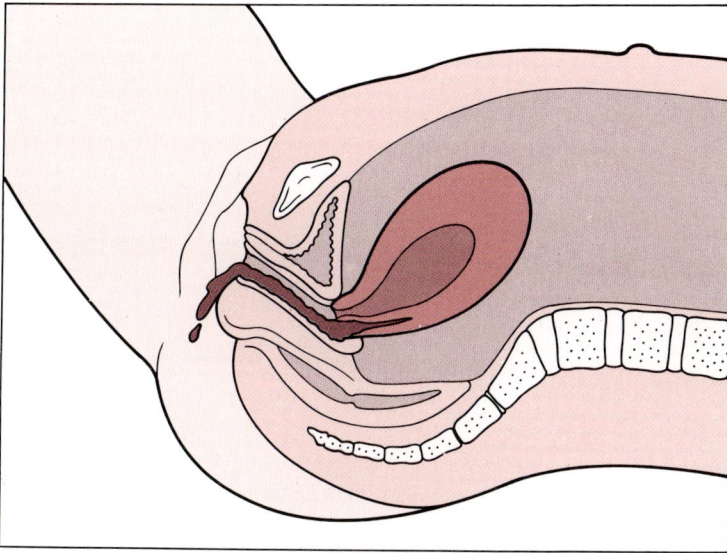

Fig.12.6   Primary postpartum haemorrhage from a cervical tear. Damage to the cervix has laid open some major blood vessels which are bleeding into the vagina.

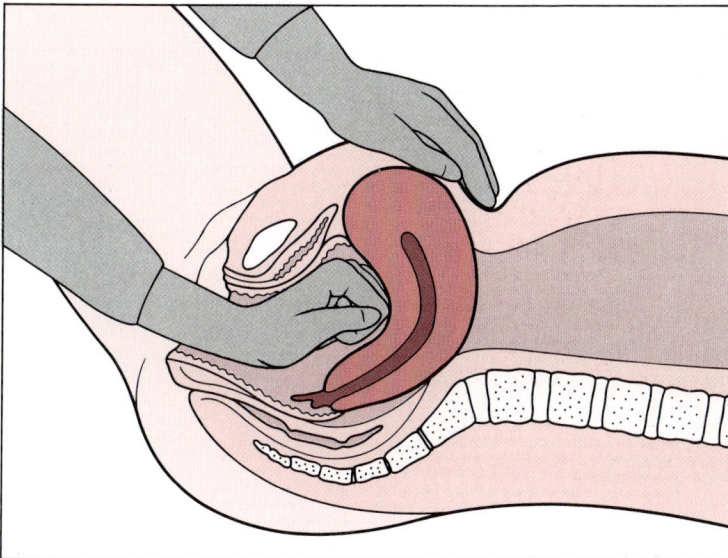

Fig.12.7   Bimanual compression of the uterus. The whole hand of the operator is introduced into the vagina. The other hand is placed on the abdominal wall and the uterus compressed firmly between them. This manoeuvre cannot be maintained for long periods but it can be life-saving if no other equipment is available.

185

(Fig.12.8). If the tear extends into the uterine body, effective suturing cannot be performed and repair will involve opening the abdomen.

If the cervix shows no tear there may be rupture of the uterus at a higher level, although this is rare. An exploration of the uterus under general anaesthesia must be undertaken if heavy bleeding continues and there is no evident site of blood loss in the vagina or cervix.

Secondary postpartum haemorrhage

Secondary postpartum haemorrhage is defined as any excess vaginal bleeding occurring from twenty-four hours to six weeks after delivery; it is most common between the eighth and the fourteenth day postpartum. The presence of a red lochial discharge may make it difficult to decide whether secondary postpartum haemorrhage is occurring, but it should be remembered that bright bleeding during the puerperium is always abnormal and should be investigated.

Secondary postpartum haemorrhage may be caused by retention of small pieces of placental tissue within the uterine cavity or by a mild infection within the cavity; sometimes the cause is not evident. If there is doubt about whether or not retained placental fragments are within the uterine cavity, an ultrasound scan will often prove helpful. If the blood loss does not stop spontaneously, the patient may be treated conservatively with antibiotics and oral ergometrine.

If the woman shows any effects of severe blood loss, it may be necessary to explore the uterine cavity under anaesthesia and remove the contents. This should always be done gently since the uterine muscle will be soft and perhaps infected, and can easily be injured by the introduction of a sharp instrument. Provided the uterus is curetted gently and no damage is done, the loss usually ceases soon afterwards and the patient may be discharged.

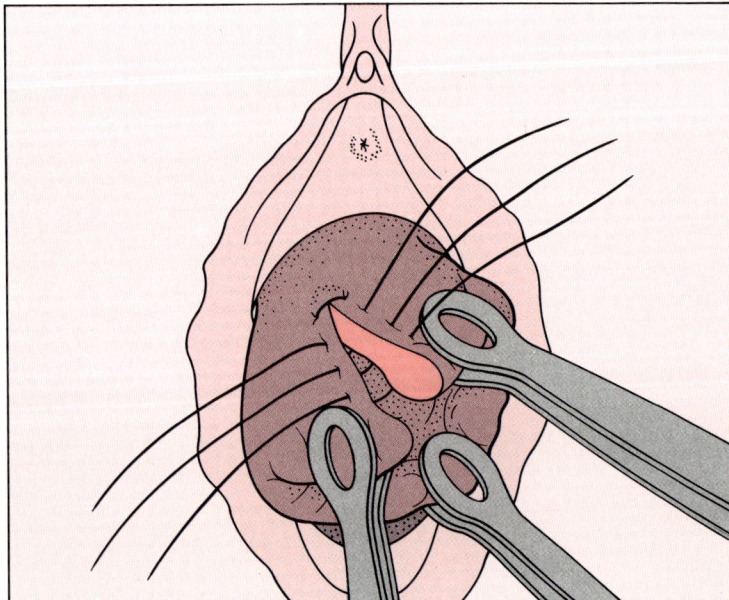

Fig.12.8 Repair of a cervical tear. Deep through-and-through stitches are inserted under anaesthesia; this ensures prompt haemostasis.

URINARY RETENTION

Urinary retention sometimes complicates the early puerperium. This may be due to bruising or oedema of the bladder base caused by stretching during delivery, or to discomfort caused by an episiotomy wound. Retention is obviously present if the woman cannot pass urine at all. However, it frequently occurs with overflow, in which case the woman passes small amounts of urine repeatedly. Palpation of the lower abdomen will reveal the uterine fundus displaced to a high level and a large palpable bladder (Fig.12.9). Catheterization is necessary and if the problem recurs, an indwelling catheter should be used for forty-eight hours and a course of antibiotics given to keep the urine sterile. After the first day without the catheter one should check the residual volume of urine, which should not exceed 150ml.

UTERINE INVERSION

An inverted uterus is one which is turned inside out. Inversion is described as incomplete when the uterine fundus comes down through the cervix, which remains in its normal position (Fig.12.10 left), or complete when the whole of the uterus and cervix are involved (Fig.12.10 right).

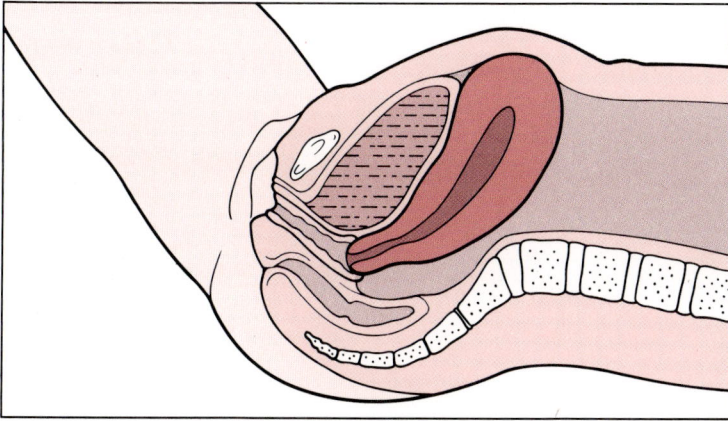

Fig.12.9 Urinary retention. This may occur after delivery, causing the uterus to enlarge and bleed.

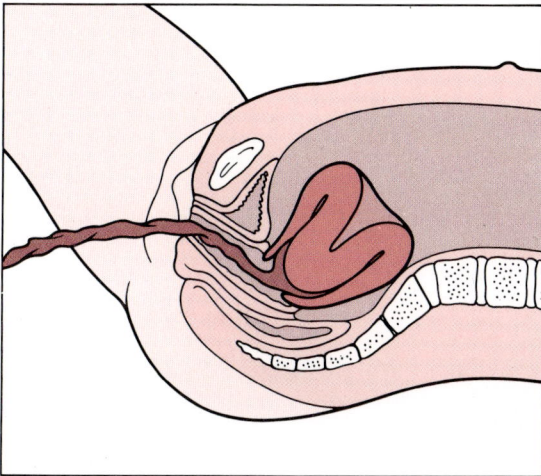

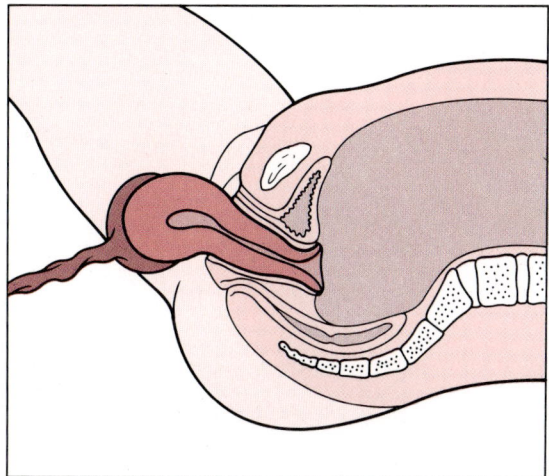

Fig.12.10 Uterine inversion. Left: incomplete inversion. The fundus is inverted but the cervix is in its normal position. Right: complete inversion. The whole of the uterus is inverted and placenta is still attached to the fundus; the woman will be severely shocked.

187

This disorder should be suspected if there is un-explained shock but no bleeding following delivery. If the inversion is incomplete, the uterine fundus may feel abnormal on abdominal examination, although it is seldom possible to detect a specific dimple. A vaginal examination must be made as soon as possible to exclude or confirm this complication. If the inversion is incomplete, the soft putty-like uterine fundus will be felt filling the upper vagina and coming through the cervix. In a complete case, the inverted uterus may be visible outside the vulva.

Uterine inversion is an extremely dangerous complication of labour. If a doctor is present when the inversion occurs, the correct management is to replace the uterus within the abdomen immediately, using upward pressure from below. It is unnecessary to scrub-up before doing this, since undue delay will result in spasm at the neck of the sac and replacement will then be very difficult. If such spasm has occurred,

the patient will very quickly become shocked, and resuscitative measures will be necessary before replacement is attempted. An intravenous line must be set up immediately and plasma expanders and dextrose saline given until blood is available.

Once treatment for shock has started, one can attend to the replacement of the inversion. This should be performed under general anaesthesia either manually or, if that fails, by the hydrostatic method (Fig.12.11). Normal saline is passed into the vagina whilst the vulva is blocked by as many pads as possible; the vagina will be felt to dilate to a large size and the gentle, even pressure produced by this procedure will often replace the inverted uterus into the abdomen. Such a low hydrostatic pressure is thought to work because it is universally applied over all surfaces of the genital tract, ballooning them out and allowing the uterus to return to its normal position.

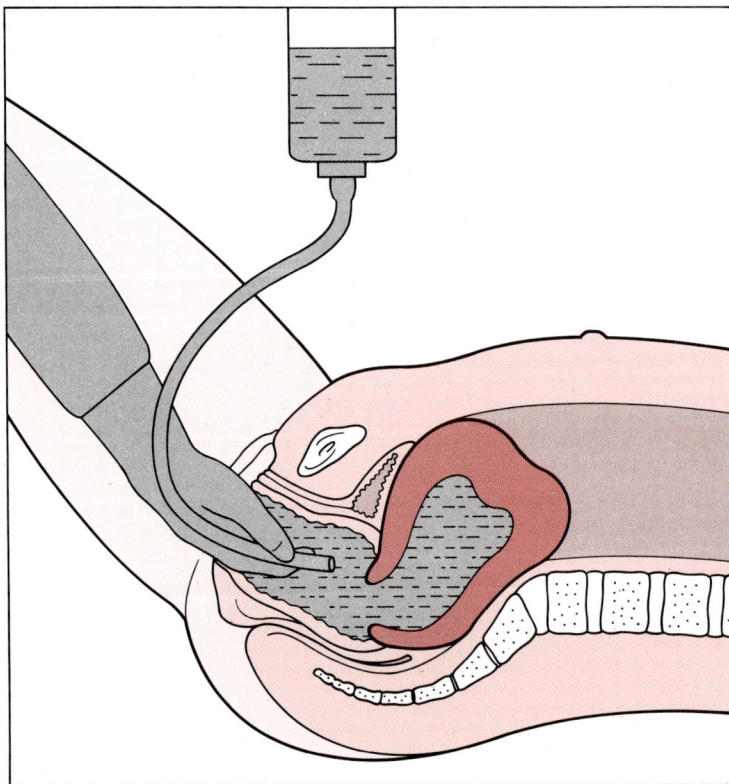

Fig.12.11 Hydrostatic replacement of an inverted uterus. The hand holds the end of a sterile nozzle in the vagina, thus plugging the lower end. With a water pressure of a few feet, a sterile saline solution is passed into the cavity, causing the uterus to return gently to its normal position.

PARAVAGINAL HAEMATOMAS

A paravaginal haematoma may form at one of two points:
- Beneath the levator ani muscles (following a vaginal tear).
- Above the levator ani muscles (following a cervical or lower uterine segment tear).

A paravaginal haematoma (Fig.12.12) is one of the conditions which must be suspected if the patient becomes unaccountably shocked soon after labour. It may be possible to see the haematoma at the lower part of the vagina and perineum, or it may become evident on examination of the vagina and uterus.

Treatment of a paravaginal haematoma is more difficult than might first be imagined. If the general condition of the patient has suffered, she will first require resuscitation with blood transfusion. The haematoma may be evacuated or, if the bleeding seems to be stopping, it may be left untreated to see if it will resolve. If the haematoma is explored, it is seldom possible to identify the bleeding point in a mass of blood clot, and deep stitches may have to be inserted into an oozing surface. A definitive tear in the lower part of the vagina causing a vulval haematoma should be firmly sutured.

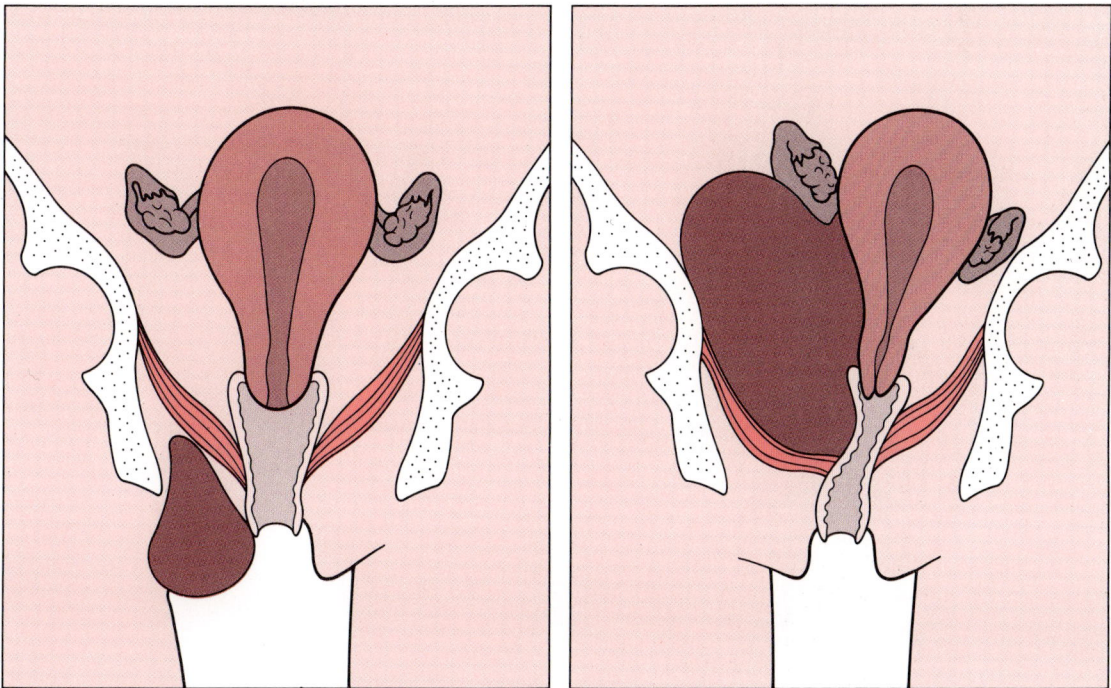

Fig.12.12 Vulval haematoma. Left: haematoma in the ischiorectal fossa. This is well below the levator ani muscles and may be very painful. Right: haematoma in the base of the broad ligament. This is above the levator ani muscles and can spread up behind the peritoneum of the anterior or posterior abdominal walls.

189

PERINEAL TEARS

Perineal tears are of three degrees (Fig. 12.13):
- First degree, involving skin and vagina only; the tear does not reach the perineal body.
- Second degree, involving the perineal body.
- Third degree, involving the perineal body and passing through the anal sphincter.

First degree perineal tears often require no management, although occasionally a single stitch may be needed.

Second degree tears should always be sutured carefully; this may be satisfactorily accomplished under local analgesia. The apex of the tear should be identified first and a continuous catgut stitch inserted in the vaginal wall, beginning above the apex of the tear and continuing to the introitus. Two or three deeper stitches should then be inserted into the torn muscles of the perineal floor to bring them into apposition. The skin of the perineum may then be brought together either by interrupted stitches or by a subcuticular stitch, which is often more comfortable.

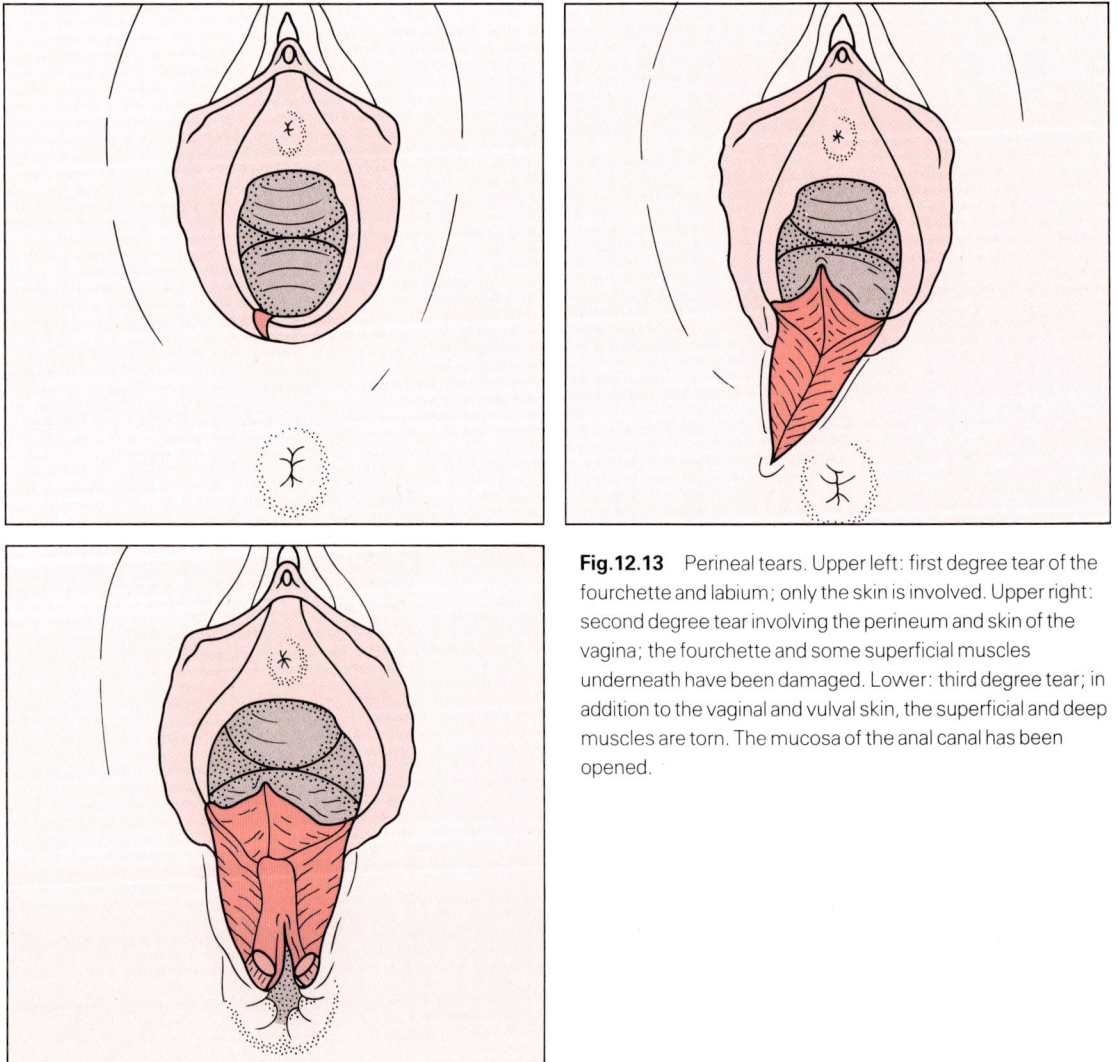

Fig. 12.13 Perineal tears. Upper left: first degree tear of the fourchette and labium; only the skin is involved. Upper right: second degree tear involving the perineum and skin of the vagina; the fourchette and some superficial muscles underneath have been damaged. Lower: third degree tear; in addition to the vaginal and vulval skin, the superficial and deep muscles are torn. The mucosa of the anal canal has been opened.

The repair of a third degree tear (Fig.12.14) is more difficult and should be carried out under general anaesthesia or epidural analgesia in an excellent light, which can best be obtained in an operating theatre. The edges of the tear through the anal sphincter must first be identified and the mucosa of the anal canal and lower rectum (if involved) approximated with fine catgut stitches. Two or three deep stitches must then be carefully placed into the torn ends of the anal sphincter and brought together in front of the anal canal. The remainder of the repair can be carried out in a similar fashion to that of a second degree tear.

INFECTION

Fortunately, puerperal infection is now less common, but it can still be a serious complication of the puerperium. Infection may involve the placental site, from which it may spread to parauterine tissue, the fallopian tubes or the pelvic veins. The parametrium may be infected following vaginal or cervical tears, or an episiotomy.

The signs will be those generalized manifestations of infection which are not specific to the site of infection, namely pyrexia and tachycardia; in more

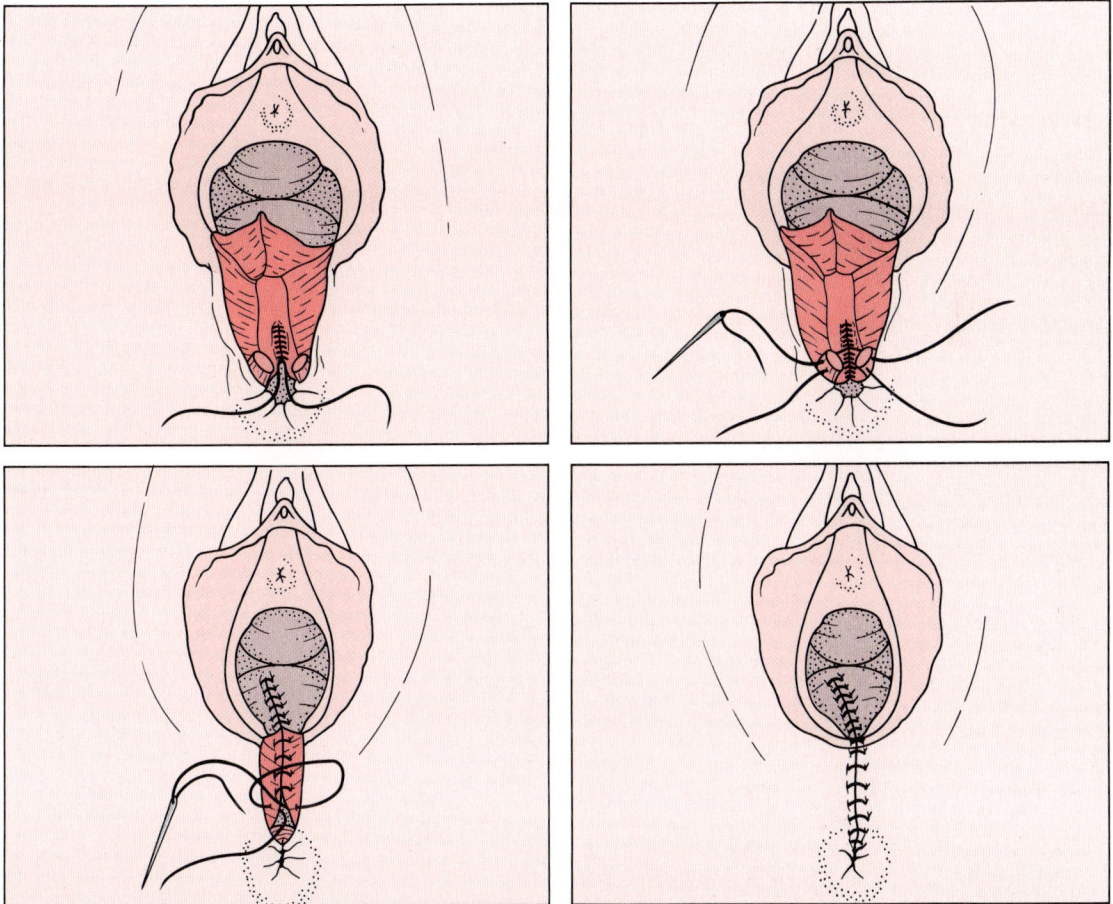

Fig.12.14 Repair of a third degree tear. Upper left: the mucosa of the anal canal is sutured with plain catgut, inverting the edges into the lumen of the canal. Upper right: the anal spincter is closed separately, with broad sutures of chromicized catgut which hold the muscle together. Lower left: the superficial muscles of the perineum are brought together and the vaginal skin closed. Lower right: the fourchette skin is closed with interrupted chromicized catgut sutures.

severe cases, the patient will appear generally ill. In addition, there may be poor involution, the fundus remaining high within the abdomen, and the lochia may remain red and may be offensive.

If there is considerable spread of the infection into the parametrium and pelvic peritoneum, it is likely that there will be high fever and toxaemia. Tenderness will be very marked in the fornices and on palpation of the uterus and, at a later stage, abscess formation may be evident. Unless the infection resolves, localized collections of pus (pyosalpinx or tubo-ovarian abscesses) may form and generalized peritonitis may occur.

Infection should always be treated promptly with antibiotics. If it is possible to identify a specific organism from a high vaginal swab, an antibiotic to which this organism is sensitive must be chosen, but such identification is not always possible. It must be remembered that infection with anaerobic organisms may occur and suitable culture conditions must be used. Most patients respond well to correct antibiotic therapy but, rarely, abscess formation may occur and drainage is then necessary.

Common extragenital sites of infection are the urinary tract and the breast.

VENOUS THROMBOSIS

Venous thrombosis may occur in the superficial or the deep veins. Superficial venous thrombosis (thrombophlebitis) is seldom serious because there is little embolic risk, although it often gives rise to discomfort or pain. A reddened, tender area is usually visible over the thrombosed vein and this generally settles well with rest.

Deep venous thrombosis is a more serious matter. This may involve the iliofemoral veins in the groin or the deep veins of the calf. Iliofemoral thrombosis arises from infection within the uterus and pelvis itself. Commonly, the leg is swollen throughout its whole length and may be cold and white or warm and blue. A cold white leg indicates that the femoral artery next to the thombosed vein has gone into spasm and considerable pain will be experienced as a result. A low grade pyrexia may have been noticed before the clinical symptoms became manifest. The woman should be treated with antibiotics for the infection and anticoagulants for the thrombosis. There is a significant risk of a pulmonary embolus occurring and, should this happen, it may be necessary to perform a Trendelenburg operation of embolectomy.

13. The Normal Newborn Baby

CHANGES AT BIRTH

The onset of respiration is probably the most important change at birth, but many others also occur as the baby changes from the role of parasite in its mother to that of an independent human being.

One of the most remarkable advances in recent years has been the rapid decrease in perinatal mortality (stillbirths and neonatal deaths in the first week of life). Statistics from the United Kingdom (see Chapter 16) show a recent decrease, which is partly the result of improved perinatal care. Unfortunately, this reduction in mortality in the United Kingdom is less striking after the first month of life. Some of these deaths are of preterm babies who survive the newborn period of the first month, but die later from infections or from sudden infant death syndrome (SIDS).

Onset of respiration

The fetus makes repiratory movements but, unlike the constant respirations that are essential after birth, movements of the fetal chest occur for about only a third of the time *in utero*. They seem to occur in rapid-eye-movement sleep, which is more common in the newborn than in adults and older children, and even more common in the fetus.

The fetus lives for nine months in a liquid environment and has to adapt to the atmosphere at birth. Amniotic fluid is produced from a number of sources including lung liquid, which is secreted from the alveoli and passed up the trachea. Lung liquid is acidic and high in chloride (Fig.13.1). The similarity in composition between this and upper gastrointestinal

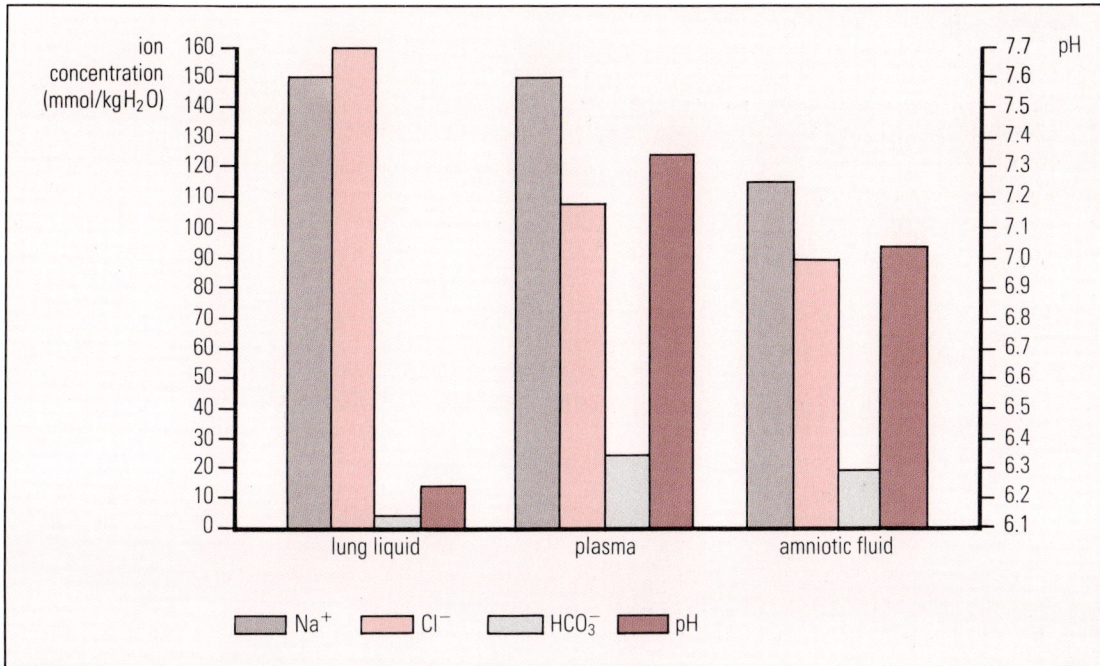

Fig.13.1 Electrolyte composition of lung liquid, plasma and amniotic fluid. The lung liquid is relatively acidic and has a higher chloride level than plasma and amniotic fluid.

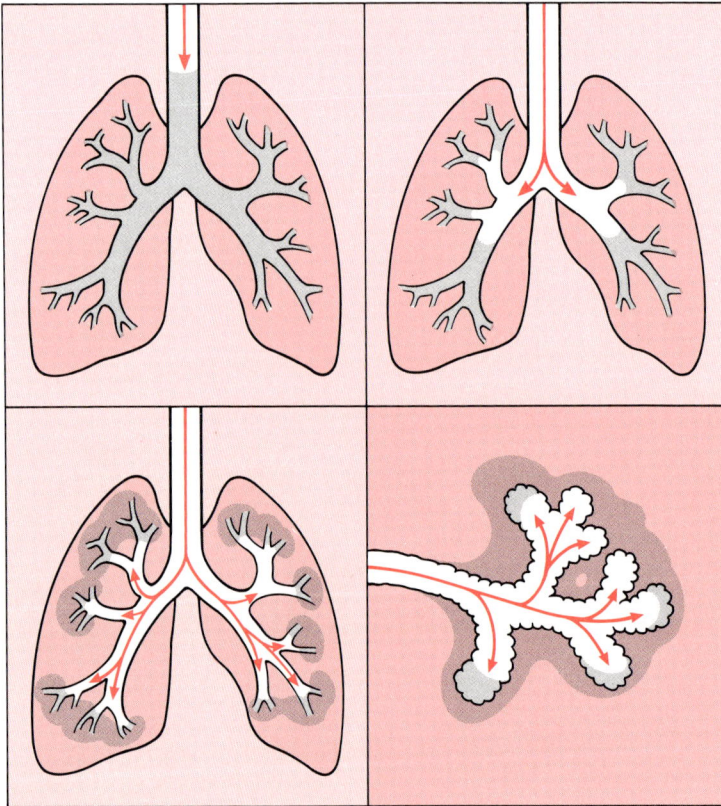

Fig.13.2 Displacement of lung fluid from the fetal lungs. Upper left: the baby has been born and negative pressure produced by the expanding chest wall causes air to be drawn into the trachea. Upper right: more air is drawn in and the lung fluid is pushed and sucked into the bronchi. Lower left: as the column of air reaches the alveoli the fluid escapes into the lung lymphatics. Lower right: most of the lung fluid is cleared into the lymphatics after a couple of breaths but it takes 10–15 minutes for all of it to be absorbed.

FACTORS STIMULATING ONSET OF RESPIRATION

$\uparrow Pco_2$

$\downarrow Po_2$

$\downarrow Po_2$ & $\uparrow Pco_2$

cold

other physical stimuli

Fig.13.3 Factors which stimulate the onset of respiration.

secretions is not surprising given that the lungs are formed from the upper gut. The production of lung liquid ceases suddenly at birth when there is a surge of catecholamines in the fetus, possibly as a result of relative hypoxia or cooling. The fluid inside the lungs is partly cleared, moving up the trachea and into the nasopharynx when the thorax is squeezed during its passage through the birth canal. The rest is absorbed in the lung (Fig.13.2), into either the blood vessels or the lymphatics. The liquid is replaced by air and the lungs expand to a great extent, something which is not seen in the post-mortem appearance of stillborn babies.

A number of factors act together to make the baby take his first breath (Fig.13.3); the most important of these are the changes in blood gases. When the umbilical cord is compressed during delivery and the placenta begins to separate from the uterine wall, the oxygen supply to the fetus and his ability to excrete carbon dioxide are reduced. Marked hypoxaemia or hypercarbia can each excite the first breath, but the more usual stimulus is probably a combination of mild hypoxia and a slightly raised Pco_2. Other stimuli

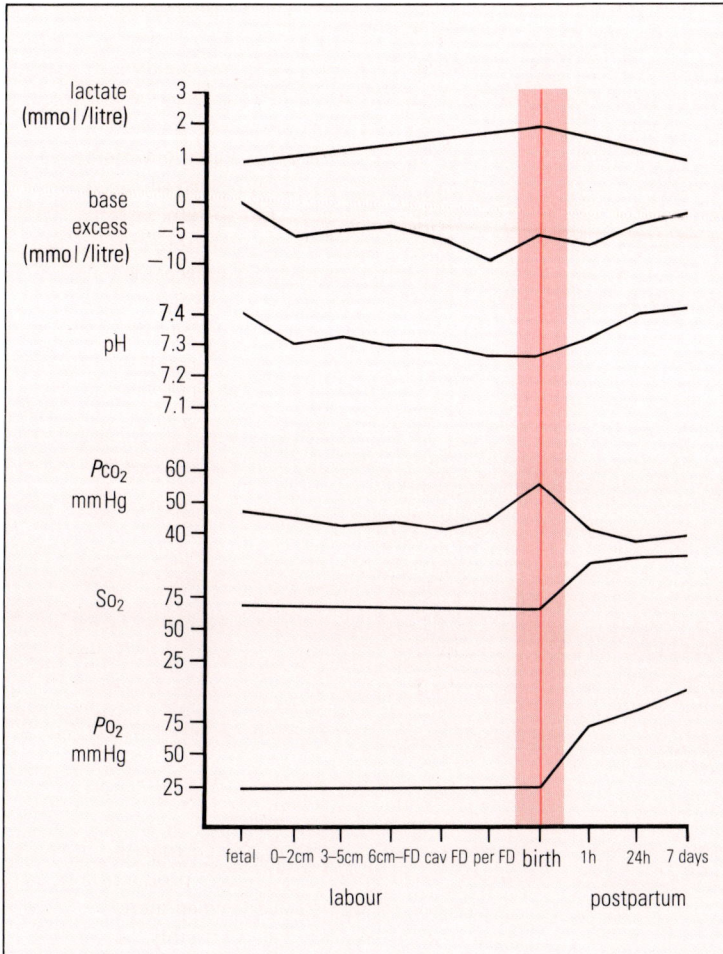

Fig.13.4 Changes in blood gases during and after birth. Base excess is a measurement of the non-volatile base (alkali) in tissue fluid — mostly bicarbonate. Fetuses and neonates tend to be acidaemic and deficient in alkali, thus the values given here are negative. FD = full dilatation; Cav = head in cavity; Per = head on perineum.

are also effective; the major drop in ambient temperature compared to the warmth inside the uterus has been shown to initiate the first breath in animals. At one time it was common to slap a baby's bottom at birth, but such an assault is unnecessary, unkind and could worsen the state of an ill baby. If any extra stimulus is needed, light tapping on the soles of the feet often makes the infant breathe.

Considerable changes occur in the blood gases during and after birth (Fig.13.4). During the first stage of labour, the pH, P_{CO_2} and P_{O_2} in fetal blood do not change a great deal; the pH and P_{CO_2} are very similar

to the values found in adult blood, but the P_{O_2} is much lower. There is a tendency for the pH to fall a little during the second stage of labour, although readings from cord blood are very variable. The most usual finding is a mild acidaemia; this results from a combination of respiratory acidaemia with a high P_{CO_2} and a metabolic acidaemia due to accumulation of lactic acid during anaerobic respiration. After birth, the P_{CO_2} drops rapidly to normal levels; it may be lower than normal for some time as the baby overbreathes to compensate for the acidaemia. The pH then rises to normal levels (about 7.4) as the P_{CO_2}

195

falls, and the baby metabolizes lactic acid with the aid of oxygen. There is a rapid rise in the Po_2 of the blood (Fig.13.5); the fetal Pao_2 is around 3kPa (22mmHg) and the neonatal Pao_2 is about 7–11kPa (55–80mmHg). These are lower than the values found in babies over one week old. The relatively low oxygen pressure in the newborn baby's blood is the result of a right-to-left shunt of blood in the first week of life. The shunt occurs at several sites; blood can bypass the lungs through the foramen ovale or the ductus arteriosus, but the shunt also occurs in areas of the lungs which are not yet properly expanded and oxygenated.

The baby's respirations change at birth to become regular and constant. The first few breaths often require a considerable effort. The pressure inside the neonatal thorax may have to be reduced to 70cmH$_2$O below atmospheric pressure before any air enters the lungs. This is often called the opening pressure. At the end of the first breath, a residual volume of air stays in the lungs and the second and subsequent breaths are then easier (Fig.13.6).

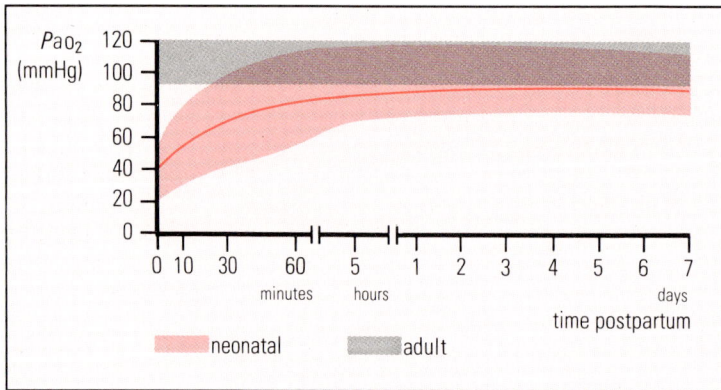

Fig.13.5 Range of Pao_2 values after birth. The normal adult range is shown for comparison.

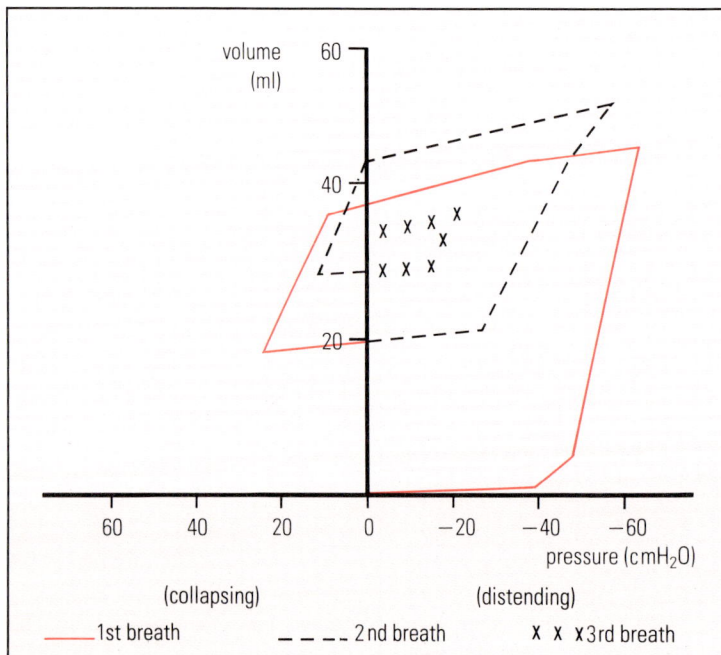

Fig.13.6 Pressure–volume relationships during the first few breaths, measured using an oesophageal catheter and reverse plethysmograph. Modified from Karlberg, P. et al. (1962) *Acta Paediat.* **51**, 121.

The stability of the alveoli depends on the presence of surfactant, a collection of phospholipid molecules which have hydrophobic and hydrophilic terminal groups and thus an affinity for an air–water interface. They reduce the surface tension at this interface, preventing the alveoli (which are lined with water) from collapsing at the end of each breath. Surfactant begins to appear in the lungs between twenty and twenty-four weeks gestation (Fig.13.7); it is this, together with the increasing structural maturity of the lungs, which allows survival of the newborn from twenty-four weeks. The preterm baby is particularly prone to hyaline membrane disease, or respiratory distress syndrome (RDS), which causes difficulty in breathing. Surfactant is deficient in the lungs of such babies, and thus the alveoli tend to collapse after expiration. During pregnancy, surfactant flows out of the fetal mouth in the lung liquid and can therefore be sampled in amniotic fluid. One of the most important components of surfactant is diphosphatidyl-lecithin; this increases in pregnancy compared to sphingo-myelin, another constituent of surfactant. A comparison is made of these two substances as a ratio (the L/S ratio), and a value of less than two in the amniotic fluid indicates a risk of RDS. Diphosphatidyl-glycerol, another surfactant component, is now also thought to be important in RDS since it is always absent from the lungs of babies with this syndrome.

Cardiovascular changes

The differences between the fetal and neonatal cardiovascular systems are discussed in Chapter 2.

Temperature changes

A newborn baby loses heat at birth and a drop in body temperature of about 1°C is inevitable. The baby is born wet and warm into a relatively cool environment; evaporation of amniotic fluid from the skin causes most of the heat loss.

The newborn baby is small with a relatively large surface area for its weight, and is therefore not so well equipped for temperature control as an adult. Like any homeothermic mammal, the human neonate can increase its metabolism when in a cool environment. This is shown by the increase in oxygen consumption at low ambient temperatures, but the body temperature will drop if the baby is not able to compensate sufficiently.

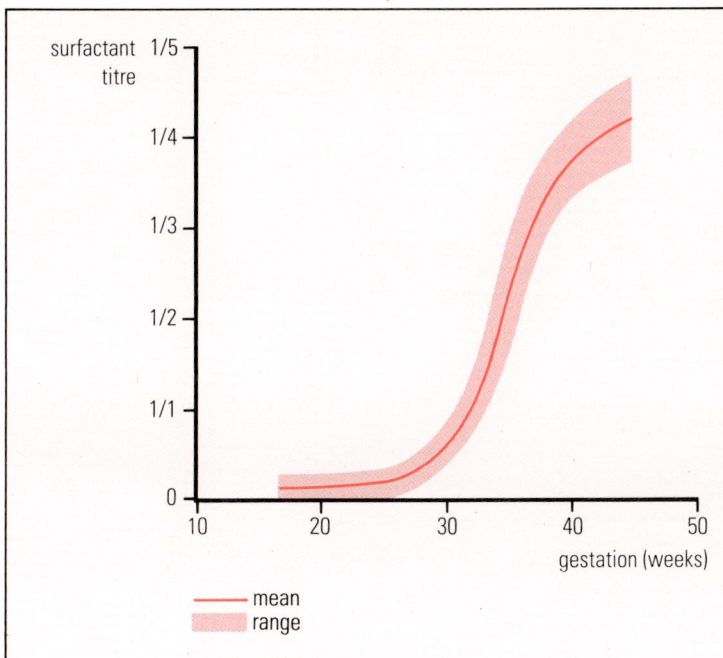

Fig.13.7 Surfactant in amniotic fluid. The titre of surfactant rises as gestation advances.

Babies do not shiver but have a large amount of brown fat around the major arteries (Fig.13.8), which becomes metabolically active and warmer when an infant is cooled. This cooling induces other changes in

the body, for example a surge of thyroid activity and a sudden rise in the plasma level of thyroid stimulating hormone, which then subsides. Since this hormone is now measured routinely as a screening test for hypothyroidism, it is important to choose the right time for the test. Cord blood can be used, but the hormone is usually measured at six days as part of the Guthrie test.

Other changes

Although the dramatic alterations in the lungs and heart are the most important events at birth, many other changes occur. The fetus is a parasite, but the neonate has an independent existence. Fetal urine is passed into the amniotic fluid, but the excretion of waste products occurs across the placenta. Thus, a fetus can survive the whole pregnancy without kidneys, but a newborn baby with this condition inevitably dies within the first week.

All nutrients pass to the fetus, across the placenta, in the form of simple chemicals. The newborn baby, however, must digest milk and absorb the products through the gut wall. The neonatal blood glucose level drops in the first few hours to a concentration which would be considered hypoglycaemic in an older child (Fig.13.9).

Normally, a baby is born microbiologically sterile,

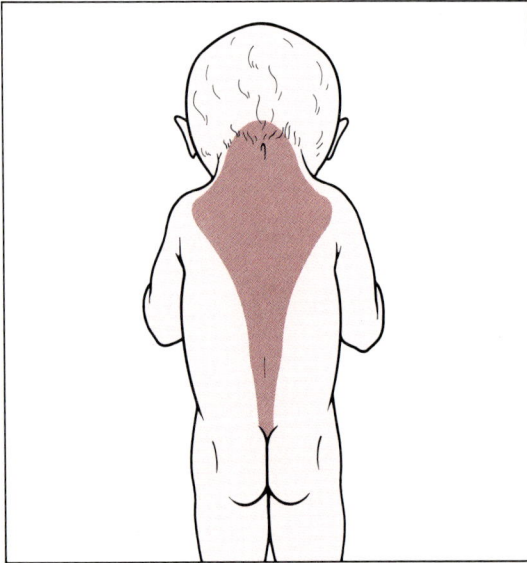

Fig.13.8 Distribution of brown fat in the neonate. Fat is present around the major arteries coming from the heart and between the scapulae.

Fig.13.9 Alteration in blood glucose level after birth.

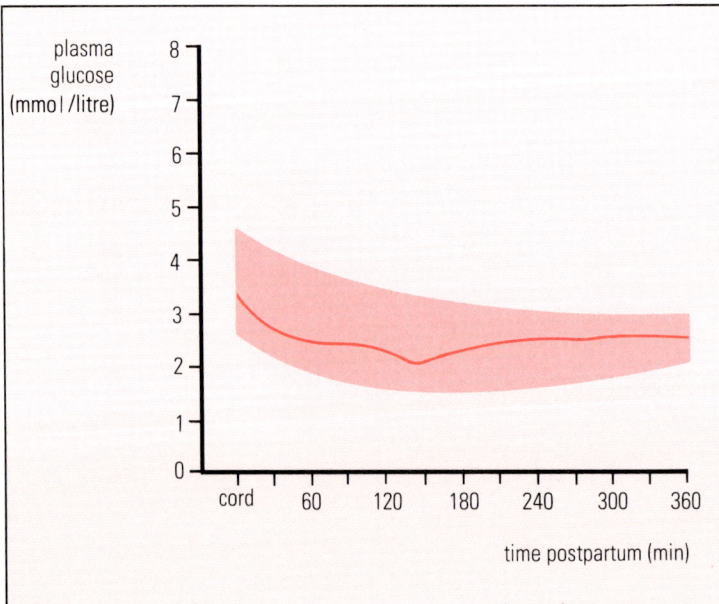

but bacteria will soon colonize the skin and spread throughout the gut. This process is distinct from infection, which involves invasion of the body by organisms.

The metabolism of bilirubin also changes at birth (Fig.13.10). Bilirubin is produced in the fetal body from the breakdown of haemoglobin and other sources. It circulates in the blood bound to albumin, from which it can be detached to cross the placenta. It is then conjugated in the mother's liver for excretion in her bile. After birth and separation of the placenta, the baby's liver must conjugate the bilirubin itself and at this time there is a slight rise in the fetal plasma bilirubin concentration; this is more marked in the baby.

Not only are there physical changes in the baby, but his whole environment changes. It is known that a fetus can hear, since the heart rate will change in response to a loud noise transmitted though the mother's abdominal wall. The baby can see at birth and has been shown to be interested in looking at a human face. He is capable of making his wishes known by crying, particularly when hungry. After a short time, the mother can distinguish the cry of her baby from that of others.

EXAMINATION OF THE NEWBORN

Ideally, every newborn baby should receive three examinations in the first week. The first inspection is made by the midwife or doctor who delivers the mother (see Chapter 7). A second and more detailed medical examination is made within the first twenty-four hours, and a third before the baby is discharged from hospital.

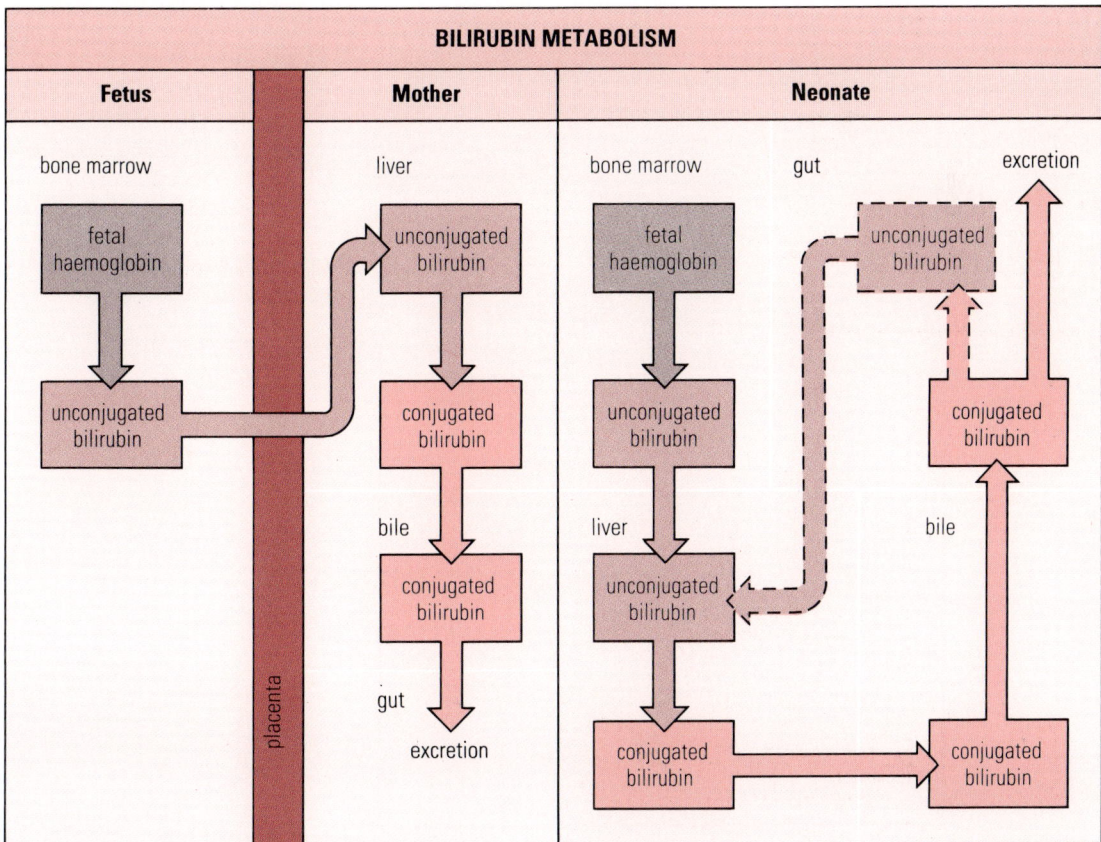

Fig.13.10 Bilirubin metabolism. Some of the fetal haemoglobin breaks down to bilirubin. This passes across the placenta, is conjugated in the maternal liver and then excreted in bile. After birth the baby starts to conjugate bilirubin in the liver.

Weight

The baby's size is one of the most important physical signs. This can be assessed using standard charts which relate gestational age to weight, length and head circumference. Most of the charts relating birth weight to gestational age have centile lines (Fig.13.11). The line for the average is the 50th centile and the limits of the normal range are often the 10th and 90th centiles as these include eighty percent of the population.

Babies who are lighter than expected are described as small-for-dates or small-for-gestational age; they are usually defined as those below the 10th centile. Such babies are at particular risk of hypoglycaemia and may need blood glucose estimations in the first two days. Babies who are born before thirty-seven completed weeks of gestation are called preterm and those after forty-two weeks are post-term. The term prematurity is being replaced; it was employed for babies weighing 2500g or less at birth, as it was thought that such babies were born early and the figures could be used for international comparisons when gestation was not known. However, it was later found in the United Kingdom that one third of such

babies were born at term. The present recommendation of the World Health Organization is that when the birth weight is less than 2500g, the infant should be called a baby of low birth weight.

Many factors are associated with low birth weight. It is much more common if the mother is short, if she has already had a small baby, if the pregnancy was complicated by hypertension, or if the baby has a congenital abnormality. Some factors are avoidable, for example smoking, which not only causes the baby to be small-for-dates (Fig.13.12) but is also associated with poor reading ability later in childhood. Babies of mothers who live at a high altitude are smaller than those born at sea level; this is not related to ethnic origin. It is known that babies in the Indian subcontinent are smaller than those in Europe or North America, but the 50th centile for those born before thirty-two weeks is the same as in developed countries. It therefore seems that something restrains the fetal growth in late pregnancy—possibly the mother's size. Multiple pregnancy is another major reason for low birth weight. Not only are the babies of such pregnancies likely to be born early, but they will probably also be small-for-dates if the gestation has lasted for more than thirty-two weeks (Fig.13.13).

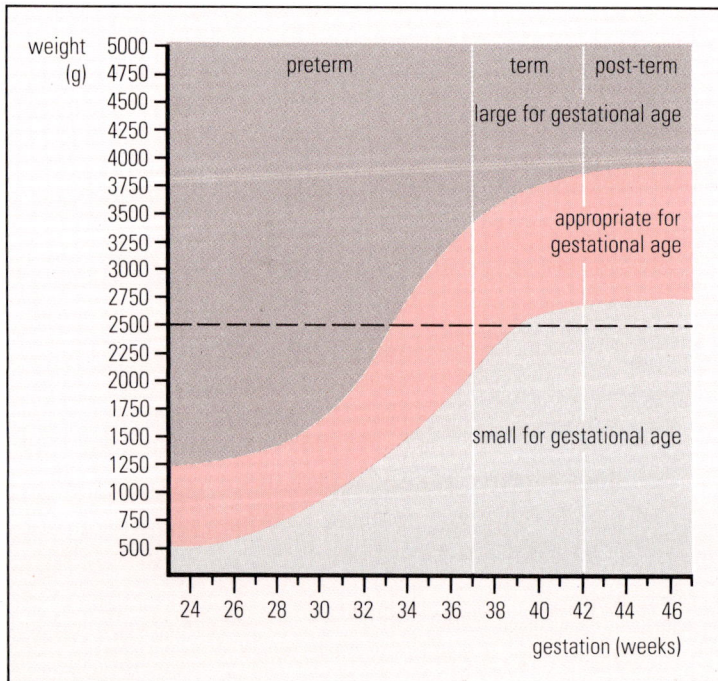

Fig.13.11 Classification of newborn babies according to birth weight and gestational age. All of those occurring below the broken line at 2500g are considered to be of low birth weight.

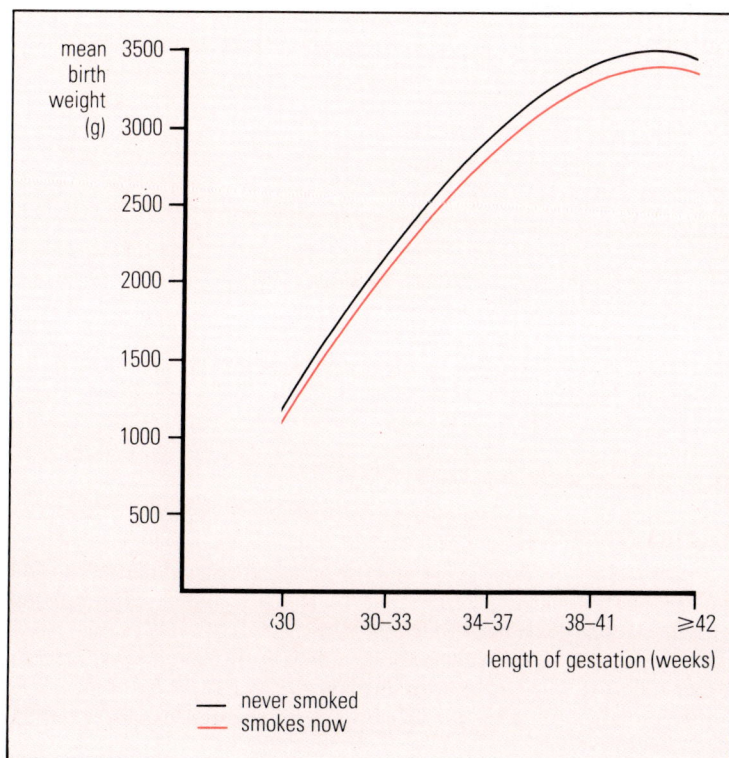

Fig.13.12 Mean birth weight for gestational age according to maternal smoking habits.

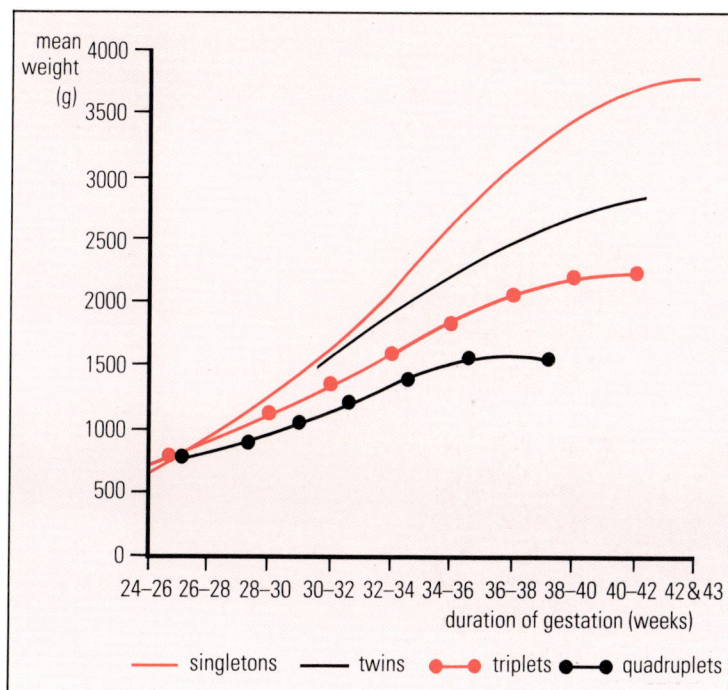

Fig.13.13 Mean birth weight of single and multiple fetuses related to duration of gestation. Modified from McKeown, T. and Record, R. G. (1952) *Journal of Endocrinology,* **8,**386.

A number of clinical tests have been described to score the gestational age of a newborn baby. The Dubowitz score is the best known and is based on a number of neurological and clinical features. External criteria include skin texture, skin colour, breast size, and ear firmness. A preterm baby has thin, red skin, soft ears and no breast tissue can be felt. A term baby has thick, cracking, pale skin, discs of breast tissue more that 1cm in diameter, and cartilage can be palpated in each pinna.

Some small-for-dates babies show dry skin, appear thin and wasted (Fig.13.14 left), and may be stained with meconium. Large-for-dates babies (Fig.13.14 right) usually have fewer problems, but they are subject to birth trauma, for example shoulder dystocia is more common. A large-for-dates baby may follow a pregnancy complicated by diabetes mellitus, particularly if it is not well controlled, and hypoglycaemia may be a problem in the first two days. Large size is also more common in babies with transposition of the great arteries.

Measurement of the crown–heel length is not possible unless it is done with a special instrument; a tape measure will produce an unreliable answer. The head circumference must be measured in every baby.

This can be done at birth as part of a routine procedure, but is better carried out two to three days later, once moulding has disappeared.

Examination after birth

The baby should be checked immediately after birth to be certain that there is no condition requiring urgent treatment and that there are no congenital abnormalities.

It is important to be sure that the airways are not blocked by mucus or other foreign material. If it is necessary to suck out the nose and front of the mouth, this must be done very gently; if a suction catheter is pushed to the back of the mouth, it is possible to induce reflex apnoea.

When the baby has been born a careful observation must be made of the respirations and heart rate. This is done at one and five minutes of age while assessing the Apgar score (Fig.13.15). It is also usual to note the time at which the baby first takes a breath and cries. If the baby is not breathing by one minute, resuscitation may be necessary (see Chapter 14).

While the baby is being assessed, he can be put flat

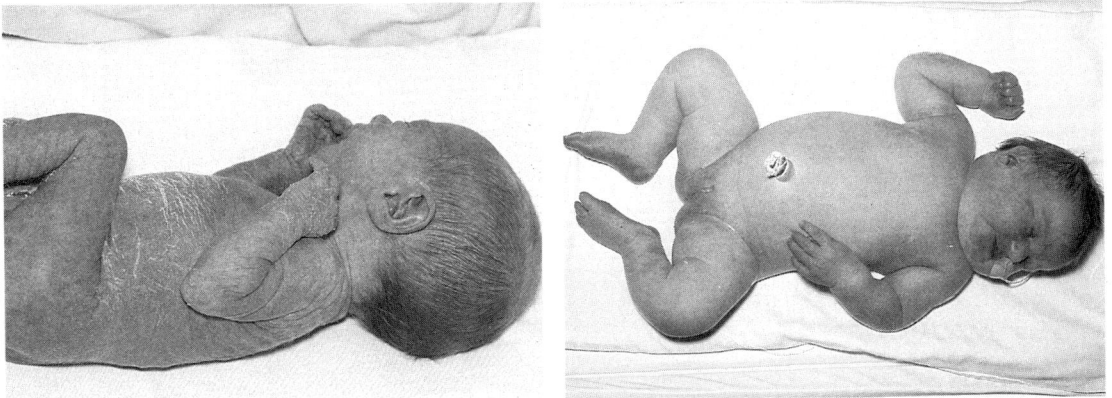

Fig.13.14   Left: a small-for-dates baby who is thin, wasted and shows dry skin.
Right: a large-for-dates baby.

on his back on a resuscitation trolley. It is not necessary to use the head-down position, which may hinder breathing. As soon as possible, the baby should be completely dried with a towel; he can then be wrapped in a blanket or an impermeable plastic sheet with a reflecting surface. In order to prevent heat loss the delivery room should be warm, if possible at a temperature of 26°C. Some hospitals use a booster heater in the delivery room, so that a part of the room can be warmed for the baby without making conditions uncomfortably hot for the mother during labour. As soon as the baby reaches the postnatal ward, the body temperature should be checked. It is not normally necessary to take the temperature rectally; it can be taken in the axilla.

If the baby is in good condition, it is not necessary to put him on the resuscitation table; the examination can be done in the mother's arms, where the baby can be unwrapped completely to allow parental contact. A short, but careful, examination for congenital abnormalities should be performed (see Chapter 7). The baby can then be held and fed by the mother.

It is very important to identify the baby properly. Labels should be completed immediately after the birth. They can be shown to the mother to check, and are then put on the baby's wrist and ankle. It is usual to check them every day, and to check them again with the mother's label before discharge from hospital.

First day examination

A full medical examination is needed within the first day. This is most efficiently done on a daily morning ward round, and it should be performed in a methodical way. Many doctors examine the baby from top to toe, but there is an advantage in listening to the heart first in case the baby becomes upset and cries.

First, the mother's notes should be read. She should then be asked again if there are any important inherited illnesses in her own or the family's medical history. A history of tuberculosis in someone living in the house is an indication for BCG vaccination. It is also necessary to know if there was any abnormality in the pregnancy and the estimated length of gestation. The routine records of birth weight and head circumference can be noted. The baby should pass urine within twenty-four hours; it is sometimes recorded as being delayed because it was passed at

APGAR SCORE			
	2	**1**	**0**
Heart rate	>100	<100	impalpable
Respiratory effort	cry	respiration alone	absent
Muscle tone	good tone	moderate tone	limp
Reflex irritability	strong withdrawal cry	some motion grimace	no response
Colour	pink	dark blue	pale

Fig.13.15 The Apgar score. The infant is checked at 1 and 5 minutes after delivery. A score of 3 or less at 1 minute indicates severe asphyxia.

birth without being noticed. Meconium, the dark-green contents of the bowel, should be passed within thirty-six hours.

The baby should be undressed completely. Any general signs such as pallor or cyanosis should be noted, and the respirations counted for any sign of tachypnoea or recession. It is then a good time to listen to the heart for abnormalities of the sounds or for a murmur.

Examination of the head may reveal a very large fontanelle with separated sutures, which would suggest hydrocephalus. A very small fontanelle with a small head circumference, indicates microcephaly. A cephalhaematoma, a collection of blood under the periosteum of the skull which is confined to one bone, may be seen (Fig.13.16).

The eyes need to be checked carefully. The eyelids should be gently retracted to look for a wide and cloudy cornea, which occurs in glaucoma. In most cases, it is possible to see the red reflex with an ophthalmoscope to exclude cataract, but the eyelids are sometimes too swollen. The attendant should check to ensure that both auditory meatus are present. Some routine hearing tests have been developed for use in the neonatal period. They vary from a simple rattle to the very sophisticated, using brain stem evoked responses and a computerized hearing cradle.

It is essential to both look at and feel the palate. A cleft of the soft palate can be missed if it is only palpated, and a submucosal cleft of the hard palate will be missed with visual inspection only. Cysts of the gums or the tongue occur quite often.

The neck should not contain any swellings; these might indicate lymphatic cysts if they transilluminate, or a goitre if present in the midline. The arms should be the same length and have no obvious deformities. The fingers should be counted and examined. It is suprisingly easy to miss syndactyly.

The abdomen should then be examined. Distension is an important sign, particularly if there is a history of bile in vomit, as this indicates intestinal obstruction. A very high obstruction, such as oesophageal atresia, presents with regurgitation of mucus and cyanotic attacks. The flanks should be palpated for enlarged kidneys. The umbilicus may show bleeding if the cord clip is not fixed properly. An inspection will have been made of the cord at birth to see if there are two arteries and one vein. In about one percent of babies, there is only one artery at the umbilicus. This is usually a harmless feature, unless other congenital abnormalities are also present.

The genitalia need careful attention. Any difficulty

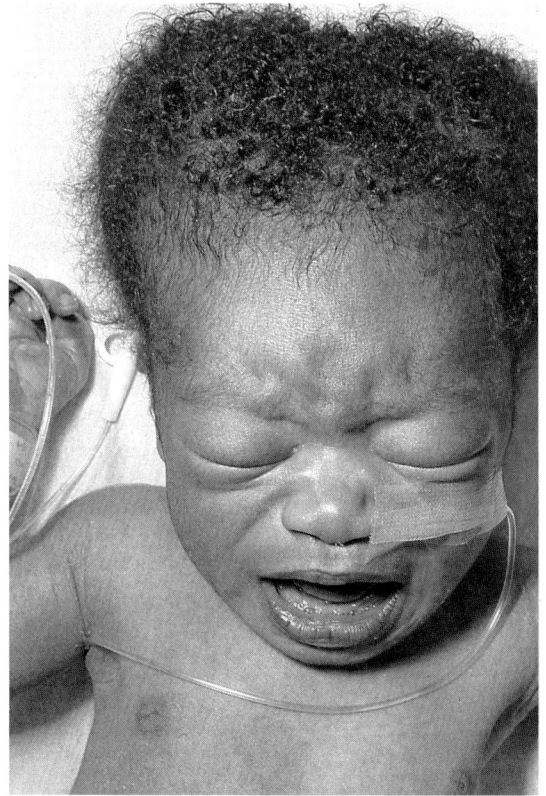

Fig.13.16 Cephalhaematomas.

in determining the sex of the baby (Fig.13.17) means that a senior opinion should be obtained immediately. The situation must be explained to the parents and a sex must not be assigned until further investigations have been performed. These may include measuring the plasma 17-hydroxyprogesterone level, which is raised in adrenogenital syndrome. This condition is due to a metabolic block in the adrenal gland, which causes virilization of females. In a boy, the opening of the urethra must be found; if it is on the ventral surface of the penis, he has hypospadias. If the testes are in the scrotum, this should be recorded carefully in case they later become retractile and are confused with undescended testes. The scrotum appears relatively large compared to later in infancy. The female

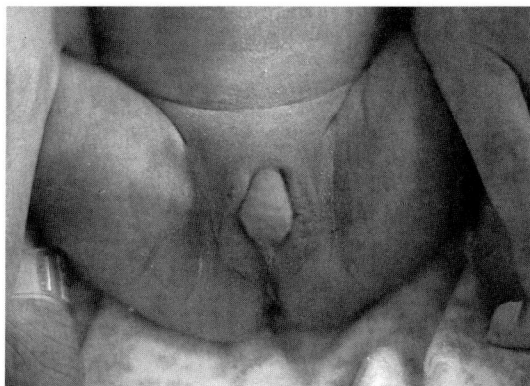

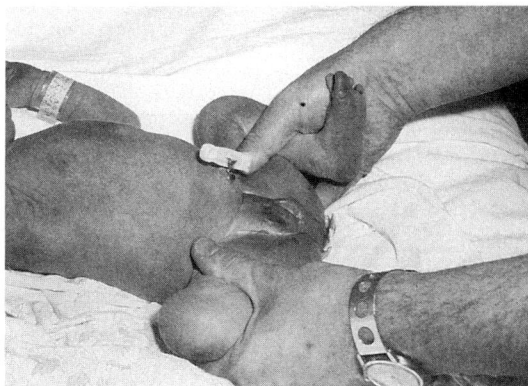

Fig.13.18 Examination of the hips. The legs are flexed at the hips and the knees and thighs gently abducted.

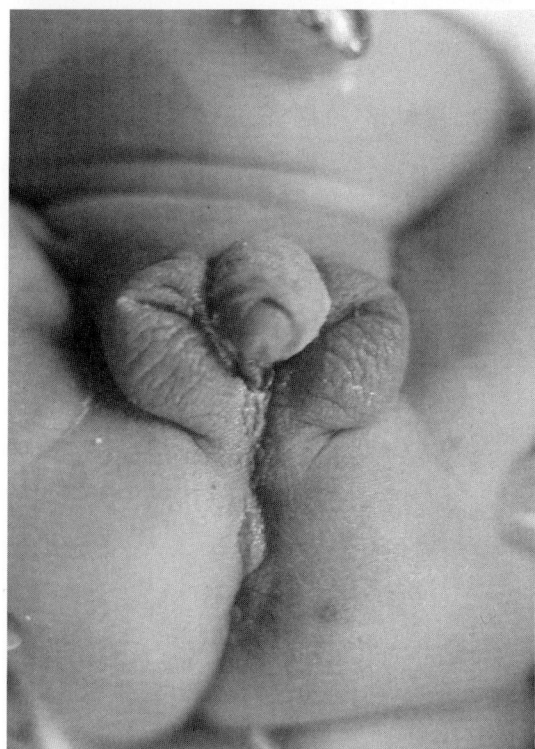

Fig.13.17 Intersex. This female baby has an enlarged clitoris — the result of adrenogenital syndrome.

genitalia also appear larger than a few weeks later, as the labia majora are very swollen. In a preterm baby, the clitoris may be rather large, but any suspicion that it is abnormal should prompt investigations for adrenogenital syndrome. It is easy to overlook an absent vagina, a very rare abnormality. An imperforate anus is much more common; the anus must be inspected carefully, wiping away any meconium before the examination.

Examination of the hips can be very uncomfortable for the baby, and should be done as gently as possible; it is conducted in two parts. The baby should be placed on a firm surface. The legs are then flexed at the hips and the knees and thighs are gently abducted (Fig.13.18); if too much force is applied in the presence of a fixed dislocation it is possible to fracture the femur. The thumbs should then be placed in front of the hips with the next two fingers behind them. When the thighs are abducted, a dislocation will be revealed by a sudden jump as the head of the femur slips back into joint. Often, a minor click is felt, even though the 'clunk' characteristic of dislocation is absent. These clicks do not indicate hip disease, but some believe that such babies should be followed up; this would best be done as part of a child health surveillance programme.

The second part of the examination involves testing whether the hips can be dislocated. With the thighs adducted, the thumbs are pressed on the upper part of the femur and the previous procedure repeated, as if ballotting the head of the femur between the thumbs and forefingers. When the hip is dislocatable, a 'clunk' will be felt over the acetabulum. This examination is particularly important after breech presentation and when there is a family history of congenital dislocation of the hips.

This is a suitable time to palpate the groins to be certain the femoral pulses are present. The legs should be the same length and should have no obvious deformities. Each foot should be reduced to a valgus position with the dorsum almost touching the shin (Fig. 13.19) to ensure that there is no talipes. Finally, the baby should be turned over. A finger can be run down the spine to feel for swellings, which might indicate a meningocele, or scoliosis.

During the examination, the attendant should take note of any birth marks and other abnormalities. An assessment can be made of tone, paricularly if there is any difference between the two sides. A number of primitive neurological reflexes have been described, of which the best know is the Moro response. If the baby's head is allowed to fall back slightly or if the cot is moved suddenly, the baby will throw out his arms in extension and then abduct them. This response can sometimes be useful to detect asymmetry, which may be due to a fractured clavicle or Erb's palsy. However, the baby usually does not like the test and cries; other physical signs will reveal the abnormality.

Discharge examination

This examination is performed to ensure that the baby is fit to go home, and is not as detailed as the first day examination. A check should be made for jaundice or other signs that the baby is ill. Examination of the heart may reveal a murmur which was not present before. The hips should be examined again.

A sample of neonatal blood is taken by heel prick between the sixth and fourteenth days of life and is tested for two unusual, but treatable, causes of mental handicap. Phenylketonuria (PKU), which occurs in approximately one in every 7000–10,000 infants, is detected by a high phenylalanine level. Hypothyroidism, due to an absent thyroid gland, occurs in one in 8000 infants and is indicated by a high level of thyroid stimulating hormone.

INFANT FEEDING

In most of the world, breast feeding is essential for the survival of the baby because there is no alternative. Artificial milk is a satisfactory food for babies in a developed country, but can be very dangerous in a society in which hygiene is inadequate and bottles cannot be sterilized.

The major difference between human milk and cow's milk is that the latter is more concentrated and contains much higher levels of protein (Fig.13.20). In cow's milk, the major protein is casein rather than the lactalbumin found in human milk; the latter is much easier for the baby to digest. Modern artificial milks for babies have a composition which is nearer to human than cow's milk. The protein and sodium content is reduced, but the protein is not human and could stimulate an allergic response.

Breast feeding has a number of advantages, the most important of which is the prevention of infection. Gastroenteritis is much less common in breast-fed babies, as is respiratory infection, although to a lesser extent (Fig.13.21). Human milk contains a number of anti-infective substances including IgA, lactoferrin, lysozymes, and antiviral agents, in addition to live leucocytes; colostrum is particularly rich in immunoglobulins.

Eczema in babies of families with a history of atopy is said to be less common in those who are breast-fed than in those who are given artificial feed. Even though the evidence for this is not conclusive, it is usual to recommend breast feeding for at least three months to reduce the incidence of atopic disorders. It has become common to use a soya formula for the prevention of asthma and eczema, but there is no evidence that this is effective, indeed a baby can become allergic to soya proteins. At one time, it was thought that breast feeding protected against cot death, or sudden infant death syndrome; although there is some effect, these tragic deaths also occur in the breast-fed.

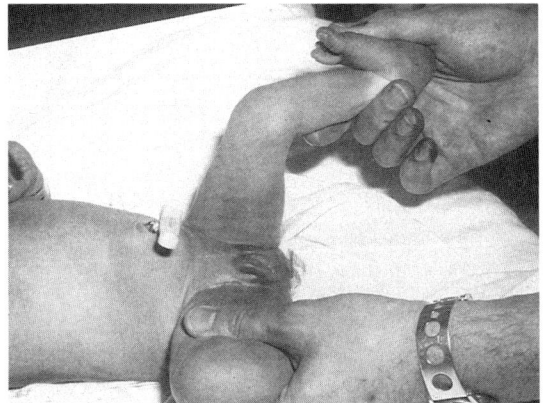

Fig.13.19 Examination of the feet. Each foot is reduced to a valgus position to ensure that there is no talipes.

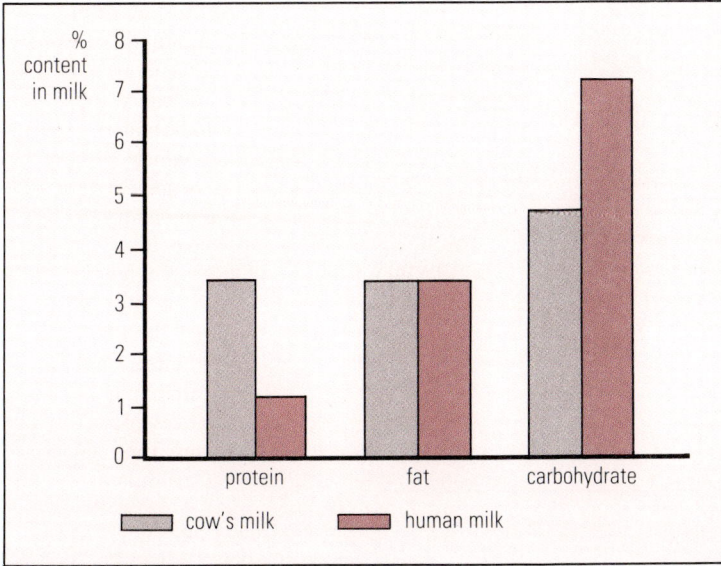

Fig.13.20 The composition of human milk and cow's milk.

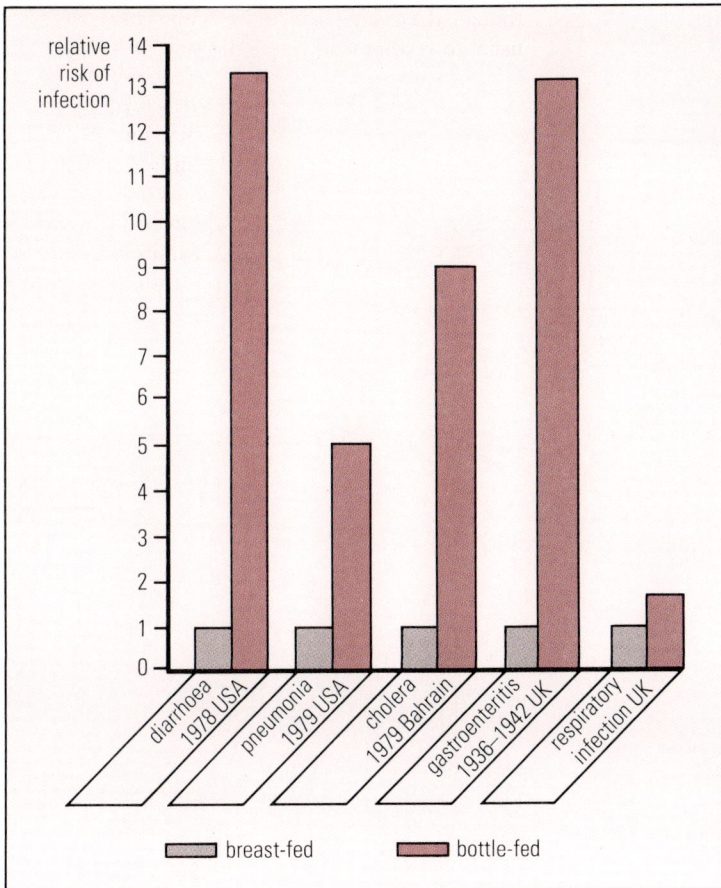

Fig.13.21 Relative risk of infection by feeding method. The relative risk is the number of cases appearing in 100 bottle-fed babies divided by the number of cases in 100 breast-fed babies from the same socioeconomic environment over the same time period. Modified from *The State of the World's Children* (1986) UNICEF.

It is believed by many that there is a special relationship between the mother and her breast-fed baby. This may be because, in our society, breast feeding usually occurs with the mother and baby by themselves, whereas bottle feeding tends to be a more social activity. Two hormones are particularly concerned with the production of milk in the mother (Fig.13.22). Prolactin from the anterior lobe of the pituitary gland stimulates the formation of milk in the breast, and oxytocin from the posterior pituitary lobe stimulates ejection of the milk. Both hormones are released when the baby sucks at the nipple. When a baby sucks at one breast, the response to oxytocin will cause some milk to flow out of the other nipple.

The number of feeds increases during the first few days. Initially, the baby obtains very little fluid and can lose up to ten percent of body weight, but towards the end of the first week, feeds are demanded frequently (Fig.13.23). The nipple is made of erectile tissue and enlarges during suckling. It is very important that the baby should get the nipple fully into the mouth; the lips and gums are then on the brown areola and form a seal, which allows the baby to draw the nipple into the mouth and extract the milk by squeezing it between the tongue and the palate. If the baby does not fix well on the breast, cracks may occur in the nipple causing bleeding and infection.

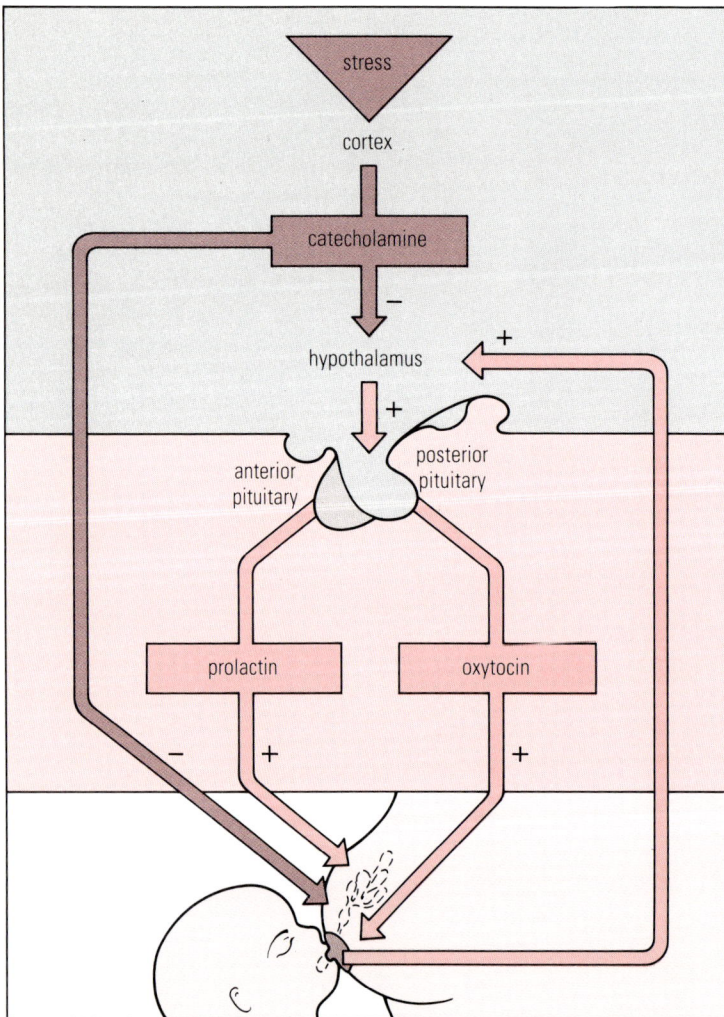

Fig.13.22 Hormonal regulation of milk production. Suckling stimulates production of prolactin and oxytocin. Prolactin stimulates milk formation and oxytocin stimulates ejection from the breast. Stress may interfere with production by stimulating release of catecholamine, which supresses the hypothalamus directly in addition to causing a reduction in blood flow within the breast.

During a breast feed, the baby obtains most of the milk within the first two minutes and almost all of it within four to five minutes. It is common for a baby to suck for much longer than five minutes; this may be for pleasure, but it will also stimulate milk formation in the breast for a subsequent feed.

Breast-fed babies are particularly prone to vitamin K deficiency. This causes a prolonged prothrombin time and thus bleeding, which may present as melaena, bleeding from the umbilical cord or an internal haemorrhage, most dangerously into the brain. Vitamin K is therefore given routinely at birth, either orally or by intramuscular injection.

Feeding with artificial milk is a satisfactory way of feeding an infant in a country with adequate hygiene, although breast feeding is more satisfactory and has become popular again in recent years. If bottle feeding is to be used, the mother should have an explanation of the need for hygiene when feeding the baby. There are two common methods of sterilizing feeding bottles — boiling for about five minutes, or soaking in a solution of sodium hypochlorite. It is essential to make up artificial milk according to the instructions on the packet. Milk which is too concentrated can be dangerous when given to a baby with diarrhoea because it may lead to hypernatraemia.

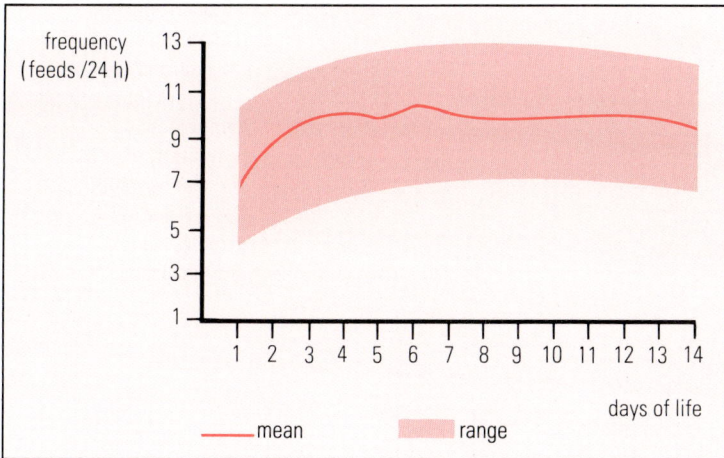

Fig. 13.23 Frequency of feeds during the first two weeks of life.

14. The Abnormal Newborn Baby

CONGENITAL ABNORMALITIES

About one in fifty babies has a serious congenital abnormality, although not all of these are detectable at birth. The incidence of different types of malformation varies from one part of the world to another. For example, neural tube defects are common in the United Kingdom (Fig.14.1), whereas cleft palate is more common in East Asia. There are many varieties of malformation; some are more important than others because they require urgent surgical treatment or because they are very severe and may be lethal. Common congenital malformations in England and Wales are shown in Fig.14.2. It is quite common to see several congenital abnormalities in one child.

Neural tube defects

Neural tube defects include spina bifida and anencephaly. They arise during the formation of the brain and spinal cord in the embryo, when the skin and other tissues fail to close over the nervous tissue. In the most severe type, anencephaly, the brain is exposed and survival is impossible; diagnosis is usually made by ultrasound in the antenatal period. There are three main types of spina bifida (Fig.14.3):
- Spina bifida occulta. The vertebrae are not fused but the skin is intact. This rarely causes any problems.
- Meningocele. A sac of cerebrospinal fluid is present over the surface of the spine.
- Meningomyelocele. The sac contains cerebrospinal fluid and nervous tissue. Usually, there is no skin cover and the spinal cord is exposed.

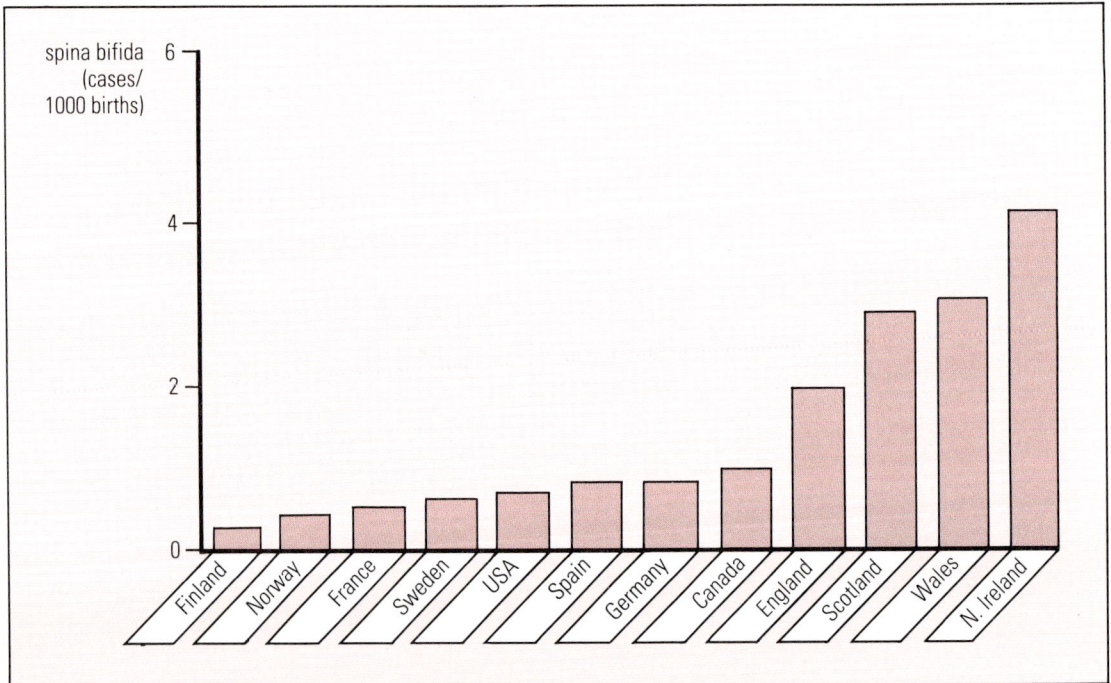

Fig.14.1 Incidence of spina bifida. This condition is much more common in the United Kingdom than elsewhere in the world.

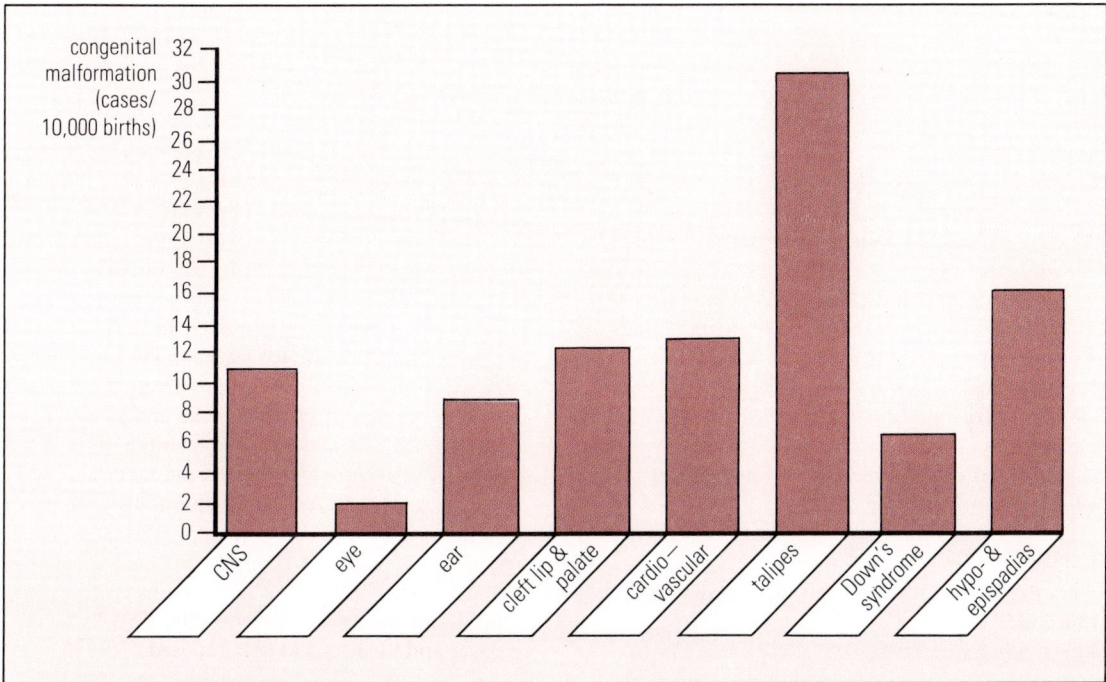

Fig.14.2   Incidence of congenital malformation in England and Wales (1986).

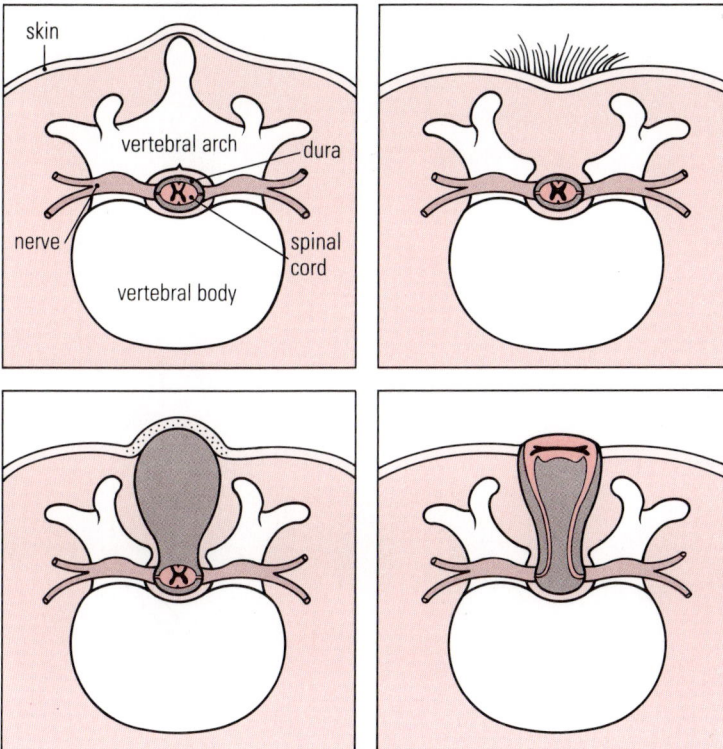

Fig.14.3   Spina bifida. Upper left: normal spine. Upper right: spina bifida occulta. The vertebrae are not fused but the skin is intact. Lower left: meningocele. A sac of cerebrospinal fluid is present over the spinal cord. Lower right: meningomyelocele. The sac of fluid also contains nervous tissue.

211

Meningoceles are found most often at the neck or thorax. They can be repaired shortly after birth and have an excellent prognosis. Meningomyeloceles are most commonly found in the lumbosacral region (Fig.14.4); the prognosis depends on the amount of nervous tissue involved. Such children are physically disabled by hydrocephalus at birth, or paralysis of the lower limbs, anus and bladder sphincters, and they are usually mentally handicapped; other congenital abnormalities may also be present. An urgent operation to close the skin over the lesion is now usually performed only if the prognosis is thought to be good. The back can always be closed later if the child survives.

In most cases of meningomyelocele, hydrocephalus (Fig.14.5) develops and is associated with an abnormality of the cerebellum (the Arnold-Chiari malformation). This can be treated by the use of a shunt with a valve to divert cerebrospinal fluid from the lateral ventricles of the brain into the bloodstream or peritoneal cavity.

A defect at the occiput usually contains brain and is known as an encephalocele. If the amount of brain involved is large the prognosis is hopeless.

Cleft lip and palate

There are two distinct types of cleft palate – a midline cleft which is not associated with a cleft lip, and a cleft on one side of the palate with an abnormality of the lip (Fig.14.6). Bilateral clefts in the palate and lip constitute a very severe abnormality. The main problem shortly after birth is feeding. Some babies

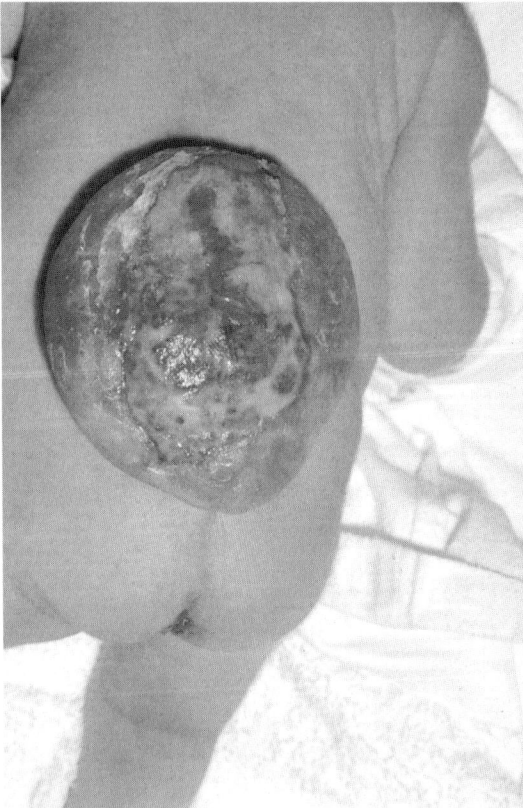

Fig.14.4 Meningomyelocele of the lumbar region; nervous tissue is probably present in the wall of this lesion.

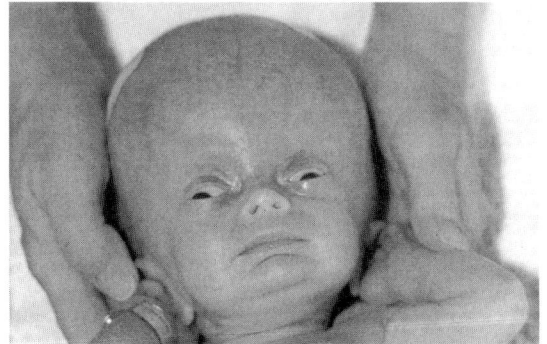

Fig.14.5 Hydrocephalus. The head is characteristically large with a prominent forehead and distended scalp veins.

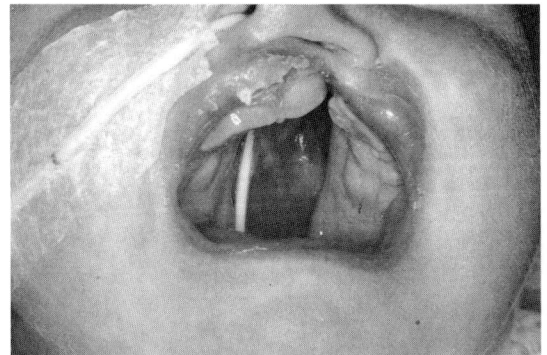

Fig.14.6 Cleft lip and palate.

will suck excellently at the breast, but many need a long teat on a bottle or even to be fed by spoon or tube.

The lip is usually closed by operation at about three months, although some paediatric surgeons will operate in the first week. The palate is repaired towards the end of the first year or during the second but again, some surgeons operate much earlier.

Oesophageal atresia

A baby with oesophageal atresia will present with regurgitation of fluid from the mouth or a cyanotic attack. A tracheo-oesophageal fistula is usually also present (Fig.14.7). Atresia may be diagnosed by passing a large nasogastric tube before offering the first feed. This is particularly important in babies born to mothers who have been diagnosed as having poly-hydramnios in pregnancy. If the condition is recognized and an operation performed early, the outlook is good.

Congenital heart disease

Not all forms of congenital heart disease produce signs or symptoms in the newborn. However, often a murmur is detected or the baby is seen to be blue. The most characteristic sign of heart failure is a large liver; a large heart may be seen on an X-ray examination of the chest.

Congenital heart disease is usually divided into acyanotic and cyanotic abnormalities. The most common acyanotic lesion is ventricular septal defect. A long systolic murmur is heard at the left sternal edge, however, this may not be diagnosed in the neonatal period because the high pulmonary arterial pressure prevents the flow from the left to the right side of the heart. The condition usually has a good prognosis; about eighty percent of these septal defects close spontaneously by eight years of age.

Cyanotic lesions are more serious. Transposition of the great arteries produces very profound cyanosis when the ductus arteriosus closes a few days after birth. A balloon septostomy is life-saving; a catheter is passed into the right atrium and through the foramen ovale into the left atrium. A balloon on the end of the catheter is inflated and the atrial wall is torn by pulling it back, thus causing an artificial atrial septal defect. It is important to get the baby to a cardiac unit urgently. As a first aid measure, an infusion of prostaglandin E_2 can reopen the ductus arteriosus temporarily and reverse the cyanosis for the duration of the journey.

Coarctation of the aorta also produces symptoms when the ductus arteriosus closes. Unlike the adult type, the proximal part of the aorta and the left ventricle are often hypoplastic. At present, there is very little prospect of long-term treatment other than heart transplant.

Recent advances in ultrasound technology allow the diagnosis of cardiac disorders in the antenatal period, so that plans can be made to deliver the baby in hospital with appropriate cardiac facilities. When ultrasound is used in the newborn, an anatomical diagnosis can often be made at the bedside.

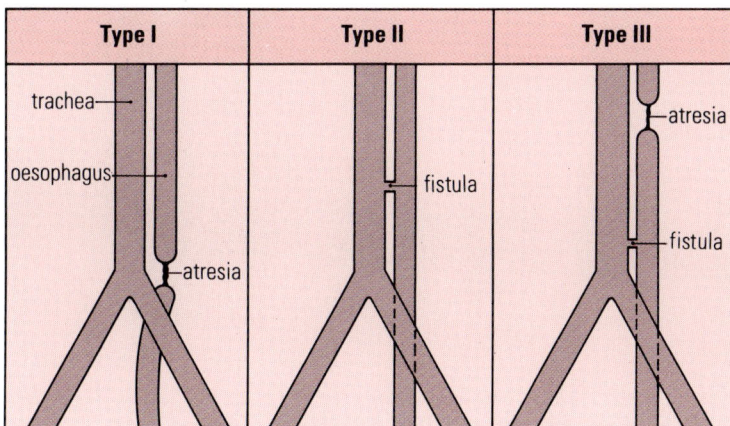

Fig.14.7 Types of tracheo-oesophageal fistula. Left: atresia only. Centre: fistula only. Right: atresia plus fistula. Types II and III allow milk and saliva to pass from the oesophagus into the trachea.

Diaphragmatic hernia

An infant with a diaphragmatic hernia remains cyanosed after birth and usually has dextrocardia. X-ray examination will show gut in the chest, almost always on the left side. Surgery is performed to repair the diaphragm and to return the gut to the abdomen. Unfortunately, the lung on the left is often severely hypoplastic and the baby does not survive. At present the standard policy is to postpone the operation for a day or so to see if the baby survives with ventilation. Since the diagnosis can be made by ultrasound before birth, it is wise for the mother to be delivered in a hospital where a paediatric surgeon can be consulted.

Obstruction of the intestine

There are several types of intestinal obstruction, one of which is associated with Down's syndrome. There is atresia of the duodenum with bilious vomiting and a characteristic X-ray appearance of gas in the stomach and duodenum alone, known as the 'double bubble'

sign. This is often diagnosed by ultrasound in the antenatal period (Fig.14.8). The prognosis is good if an operation is performed.

Obstruction lower in the small intestine, for example atresia in the ileum, causes abdominal distension as well as bile-stained vomiting. Intermittent or partial obstruction may occur with a volvulus, where the gut twists on itself.

Atresia is also common at the anus; this is often diagnosed when the midwife attempts to take the baby's temperature in the rectum. An X-ray examination is performed with the baby upside down. This allows air to reach the rectum, revealing how big a gap is present between the anal dimple and the blind end of the rectum. Several operations are necessary to correct this defect.

Hirschsprung's disease causes spasm of the anal wall. There is delay in passing meconium and the anus feels tight on digital examination. The condition is more common in boys than girls. The diagnosis is made by rectal biopsy, which reveals absence of ganglion cells in the muscle. A colostomy is necessary in the neonate before definitive surgery.

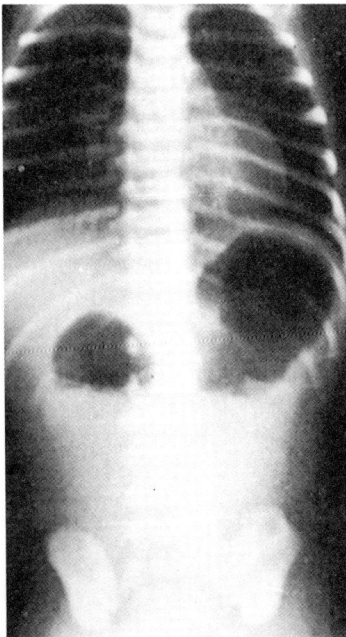

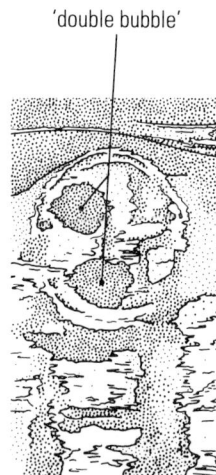

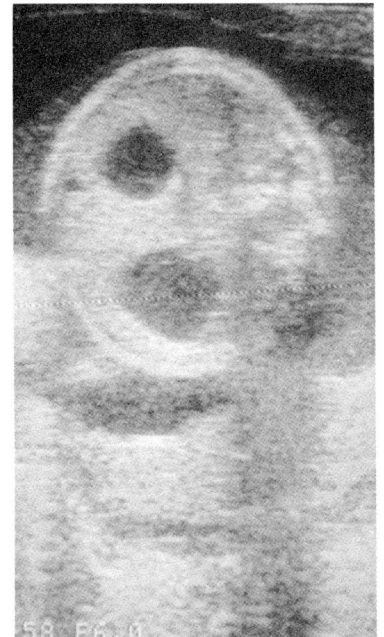

Fig.14.8 Duodenal atresia. Left: X-ray (anteroposterior view) showing characteristic 'double bubble'. Right: antenatal ultrasound (cross-sectional view) showing 'double bubble'. Ultrasound courtesy of Dr. R. Patel.

Exomphalos

In exomphalos the gut protrudes from the umbilicus in a sac. If the lesion is small an operation will correct it but treatment is more complicated with a very large lesion. The latter is now often covered with a special bag which is tightened slowly over a period of time to reduce the gut into the abdomen; an operation can then be performed to close the defect.

Some babies have gastroschisis, in which a defect is present alongside the umbilicus and the protruding gut is not covered in a membrane. This condition has a worse prognosis than exomphalos.

Hypospadias

In this condition, the urethra does not open on the tip of the penis, but on the ventral surface (Fig.14.9). If the opening is on the glans, there should be no functional problem. An opening further down will require surgery.

Renal abnormalities

Renal abnormalities include polycystic disease and obstructive lesions. Ultrasound frequently detects such abnormalities both antenatally and after birth. A large kidney may be found on clinical examination.

Urethral valves may cause obstruction in a boy; the characteristic sign of this is a poor stream of urine. Absent kidneys are invariably fatal, death occurring shortly after birth. In such cases, there is oligohydramnios and the signs of Potter's syndrome from fetal compression – the face is squashed and other deformities, such as talipes, are also present.

Undescended testes

This is very common in preterm babies and may be accompanied by an inguinal hernia; the testes will descend later. In a term baby, an undescended testis may be expected to descend by three months. After this time, referral to a surgeon should be considered because early orchidopexy is thought to reduce the risk of infertility.

Dislocation of the hips

A dislocatable hip detected at the first-day examination needs careful re-examination later in the first week. In many cases it is then found to be normal, but it is important to arrange follow-up, including an X-ray film at about five months of age. The same procedure should be followed for a dislocated hip, but this is less likely to become normal in the first week.

If a dislocatable hip does not return to normal, it

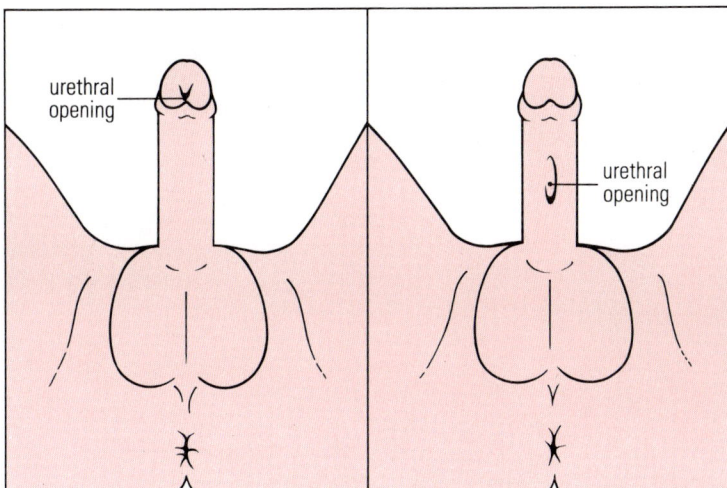

Fig.14.9 Hypospadias. Left: the urethral opening is on the glans. Right: the urethral opening is further down the penis. This is more serious than the first type and requires surgery.

will need to be held in abduction by splinting or a harness. The purpose is to prevent late dislocation, which occurs in about one in a thousand babies and which is more difficult to treat. Dislocation in the neonatal period is much more common (about one in a hundred babies), but treatment at that time should reduce the chances of permanent dislocation. A number of cases of late dislocation still occur; it seems that a shallow acetabulum may not be detectable by clinical examination in the first week, but it is hoped that ultrasound examination will improve the chances of early detection.

Talipes equinovarus

This is by far the most common ankle deformity seen in the newborn. The feet are twisted inwards and

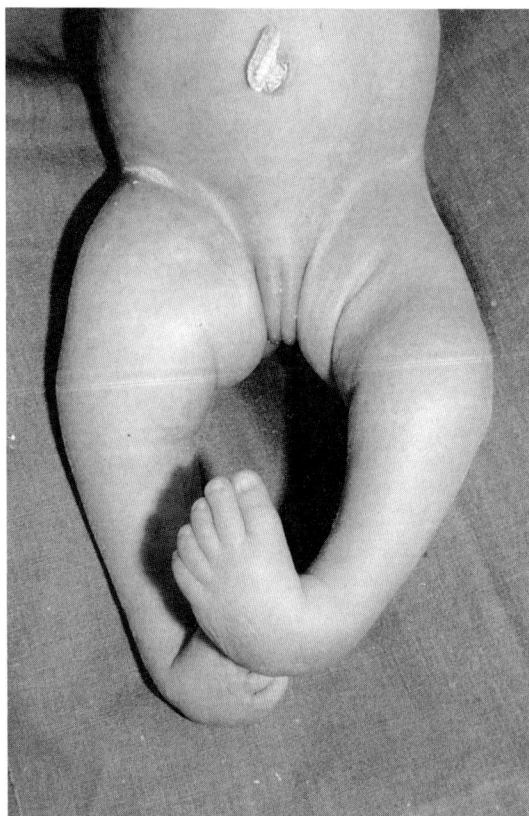

Fig.14.10 Talipes equinovarus. The feet are twisted inwards and downwards.

downwards (Fig.14.10). They cannot be reduced by pressing the sole upwards to make the dorsum of the foot touch the skin of the shin, a manoeuvre which can be performed in babies with normal feet in the position of talipes. It is important to start treatment early by strapping the feet in a good position. A number of babies will need operative treatment later.

Chromosomal disorders

The most common chromosomal disorder is Down's syndrome. It is diagnosed by crowded features in the face, upward slanting eyes (Fig.14.11), Brushfield's spots on the iris, a flat occiput with loose folds of skin behind the neck and small ears. Other characteristic features include hypotonia, a single transverse crease in each palm, a short curved little finger and a longitudinal crease in the sole.

The disorder is more common in babies from older women (see Chapter 3) and it is confirmed in the newborn by chromosomal analysis of white blood cells. Analysis shows an extra chromosome, trisomy 21 (see Fig.3.33). It is important to recognize that in a few cases the extra chromosome comes from the father; the condition should not be blamed on the mother. Breaking the news of the diagnosis requires skill and compassion. It is best to tell both parents together, with only a few people present, and to explain clearly what the future holds. Many people do not realize that a child with Down's syndrome may go to school, but think that they are all very severely mentally retarded. Many parents will want antenatal diagnosis for chromosome disorders in the next pregnancy; the recurrence rate is thought to be about one percent.

Other chromosomal disorders are less common, but often more severe. Trisomy of chromosomes 13 or 18 produces a number of severe congenital abnormalities including heart defects and very severe mental handicap. All of these babies die before two years of age.

Many congenital malformations and inborn errors of metabolism are inherited according to Mendelian principles. Inborn errors are particularly likely to be inherited in an autosomal recessive fashion: minor congenital abnormalities, such as extra digits on the ulnar side of the hands, are likely to be autosomal dominant conditions (Fig.14.12). Many abnormalities appear to be the result of polygenic inheritance, that is, inheritance influenced by several genes as well as environmental factors.

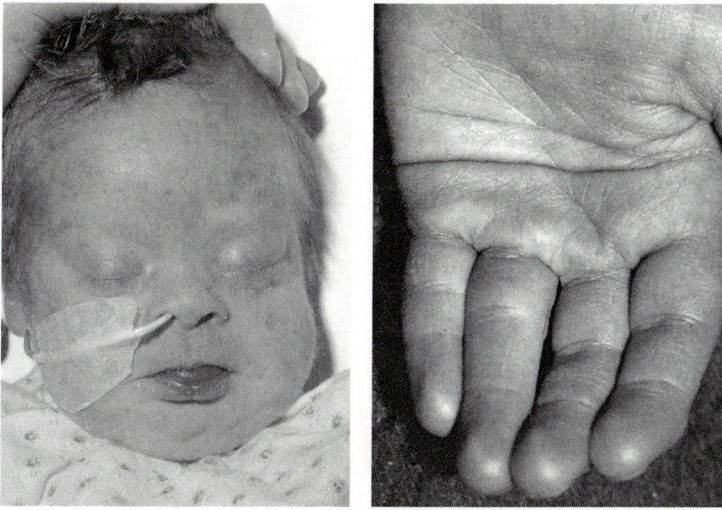

Fig.14.11 Down's syndrome. Left: the features are crowded and the eyes slant upwards. Right: a single transverse crease is present in each palm.

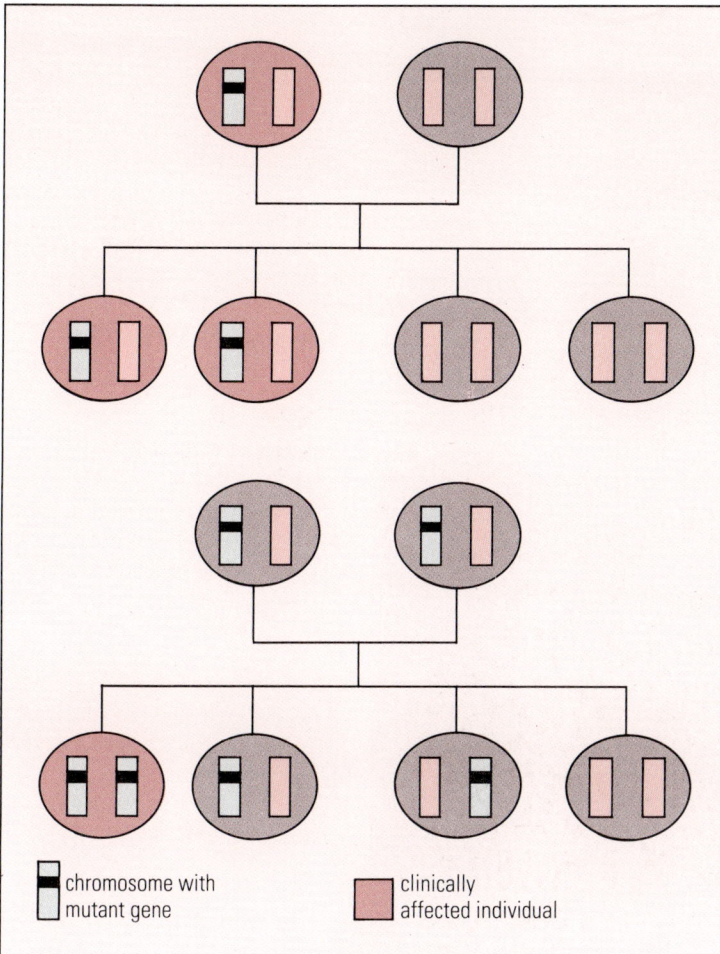

Fig.14.12 Inheritance of congenital disorders. Upper: autosomal dominant condition. The mutant gene is always expressed; the condition can be passed on from mother or father to daughter or son. Lower: autosomal recessive condition. The condition arises only when 2 mutant genes occur together. The parents are apparently normal; 1 in 4 of their children is affected.

chromosome with mutant gene

clinically affected individual

Birth trauma

Physical injury to the baby at birth in the United Kingdom is now less common since fewer women deliver without a skilled attendant. Brain damage from traumatic intracranial haemorrhage after a difficult forceps delivery is rare, and damage to the spinal cord during breech delivery is now almost unknown.

Soft tissue injuries

Bruising may be seen over the presenting part, for example over the buttocks after breech delivery or on the head following vacuum extraction. Sometimes there is an abrasion of the skin caused by forceps, but this rarely leaves a scar.

Necrosis of the subcutaneous fat sometimes occurs at a pressure point. Hard, mobile lumps appear under the skin on the cheeks, over the parietal bones, or on the elbows a few days after birth; they resolve within a few weeks.

Bruising under the periosteum of the skull bones results in a cephalhaematoma. The swelling is confined to the area of the bruising (Fig.14.13) and, since it is under the periosteum, to the parietal bone, or the occipital bone.

Fractures

The clavicle may break when the shoulders are delivered (Fig.14.14). It is usually not noticed at the time, but a lump is found on the clavicle a couple of weeks later. Careful examination in the first week may show that the baby is moving the arm less on the side of the fracture.

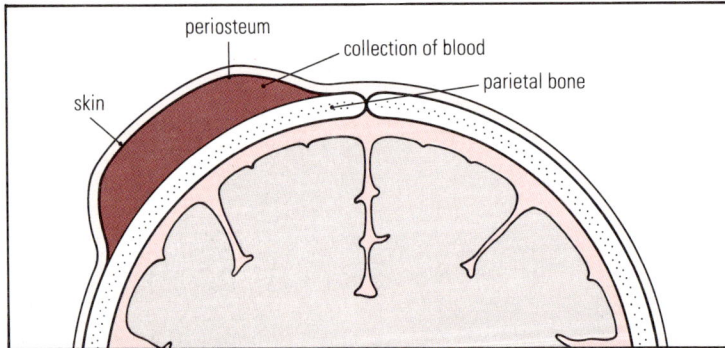

Fig.14.13 Cephalhaematoma. Blood is present under the periosteum and is therefore confined to the area of the parietal bone.

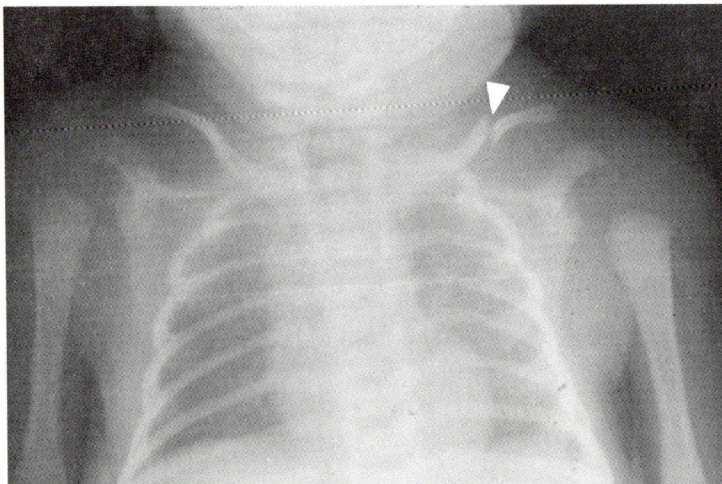

Fig.14.14 Fractured clavicle (arrow). Callus usually forms within days.

Lack of movement is more obvious when the humerus fractures. This happens when the arm is brought down in breech delivery. Fracture of the femur may occur in a breech birth, but may also happen without any history of trauma.

Nerve injuries

The facial nerve can be damaged by pressure on the cheek during forceps delivery, but damage can also occur at a normal birth. The mouth is drawn to one side when the baby cries (Fig.14.15) and there is difficulty in closing the eye on the paralysed side, however, the facial nerve usually recovers completely.

Damage to the brachial plexus occurs during shoulder dystocia and is likely to happen when the baby is large. Damage to the nerves occurs when the head is pulled in an attempt to deliver the shoulders.

With damage to the upper part of the plexus (Erb's palsy), the arm is held in the waiter's tip position (Fig.14.16). Most cases recover completely, but a few children remain unable to lift or abduct the arm.

Birth asphyxia

Hypoxia is present to some extent at every birth. In severe asphyxia there is apnoea and bradycardia, or even cardiac arrest. In mild cases the baby is cyanosed, but in severe cases he is pale from shock. Blood gas analysis reveals a marked metabolic and respiratory acidaemia. The effects are more severe in a preterm baby.

The baby is assessed with the Apgar score (see Chapter 13). A score of three or less at one minute indicates severe asphyxia, but the most important parts of the score are heart rate and respiration.

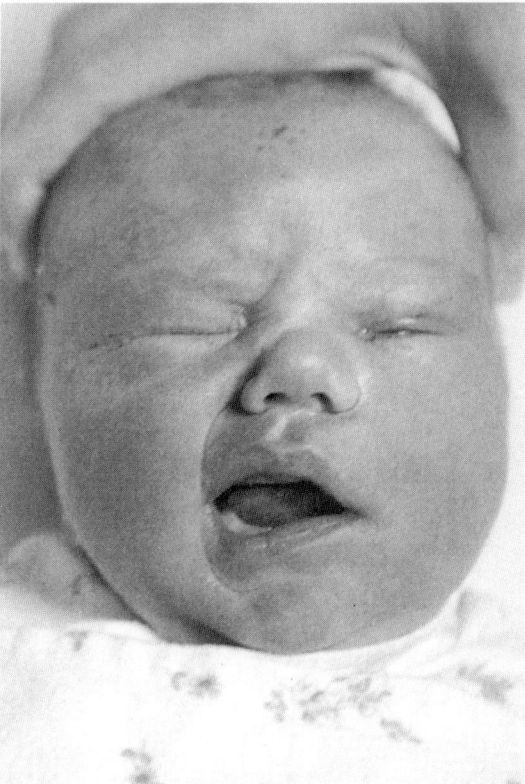

Fig.14.15 Left facial nerve paralysis. The lower face is affected so that the mouth is drawn to one side when the baby cries.

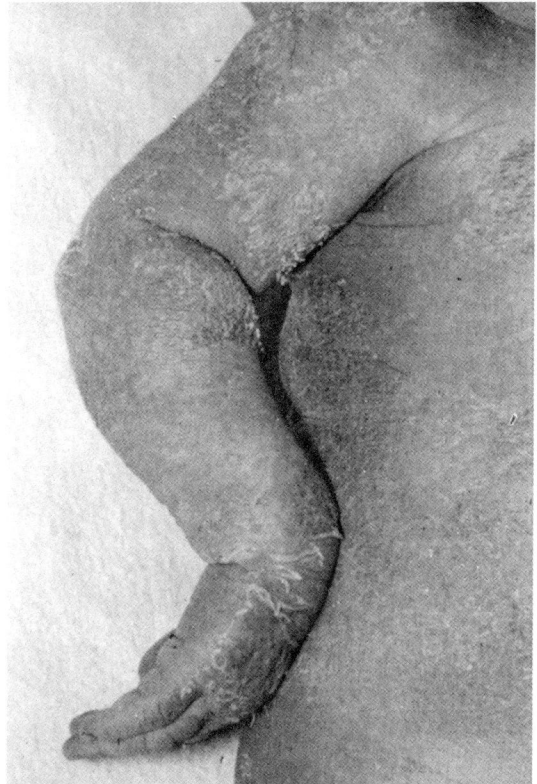

Fig.14.16 Erb's palsy. The arm is adducted at the shoulder, extended at the elbow, internally rotated and flexed at the wrist.

219

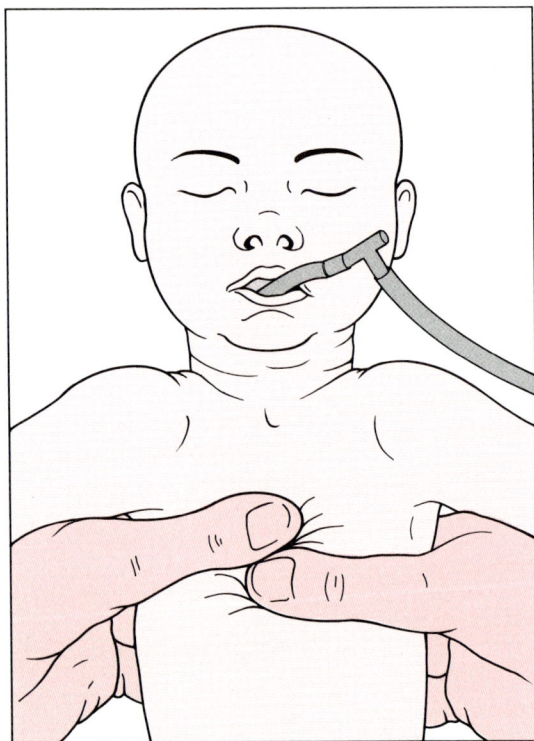

Fig.14.17 Technique for external cardiac massage. The baby is held around the chest with both hands while both thumbs are used to massage the heart.

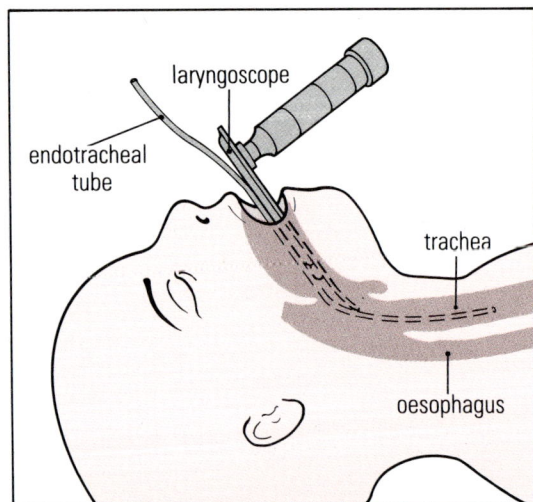

Fig.14.18 Technique for intubation. A laryngoscope is passed into the mouth, allowing visualization of the larynx. An endotracheal tube is then inserted into the larynx and the laryngoscope is withdrawn.

Cardiac arrest

If cardiac arrest occurs the baby must be given cardiac massage. This can be done by pressing regularly on the sternum (Fig.14.17); intubation and ventilation of the lungs must also be performed. If the heart rate is very slow (less than 60 beats/minute) at birth, repeated cardiac massage will often cause it to speed up.

Apnoea

A baby who is not breathing by one minute will need some form of artificial ventilation. This can be done with a bag and mask, but the mask should be circular in order to provide a good seal on the face. Slow, long inflations should be used and the chest must be observed to be certain that air is entering the lungs.

A term baby who has not breathed by two or three minutes and whose heart rate and colour are not responding to bag and mask ventilation will need intubation of the trachea (Fig.14.18). A laryngoscope is passed into the mouth so that the larynx can be seen and any mucus or meconium is carefully aspirated. A tube is then passed into the trachea and the lungs are inflated. Inflations at least one second long are used; they must be carefully controlled to avoid excessive pressure. The pressure is limited to $30 cmH_2O$ by the use of a blow-off valve or a bag appropriate for inflating the lungs of the newborn.

Endotracheal intubation is particularly important for a preterm baby of under thirty weeks gestation. If asphyxia is not treated promptly, the baby is likely to suffer severe respiratory distress and will need prolonged ventilation.

The respiratory acidaemia is improved by the ventilation, and the metabolic acidaemia will improve when the baby is properly oxygenated. When a baby is profoundly asphyxiated, sodium bicarbonate will improve the metabolic acidaemia.

Babies who have not breathed spontaneously by twenty-five minutes of age are likely either to die or to suffer brain damage.

Meconium aspiration

During intrapartum hypoxia, meconium is passed into the amniotic fluid and is aspirated during the respiratory gasps which occur in the uterus as a result of asphyxia. This can lead to severe respiratory distress. After birth, any meconium must immediately be aspirated from the mouth; the larynx should be inspected and the trachea aspirated if there is any evidence of meconium inhalation. Since meconium is thick, it is often best to apply mechanical suction to the endotracheal tube, which is then removed with the aspirated meconium inside and on the end (Fig.14.19). Some believe that the chest should be held tightly until this has been done to prevent inspiration,

which would draw the meconium down into the lungs.

JAUNDICE

Almost every newborn baby becomes jaundiced to some extent; this may be due to several factors (Fig.14.20). The baby has to switch from the excretion

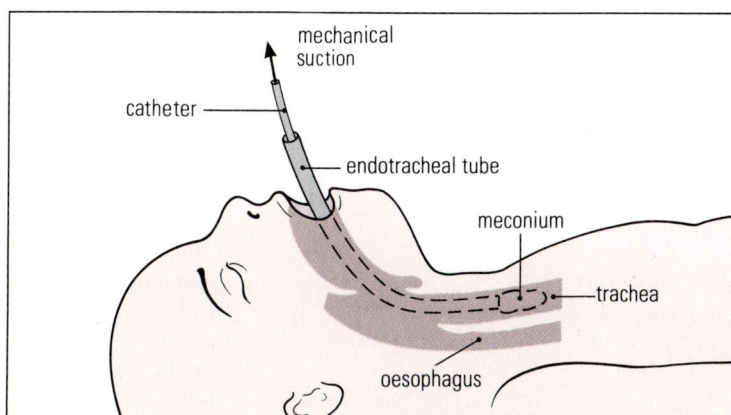

Fig.14.19 Removal of aspirated meconium. This used to be done by the operator sucking on the tube, but is now considered dangerous because of the risk of infection. Gentle mechanical suction is therefore applied to the pharynx and down into the endotracheal tube if there is any suspicion that meconium has been aspirated into the trachea.

| CAUSES OF JAUNDICE ||
Unconjugated bilirubin	Conjugated bilirubin

Haemolytic disorders
  rhesus isoimmunization
  ABO incompatibility
  red cell enzyme defects
  (glucose-6-dehydrogenase deficiency)
  hereditary spherocytosis
Infections
  septicaemia
  urinary tract infections
Bruising/haematomas
  cephalhaematoma
  bruising in breech delivery
Polycythaemia
  twin transfusion syndrome
  delayed cord clamping
Deconjugation in gut
  breast milk jaundice
Failure of conjugation
  preterm birth
	Extrahepatic obstruction
	  congenital biliary atresia

Fig.14.20 Causes of jaundice. Jaundice occurs when the production of bilirubin exceeds the liver's ability to conjugate bilirubin. Bilirubin levels are increased in haemolytic disease, infection and polycythaemia. Preterm birth is a common cause of jaundice since the liver is not yet ready for conjugation. Jaundice also occurs in some breast-fed babies because it is thought that conjugated bilirubin is converted to the unconjugated form and reabsorbed.

of unconjugated bilirubin through the biliary tract; there is therefore a rise in plasma bilirubin (Fig.14.21) and about fifty percent of newborn babies appear clinically jaundiced. It is thought that the enzyme glucuronyl transferase, responsible for the conjugation of bilirubin in the liver, is often not fully functional at birth. This phenomenon used to be called physiological jaundice. The condition appears slowly after the first day, reaching its peak at about five or six days postpartum.

The most important influence on jaundice is gestational age (Fig.14.22). Higher plasma bilirubin concentrations are much more common in the preterm baby and are dangerous because of the risk of brain damage. Like most illnesses in the first week of life, jaundice is more common in boys than girls.

Any factor which increases the production of bilirubin in the baby's body will cause jaundice. Most bilirubin is produced from haemoglobin contained in the red blood cells; haemoglobin is released when the red blood cells break down, so haemolysis causes the plasma bilirubin to rise rapidly. Jaundice in the first twenty-four hours of life is a serious sign and must be investigated.

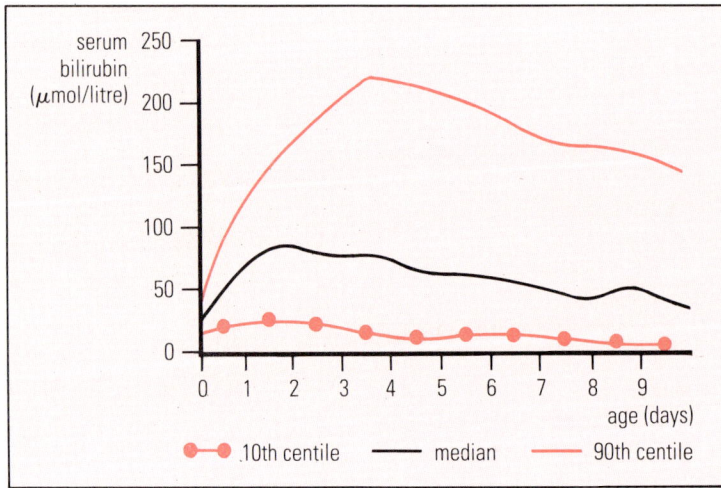

Fig.14.21 Serum bilirubin concentrations in newborn infants.

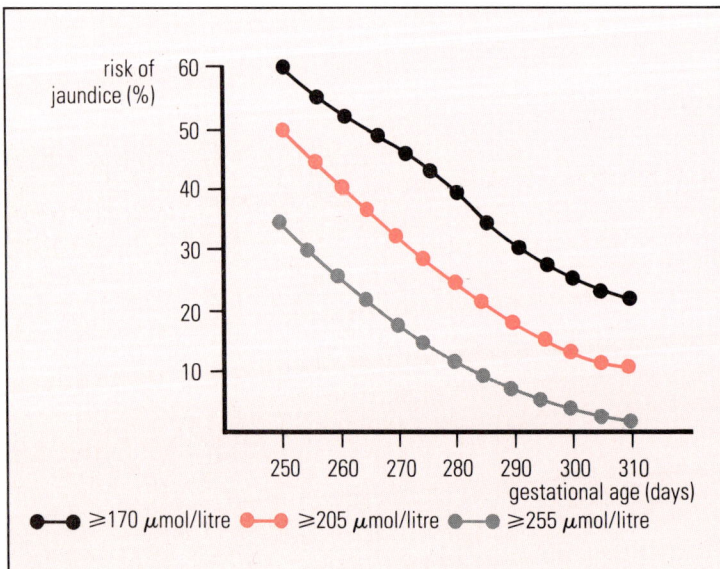

Fig.14.22 Risk of jaundice with gestational age. Each trace shows the percentage of babies reaching a particular plasma bilirubin concentration.

Rhesus isoimmunization

In Europe, rhesus isoimmunization has become less common in the last decade because of the use of anti-D antibody. This is given to Rh-negative women after the birth of an Rh-positive baby (see Chapter 5) and after any event in early pregnancy which might have facilitated transfusion of fetal blood into the mother (for example amniocentesis). There are three major rhesus groups, but anti-D and anti-c are the most commonly found antibodies and produce the most severe effects. In many parts of the world rhesus disease is almost unknown, for instance, in China almost everyone is Rh-positive.

An Rh-negative mother can be sensitized by fetal Rh-positive red cells which may leak into her circulation, usually at delivery. This transplacental haemorrhage can occur during pregnancy and anti-D may be given at twenty-eight and thirty-six weeks. A woman with rhesus isoimmunization is monitored during pregnancy by measuring the titre of antibodies in her blood and, if this rises, the level of bilirubin is measured in a sample of amniotic fluid obtained by amniocentesis. Treatment in pregnancy of a severely affected fetus by intraperitoneal, and now intravascular, transfusion greatly improves the baby's condition at birth.

The main signs of rhesus disease are anaemia, oedema and jaundice. The state of the baby at birth is assessed by clinical examination, which will show oedema (hydrops fetalis) and pallor, and by tests on cord blood (blood group, Coombs' haemoglobin and plasma bilirubin). The Coombs' test is positive when there are anti-D antibodies on the baby's Rh-positive red cells. The test may be falsely negative, and the blood group apparently Rh-negative, if the baby has received a transfusion of Rh-negative blood before birth.

If haemoglobin is low at birth (less than 12g/dl), an immediate transfusion is indicated. This will also be necessary if the baby is very ill with severe hydrops; such cases usually also need intensive care (Fig.14.23), including ventilation, because of pulmonary oedema. Jaundice is not present at birth because the bilirubin produced by the fetus is cleared through the placenta, but it will develop rapidly thereafter and become severe if action is not taken.

Other causes of haemolysis

ABO incompatibility probably occurs quite often, but may not be recognized because it produces a milder illness than rhesus isoimmunization; the first baby is often affected. It is likely that there are natural antigens in food which can cause sensitization. The mother is group O, and the baby is A or B. Anaemia is not common, but there can be severe jaundice.

Glucose-6-phosphate dehydrogenase deficiency is a sex-linked disorder which is carried by the mother and passed on to half of her sons. It can produce severe neonatal jaundice in males and a milder condition in female carriers. When the enzyme is absent from the red cell envelope, haemolysis occurs; the condition is aggravated by the presence of substances such as naphthalene or sulphonamides. In some parts of the world cord blood is screened for the condition, which is common in South-East Asia, the Caribbean and the Mediterranean.

Congenital spherocytosis is not common, but it is important to make the diagnosis as the affected child will probably need splenectomy later. It is an autosomal dominant condition, so one of the parents is usually affected. A blood film will show red cells which are spherical instead of the usual disc shape.

Other causes of jaundice

Extravasated blood is a frequent cause of jaundice. It is seen in a preterm baby after breech delivery where there is bruising of the buttocks and legs. It is also common with a cephalhaematoma.

Thyroid hormones increase the conjugation of

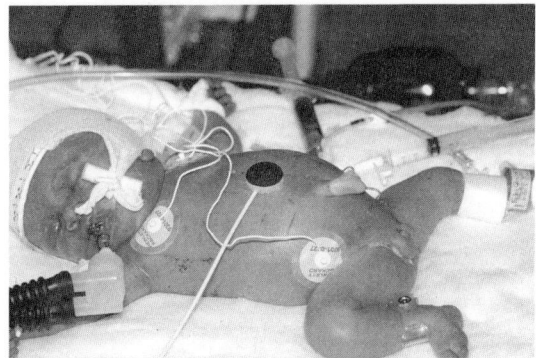

Fig.14.23 Rhesus affected baby with gross oedema receiving intensive care.

bilirubin in the liver, and hypothyroidism is a cause of prolonged jaundice. Since there is now a screening test for the condition, it is usually diagnosed.

Another cause of jaundice prolonged beyond two weeks of age is breast feeding. The milk of some women contains an enzyme which unconjugates the bilirubin that has been excreted into the baby's gut. This bilirubin is then absorbed into the enterohepatic circulation and causes jaundice.

Kernicterus

The main problem in neonatal jaundice is kernicterus, where bilirubin stains and damages basal ganglia in the brain. This results in athetoid cerebral palsy, sensorineural deafness and mental handicap. When it occurs in the newborn, there are often convulsions, abnormalities of tone such as opisthotonos, and an abnormal Moro reaction, in which repeated extension of the arms occurs.

Kernicterus is believed to occur most frequently in babies who are acidaemic and preterm. Most unconjugated bilirubin is bound to albumin in the blood. However, if the albumin is saturated because the plasma bilirubin is very high, free bilirubin will be circulating; this can then cross into the brain cells. It is also likely that the blood–brain barrier may be made more permeable by insults such as asphyxia.

The principles of treatment are to keep the baby in a good general condition and to prevent the plasma bilirubin from reaching dangerously high concentrations. These are around 350–380μmol/litre for a baby at term and 250μmol/litre for those of less than thirty weeks gestation. Intermediate values are chosen for babies who are only a few weeks preterm. Lower values are used for ill babies who are at greater risk of suffering brain damage.

Conjugated bilirubinaemia

Jaundice sometimes occurs at the end of the first week of life and appears more green than the sunny orange of unconjugated bilirubinaemia. This may be obstructive jaundice and will need careful investigation and perhaps surgical treatment. Conjugated bilirubinaemia sometimes occurs in rhesus disease, but the two main causes are congenital biliary obstruction and hepatitis.

Treatment

It is possible to encourage the conjugation of bilirubin with drugs; phenobarbitone is known to do this, but is not commonly used because of the sedation it produces.

Phototherapy

The most commonly used treatment for jaundice is light, which acts on the bilirubin in the skin and converts it into photobilirubin, a harmless pigment. Blue light is the most effective, but it is usual to use white light (which includes the blue end of the spectrum) as it is more comfortable for those nursing the baby and does not give the appearance of cyanosis. It is administered using a strong light source above the incubator or cot in a dose which is greater than 0.1mW/cm^2. Because it is so bright and uncomfortable, it is usual to cover the baby's eyes with a mask, even though there is no evidence that they can be damaged by the light.

Phototherapy is usually started as soon as jaundice appears in a rhesus baby or in a preterm baby in an incubator. Otherwise, the indication is a plasma bilirubin level about 50–80μmol/litre below the estimated danger level for kernicterus.

Many babies become irritable under phototherapy and have loose dark-green stools. Water loss through the skin is increased and so frequent suckling at the breast should be encouraged. When groups of babies receiving light therapy have been compared with controls, it has been shown to be a very effective method of treatment for neonatal jaundice (Fig.14.24).

Exchange transfusion

Plasma bilirubin levels can be reduced very rapidly by exchange transfusion. A catheter is passed into the umbilical vein and samples of 10ml of blood are removed and replaced with fresh blood (Fig.14.25). Rh-negative blood is used in rhesus disease to prevent the Rh-antibodies from causing more haemolysis. The baby's estimated blood volume is 80–90ml/kg; twice this volume is used during the exchange transfusion, which is performed over a period of two hours. The treatment causes a sudden drop in the plasma bilirubin, but there is a tendency for it to rise again in the first few hours after transfusion.

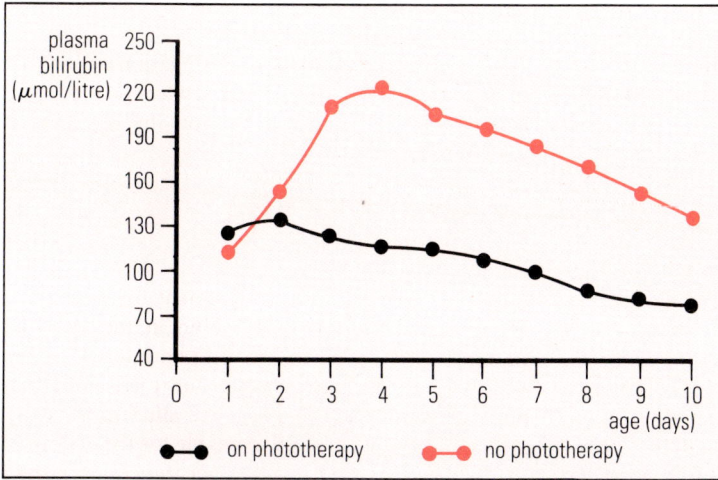

Fig.14.24 The effect of phototherapy on plasma bilirubin levels in jaundiced babies.

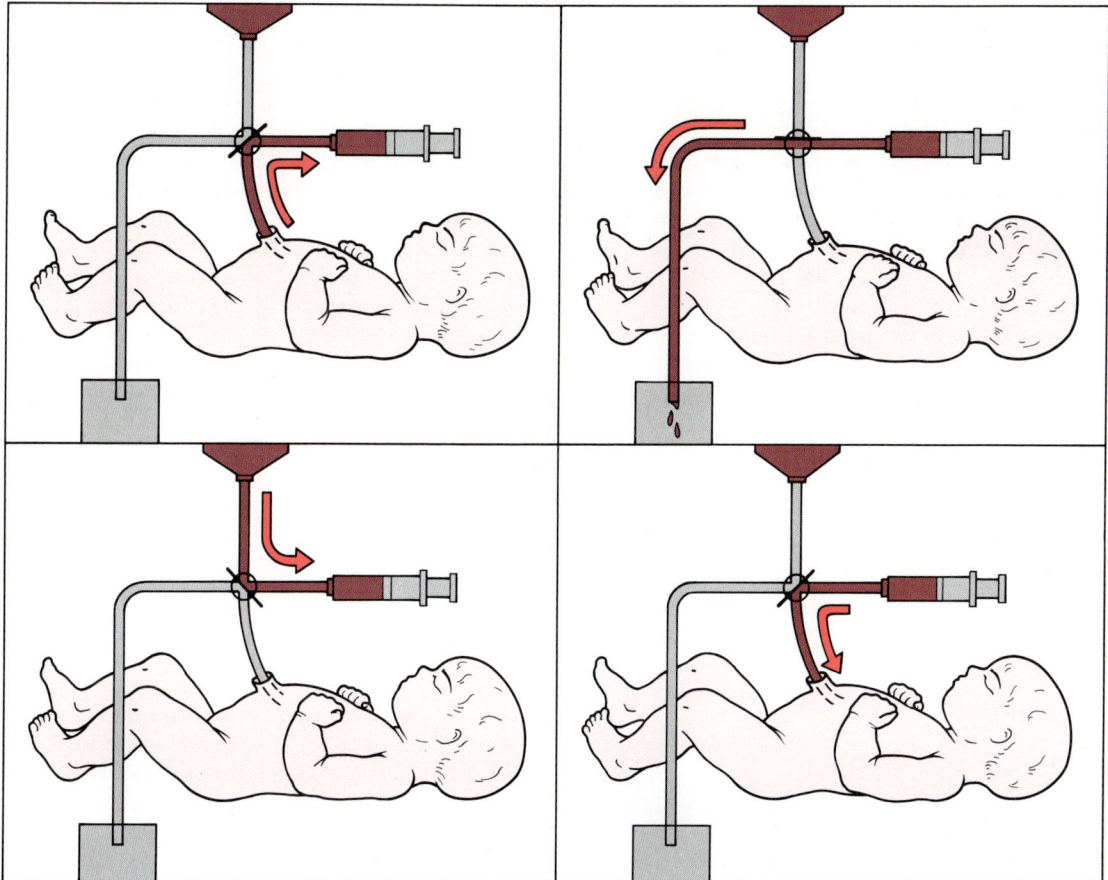

Fig.14.25 Exchange transfusion. Upper left: blood is drawn into the syringe via an umbilical vein catheter. Upper right: this blood is then discarded into a waste container. Lower left: fresh blood, warmed to body temperature, is drawn into the syringe. Lower right: this blood is slowly injected into the baby.

The indication for exchange transfusion is to prevent the plasma bilirubin concentration from approaching a level where kernicterus is likely to occur.

INFECTIONS

Newborn babies, not having the same defences as older children or adults, are particularly prone to infection and the infecting organisms are unusual. It is important for every hospital to monitor the bacterial flora of newborn babies, as this has shown a number of changes over recent decades. Infections with group A haemolytic streptococci are now rare. Serious sepsis due to *Staphylococcus aureus* is now less common than before, although minor skin sepsis is common and methicillin-resistant organisms are found in some infants. *Escherichia coli* and group B β-haemolytic streptococci (GBS) are relatively common; in some neonatal units *Pseudomonas aeruginosa* is a problem. *Staphylococcus epidermidis* has recently emerged as a common cause of neonatal septicaemia throughout the world. In some countries, *Listeria monocytogenes* is common as a cause of meningitis; in other countries, such as the United Kingdom, it is uncommon, although the number of cases has recently increased.

Prolonged rupture of the amniotic membranes allows the baby to be infected before birth, but both *Listeria* and GBS can cross intact membranes. Fever of the mother during late pregnancy or early labour is a sign of infection. Careful hygiene, especially hand-washing by staff, is the most important factor in preventing cross-infection.

Umbilical infection

A baby is usually born microbiologically sterile, but the body is quickly colonized and the umbilical cord stump is a favourite site of infection. After birth it is usual to leave the umbilicus uncovered, but many neonatal units apply a small amount of disinfectant such as hexachlorophane powder or chlorhexidene. When the cord separates at three to seven days after birth, the stump is often rather sticky. If an area of inflammation occurs around the stump it will need treatment with antibiotics. There is a danger that infection may spread up the umbilical vein to the liver and peritoneum.

Conjunctivitis

A sticky eye is very common and can be treated with saline swabbing, but serious purulent conjunctivitis (neonatal ophthalmia) needs urgent investigation and treatment. Gonococcal infection of the eye (see Chapter 6) is now uncommon, but chlamydial infections (Fig.14.26) are seen more frequently. Penicillin is used locally and systemically for gonorrhoea. Chlamydial infection is treated with local tetracycline and systemic erythromycin; local neomycin is used for other bacterial infections.

Staphylococcal infections

Although these are now less common than in the 1950s, they are often seen in a minor form. Pustules may appear around the neck or in the groins. They usually appear in infants who are over three days old, unlike the pustules of the eosinophil rash which occur in the first few days and in which the pustule fluid contains eosinophils and not neutrophils; urticarial papules and salmon-pink patches may also be present. A staphylococcal infection needs treatment with flucloxacillin, whereas the eosinophil rash is quite harmless and does not. More serious infections with *Staphylococcus aureus*, such as subcutaneous abscesses, pneumonia, and osteomyelitis are uncommon. Septicaemia with *Staphylococcus epidermidis* can be difficult to treat as many strains are

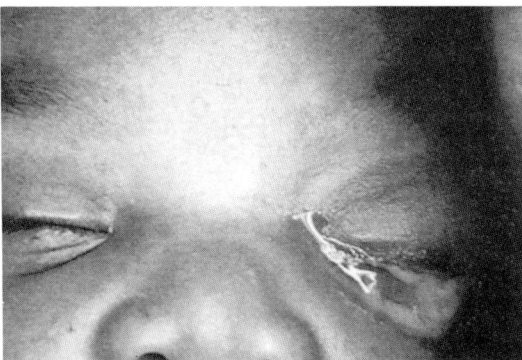

Fig.14.26 Neonatal ophthalmia due to chlamydial infection.

resistant to flucloxacillin. Other drugs, such as vancomycin, may be needed.

Septicaemia and meningitis

These are usually considered together because septicaemia is always a precursor of meningitis. The signs are frequently non-specific, since neonatal infection often does not show any localizing signs. Hypothermia is as common as fever. The baby may show poor peripheral circulation, acidaemia, jaundice, vomiting or general signs of ill health. Neck stiffness is very unusual in meningitis, so a lumbar puncture is indicated whenever a serious infection is suspected. In the first three days of life, the white blood cell count may normally be very high (up to 30×10^{-9} cells/litre), so a very low count is often more indicative of infection than a high one.

The essential investigation is a blood culture. This is supplemented by a skin swab (usually from the axilla) and a mouth or nose swab to show which micro-organisms have colonized the baby. If congenital infection is suspected, a swab from the ear will reflect any organisms present in the amniotic fluid.

Antibiotic therapy must be started as soon as serious infection is suspected, while awaiting the results of the cultures. The antibiotics must be chosen with knowledge of the bacterial flora in the neonatal unit; penicillin or ampicillin with gentamicin are commonly used. Alternatively, one of the newer cephalosporins, such as cefotaxime, may be chosen. The policy of starting treatment whenever there is any suspicion of infection means that many babies will be treated unnecessarily. If a baby is well and the cultures are negative after forty-eight hours, treatment can be stopped.

Meningitis may be caused by GBS or *E. coli*, and is a very difficult condition to treat. Chloramphenicol has been used in the past, but this requires very careful monitoring of blood levels; the cephalosporins are now more commonly prescribed.

Urinary tract infection

The first month of life is the only time when these infections are more common in males than females. They present like septicaemia with non-specific signs such as general illness, vomiting and jaundice. A culture of an uncontaminated specimen of urine is essential; it is often necessary to take a specimen by suprapubic puncture to confirm the diagnosis. All proven cases must be investigated by ultrasound and radiology.

Necrotizing enterocolitis

This mysterious and serious illness has become a major problem in neonatal units. Cases occur in clusters so it appears to be an infection, but no causative organism has been discovered. The condition usually occurs in a baby who has received intensive care. The infant appears generally unwell, has abdominal distension, bilious vomiting and blood in the stools. X-ray examination shows a characteristic picture, with gas in the bowel wall or portal tract (Fig.14.27). The most feared complication is intestinal perforation; the X-ray film then shows gas in the peritoneum.

Necrotizing enterocolitis is usually treated with penicillin, gentamicin and metronidazole. However, vancomycin has been used recently and there is now doubt about whether metronidazole need be given. Surgery is often needed to resect the abnormal gut, but many babies die.

Neonatal tetanus

Although now almost unknown in industrialized countries, umbilical stump infection with tetanus is very common in many parts of the world where the umbilical cord is prone to contamination. The baby becomes ill towards the end of the first week of life; poor feeding is commonly the first sign, and is followed by characteristic spasms and *risus sardonicus*. Tube feeding and sedation are necessary, with ventilation where available. The infection can be prevented by good hygiene at birth and immunization against tetanus, either in infancy or by giving two injections of the toxoid in pregnancy.

Congenital viral infections

Congenital rubella still occurs, although it could be prevented by universal immunization. The most dangerous time for the mother to have the infection is in the first trimester when abortion or congenital abnormalities, such as patent ductus, cataracts, or microcephaly may result. Mental retardation is also a

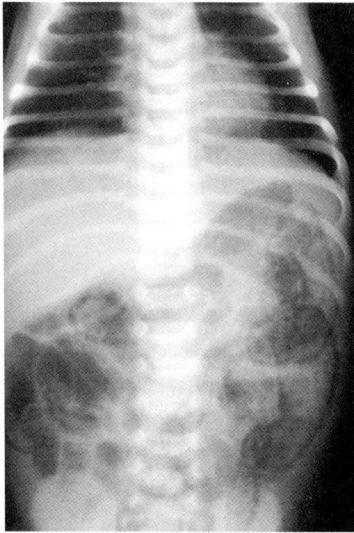

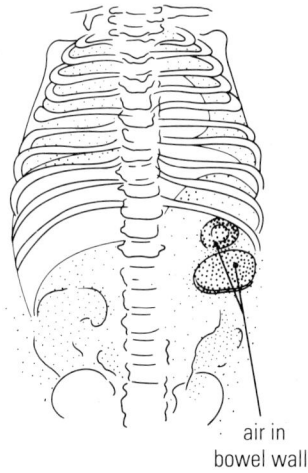

Fig.14.27 Necrotizing enterocolitis. X-ray examination reveals a characteristic picture of air in the bowel wall.

air in
bowel wall

common complication. Even when infection occurs late in pregnancy, nerve deafness may result.

Congenital cytomegalovirus infection is more common than rubella, and may also have serious consequences for the baby, with mental handicap as one of the results. Such a congenital viral infection should be suspected when a baby is born with hepato-splenomegaly, purpura and anaemia. Jaundice is also a common sign. Most children with the infection do not show any signs at birth. Blood products are now screened to reduce the risk of infection by transfusion.

Toxoplasmosis, a protozoal infection which occurs much more commonly in Europe than in Britain, produces a similar syndrome of congenital infection. It also produces hydrocephalus and choroiditis. Pregnant women should avoid contact with cat faeces, which are often contaminated with cysts.

Herpes simplex causes a generalized infection with encephalitis; those infants who survive are often profoundly mentally and physically handicapped. The disease may result from a primary infection in labour while passing through an infected vagina, but can also be caught from a skin lesion on the mother or staff in the maternity unit.

Congenital chickenpox can cause serious illness if the lesions appear on the mother at about the time of delivery. Infection with coxsackie B virus can cause myocarditis.

Carriage of the hepatitis B virus is common in many parts of the world, particularly in East Asia and Africa. A screening test for the hepatitis B antigen is performed on pregnant women in many developed countries. A baby can be infected with hepatitis B at birth, which may result in liver cancer in middle age. The mother is infectious if her blood is positive for the E antigen. In this case, the baby is given immuno-globulin to protect against immediate infection and immunization for long-term protection.

15. The Preterm Baby

The three major causes of death and morbidity in the neonatal period are:
- low birth weight
- congenital abnormalities
- birth asphyxia

Of these, the first is the most common. Although a baby who is small-for-dates may have hypoglycaemia, there are rarely many problems. The small preterm baby has many more difficulties; the two main hazards are respiratory distress syndrome and periventricular haemorrhage. With modern intensive care (Fig.15.1), it is expected that over ninety percent of babies at twenty-eight weeks and over fifty percent at twenty-six weeks gestation will survive (Fig.15.2). At present, the lower limit of gestation at which survival is possible is twenty-four weeks.

The principles of the care of the newborn are:
- adequate respiration
- warmth
- nutrition
- freedom from infection (see Chapter 14)
- love

All the hazards of birth, particularly asphyxia and hypothermia, are worse for a preterm baby.

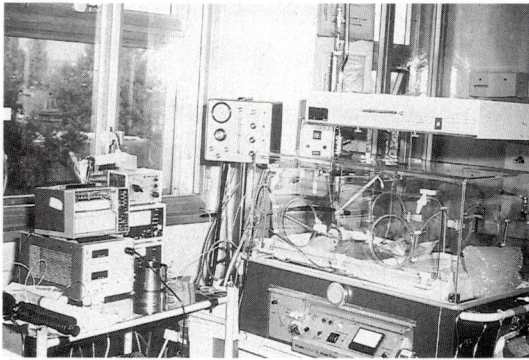

Fig.15.1 Infant in intensive care unit. Note the large amount of equipment needed to monitor the baby and sustain life.

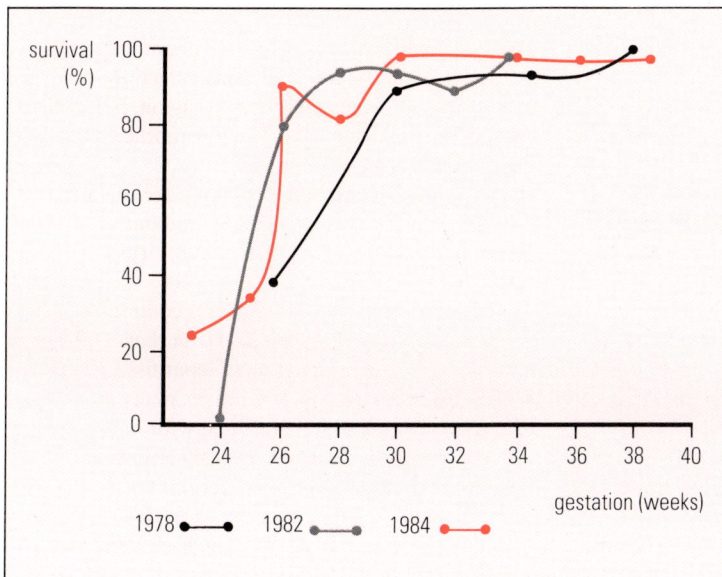

Fig.15.2 Percentage survival of infants according to gestational age (excluding lethal malformations). More babies are now surviving at gestations which were once thought to be incompatible with life. Redrawn from Fleming, P.J. *The management of the preterm baby at birth.* In Beard, R.W. & Sharp, F. (1985) Preterm labour and its consequences. London: RCOG.

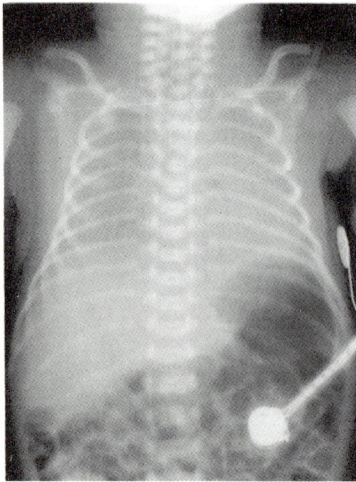

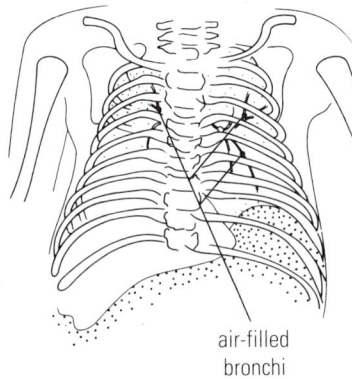

Fig.15.3 Respiratory distress syndrome. X-ray showing characteristic ground-glass appearance caused by collapse of some of the alveoli. An 'air bronchogram' appearance, caused by the contrast of air-filled bronchi against collapsed lung, is also shown.

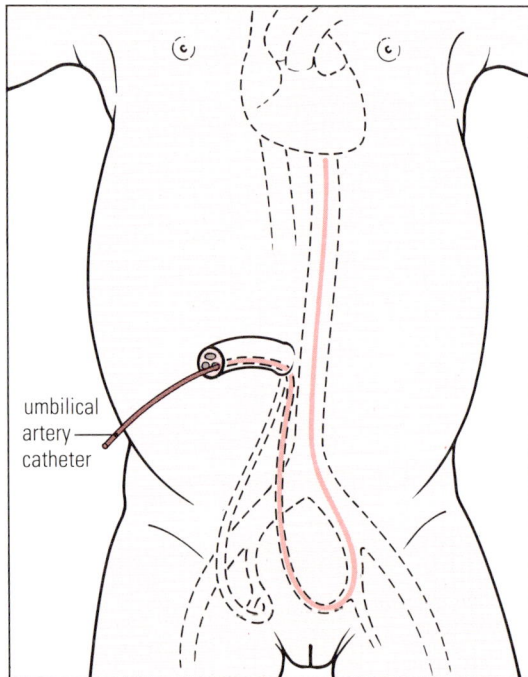

air-filled bronchi

umbilical artery catheter

Fig.15.4 A catheter placed in the aorta via an umbilical artery allows blood samples to be taken for Pao_2 assessment.

ADEQUATE RESPIRATION

Respiratory distress syndrome is now less common because of good resuscitation at birth, but is still the major problem for very low birth weight babies. The baby with respiratory failure presents with a high Pco_2, a low Po_2 and a mixed acidaemia. The clinical signs are cyanosis, sternal or chest wall recession, expiratory grunting, and tachypnoea. The chest X-ray has a characteristic ground-glass appearance (Fig.15.3). An 'air bronchogram' effect is also evident on the X-ray. This is caused by the contrast of air-filled bronchi against partly collapsed lungs. The post-mortem appearance of pink material in the terminal bronchioles has given the condition its alternative name of hyaline membrane disease.

Treatment consists firstly of giving adequate amounts of oxygen to prevent hypoxaemia. However, excess oxygen may cause blindness from retinopathy of prematurity (see Fig.15.10). Hence, careful monitoring of both the oxygen the baby is receiving and the Pao_2 is essential. The blood can be sampled from a catheter placed in the aorta via an umbilical artery (Fig.15.4) or from a radial artery. The usual aim is to keep the Pao_2 between 7 and 10kPa.

Very often, this treatment is not sufficient and respiratory support is necessary. This can be achieved by artificial ventilation using an endotracheal tube, but some babies are improved by 3–4cmH$_2$O constant pressure in the tube. Since respiratory distress syndrome is thought to be due to lack of surfactant, this pressure at the end of expiration probably prevents the lungs from collapsing. Otherwise, a baby has to make great efforts to reinflate the lungs each time a breath is taken (Fig.15.5). In the absence of surfactant, grunting is a mechanism to try to maintain alveolar patency at the end of expiration.

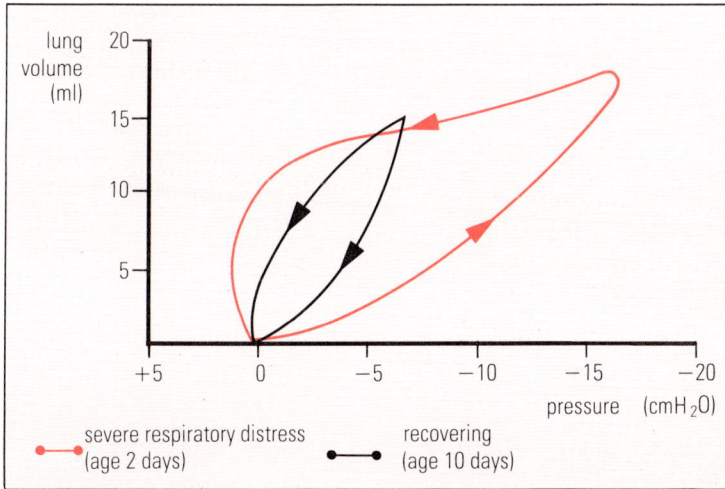

Fig.15.5 Pressure–volume curves in respiratory distress syndrome. The infant must make major respiratory efforts to inflate the lungs.

severe respiratory distress (age 2 days)   recovering (age 10 days)

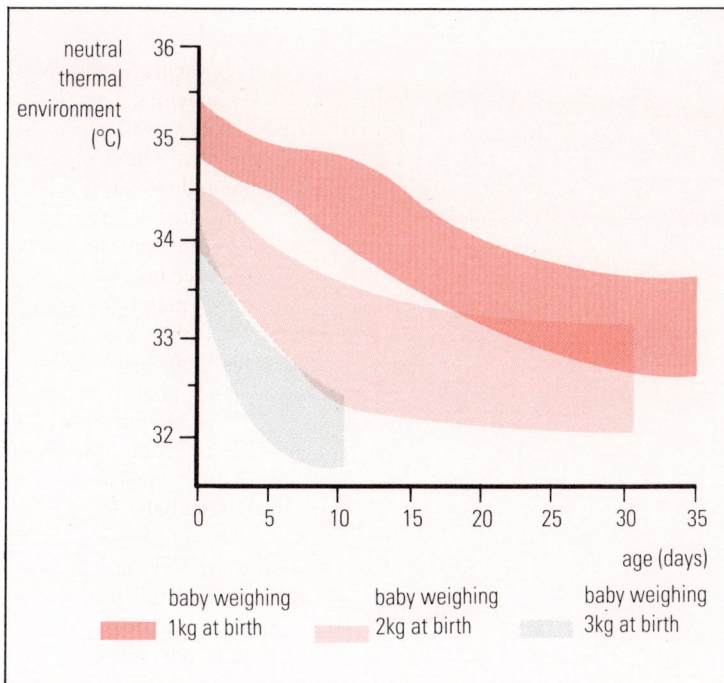

Fig.15.6 Optimal environmental temperature ranges for preterm infants. These temperatures would be needed for a naked baby in an incubator. A cooler environment is needed as the baby gets older. Modified from Hay, E. N. and Katz, G. (1970) *Archives of disease in Childhood.* **45**, 328.

baby weighing 1kg at birth   baby weighing 2kg at birth   baby weighing 3kg at birth

WARMTH

A small baby is liable to become chilled and a high environmental temperature is necessary; the incubator may need to be kept as hot as 36 or 37°C (Fig.15.6). A plastic heat shield placed inside the incubator will help to prevent radiant heat loss.

Temperature control is made more difficult by the great permeability of preterm skin to water. Infants under thirty weeks may lose a lot of water by this route (Fig.15.7) and therefore lose heat by evaporation. A humid environment in the incubator can improve temperature control.

231

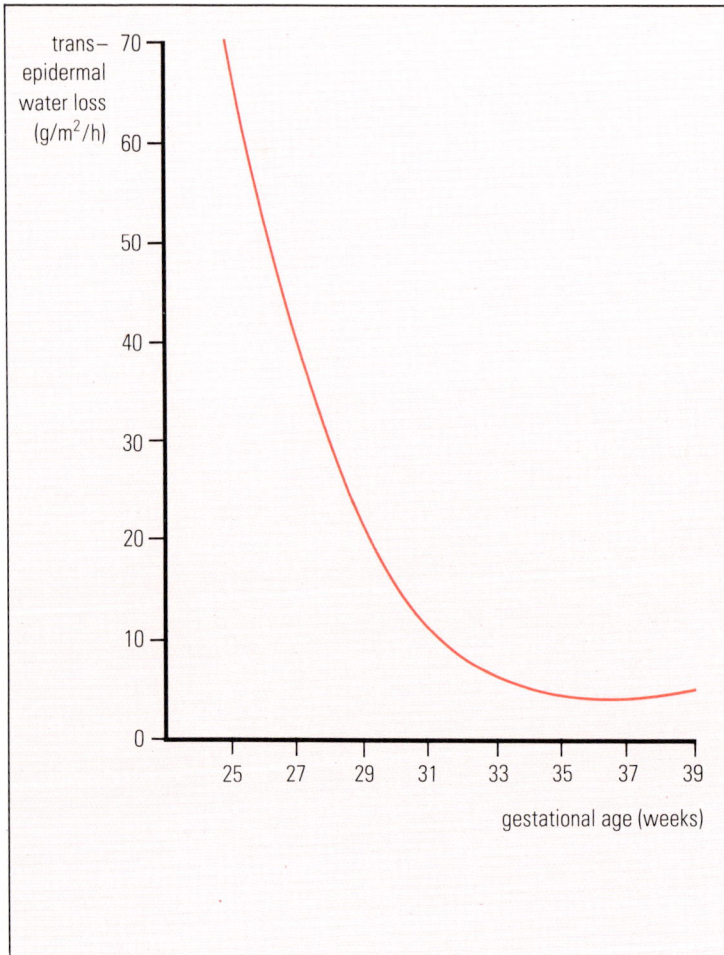

NUTRITION

This can be a problem since a baby under thirty-four weeks rarely sucks adequately. Milk can be given by a tube passed through the nose into the stomach. Fresh breast milk expressed by the mother or pasteurized supplies from a milk bank can be used. In some cases, human milk does not contain enough energy for growth, so supplements of carbohydrate are often added or an artificial milk may be used. In very small babies, intravenous nutrition may be needed or special techniques, such as nasojejunal feeding, required.

LOVE

The birth of a preterm baby is a great crisis for the parents. The small baby looks thin and quite unlike the anticipated chubby term infant. Several weeks of special care or even intensive care are needed, and this can put a great strain on the family. The staff must help the parents during this difficult period and answer all questions honestly. Whenever possible special care procedures, such as tube feeding, should be performed beside the mother's bed.

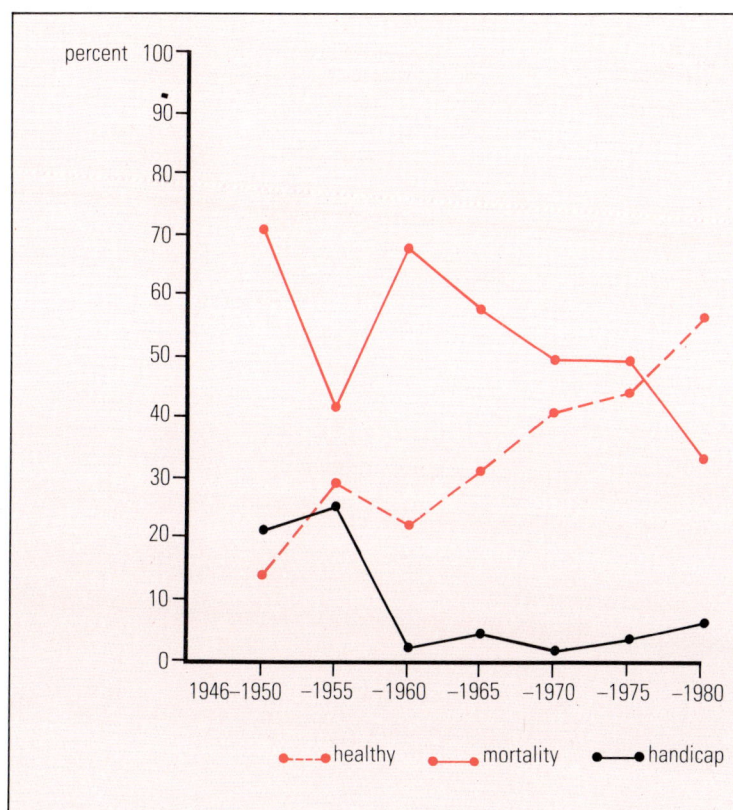

Fig.15.8 Numbers of handicapped infants in association with decreasing mortality rates. Modified from Stewart A.L., Reynolds, E.D.R. & Lipscomb, A.P. (1981)*Lancet,* **1**, 1038.

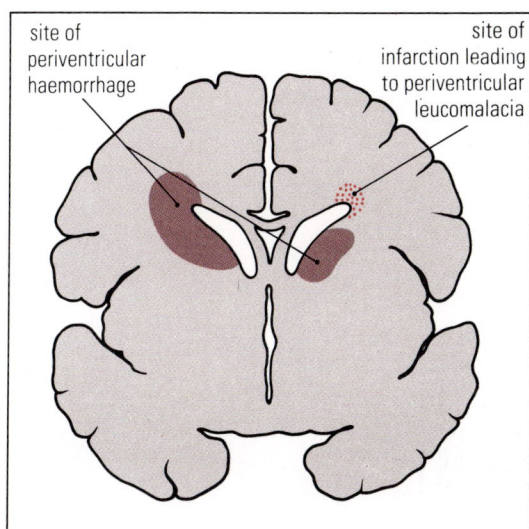

Fig.15.9 Distribution of damage in periventricular haemorrhage. Haemorrhage occurs in the germinal layer just below the lateral ventricles. Infarction may occur lateral to the ventricle.

OUTCOME

A preterm baby has a greater risk of disability than a normal baby. In recent years, the survival of such babies has improved without any attendant increase in the numbers of handicapped infants (Fig.15.8), but there is still anxiety about the survival of very small babies born at under twenty-six weeks gestation.

Periventricular haemorrhage occurs in about half the babies born at under thirty weeks gestation. The bleeding occurs near the lateral ventricle of the brain and can spread into the ventricle itself and the nearby brain substance (Fig.15.9). In most cases the haemorrhage resolves without problem, but hydrocephalus may result from blood obstructing the circulation of cerebrospinal fluid. Periventricular leucomalacia has recently been recognized. This follows infarction lateral to the ventricles with subsequent cyst formation; it has a bad prognosis, and cerebral palsy and mental handicap may result. These diagnoses can now be made by the use of ultrasound.

Retinopathy of prematurity (Fig.15.10), previously known as retrolental fibroplasia, was seen in the 1950s as a result of uncontrolled oxygen therapy. With more careful management of oxygen it became unusual, but is now becoming more common with the increasing survival rates of tiny babies. Total blindness may result.

FOLLOW-UP

Preterm babies need to be seen frequently in child health clinics. Their growth should be monitored (Fig.15.11) and they should receive supplements of iron and folic acid in their diet. They are also at great risk of developing rickets, but ordinary vitamin D often fails to prevent this.

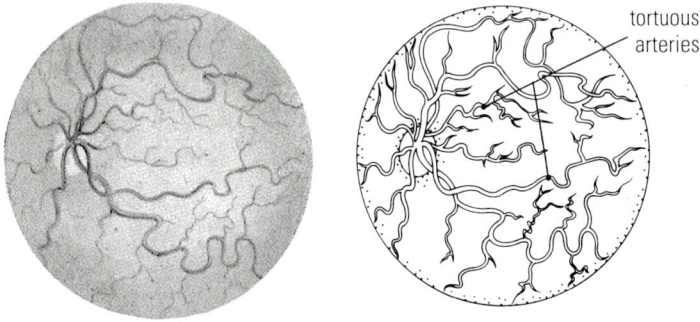

Fig.15.10 Retinopathy of prematurity. New vessel formation occurs in the retina with haemorrhage and retinal detachment. This relatively mild case shows tortuous arteries.

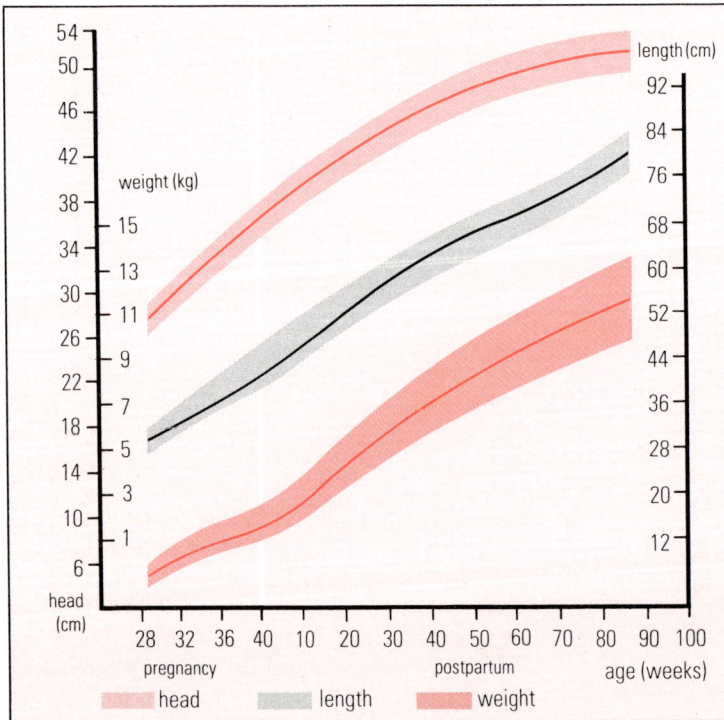

Fig.15.11 Growth charts for preterm infants. Redrawn from the charts available from Castlemead Publications, Ware, Herts.

16. Epidemiology in Obstetrics

Obstetricians deal in the vital statistics of life and death which, in epidemiological terms, are relatively hard data. Since the diagnosis of birth or death is usually obvious, these statistics are more valid and reproduceable than the subjective data of morbidity. Most doctors would agree about an event such as a birth or a death, whereas they would not necessarily agree about the presence or severity of an illness such as pneumonia or peptic ulceration.

There is a statutory obligation on doctors and midwives to collect data on births and deaths; these are passed centrally to government sources. In England and Wales this process is carried out through the Office of Populations, Censuses and Surveys (OPCS), previously the Registrar General's Office. Such data have been supplemented by national and regional surveys on births and deaths. These are special research studies mounted for a short time to answer specific questions and include, for example, the National Birthday Trust's surveys, performed in 1946, 1958 and 1970, which recorded all births during one week in the United Kingdom. Scotland and Northern Ireland collect their vital statistics separately.

BIRTH RATES

The birth rate is obtained from data at the Office of Populations, Censuses and Surveys. Every birth has to be registered by the parents at a local Registry Office within forty days of delivery. In addition, it is mandatory that any midwife attending a birth notifies the District Medical Officer within thirty-six hours, so that birth registrations and birth notifications can be checked against each other.

The birth rate (Fig.16.1) is defined as the number of viable births in a unit of time per thousand of the total population, counted ideally at the middle of that unit of time (usually mid-year or mid-quinquennium).

$$\text{Birth rate} = \frac{\text{No. of births in the year}}{\text{Mid-year population}} \times 1000$$

Both the numerator and denominator of this rate can be determined from statutory information. However, no men and few girls or older women have babies and therefore the denominator may mask information about births among the potentially fertile population.

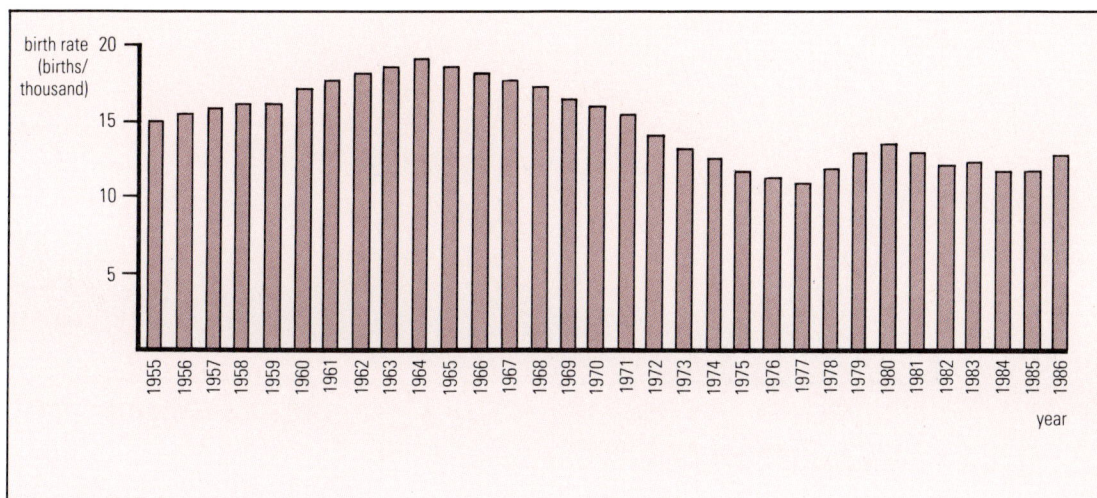

Fig.16.1 Birth rate in England and Wales (1955–1986).

Consequently, the general fertility rate (Fig.16.2) has been derived; this is defined as the number of viable births per unit of time per thousand women aged fifteen to forty-four.

$$\text{General fertility rate} = \frac{\text{No. of births in the year}}{\text{No. of women aged}\ 15\text{--}44} \times 1000$$

In the United Kingdom, the denominator can easily be obtained from census data, but in other countries this may be rather more difficult.

In addition, a coarse measure of the births in a country can be obtained from completed family size (Fig.16.3). This relates to the birth rate but must be retrospective, for it has to (in theory) await the completion of the family by the woman; thus the data will be years out of date for any given year.

Population control

The classical restrictions on population are:
- Famine
- War
- Disease

To these, Malpas (a nineteenth century scientist) added:
- Restraint
- Celibacy

The first three are being reduced by variable degrees and, in the latter part of the twentieth century, restraint and celibacy have been augmented by contraception. Undoubtedly, the wider use of contraception, particularly in developing countries of the world, would help total health much more than restricted medical improvements.

Variation in birth rates

United Kingdom

The birth rate has dropped considerably in all developed countries since the Second World War (Fig.16.4). Looking back further, this trend relates to the whole century. Since 1900, the birth rates in the United Kingdom have been at their lowest levels in the late 1930s and the late 1970s.

In general, the poorer sections of any community have a higher birth rate than rich sections, and the birth rate declines faster in towns than in the country.

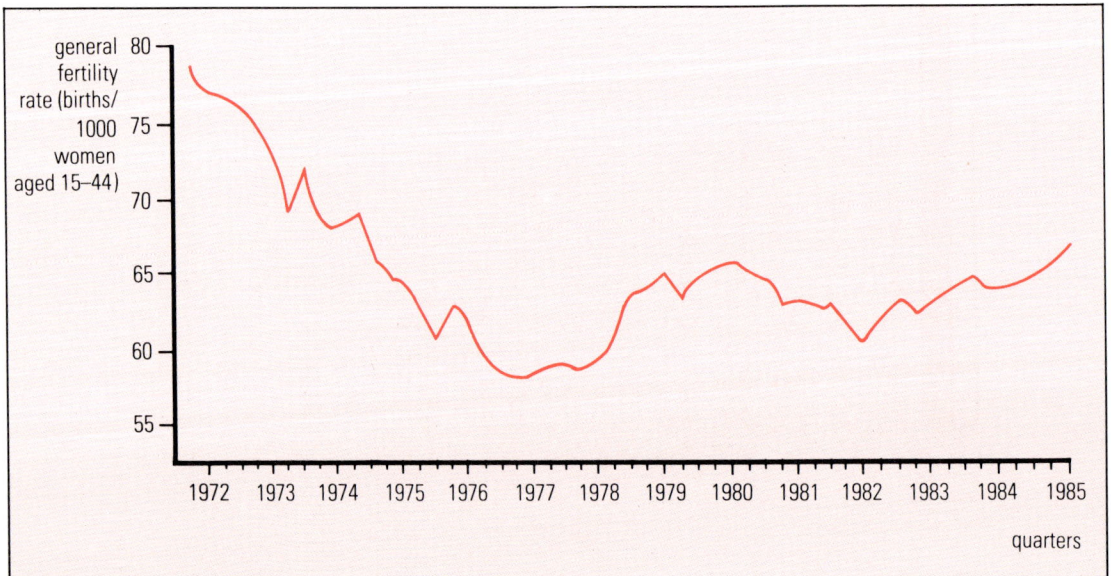

Fig.16.2 General fertility rate in England and Wales (1972–1985).

236

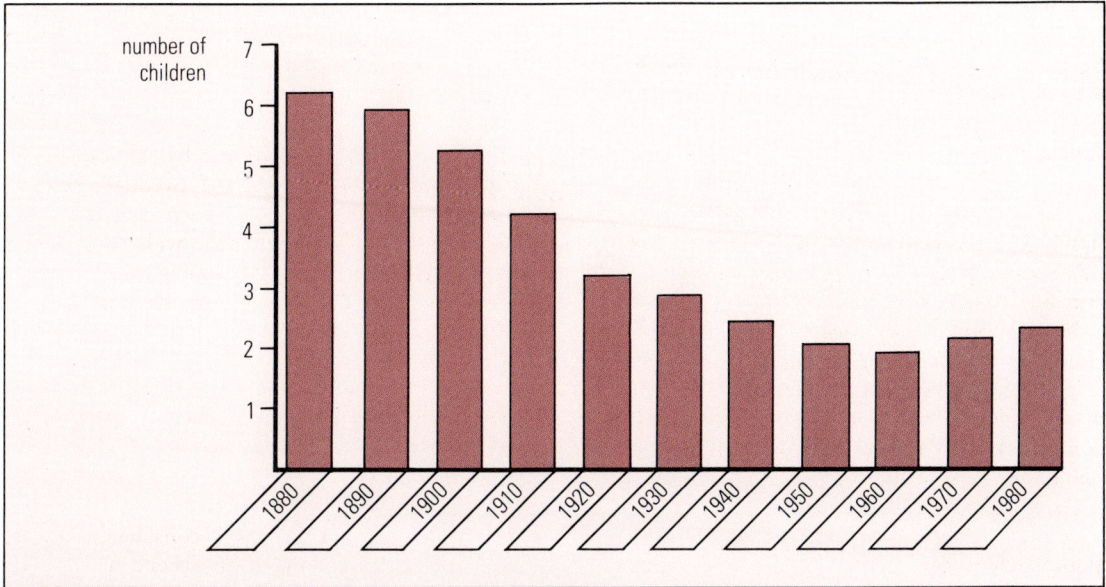

Fig.16.3 Completed family size in England and Wales (1880–1980).

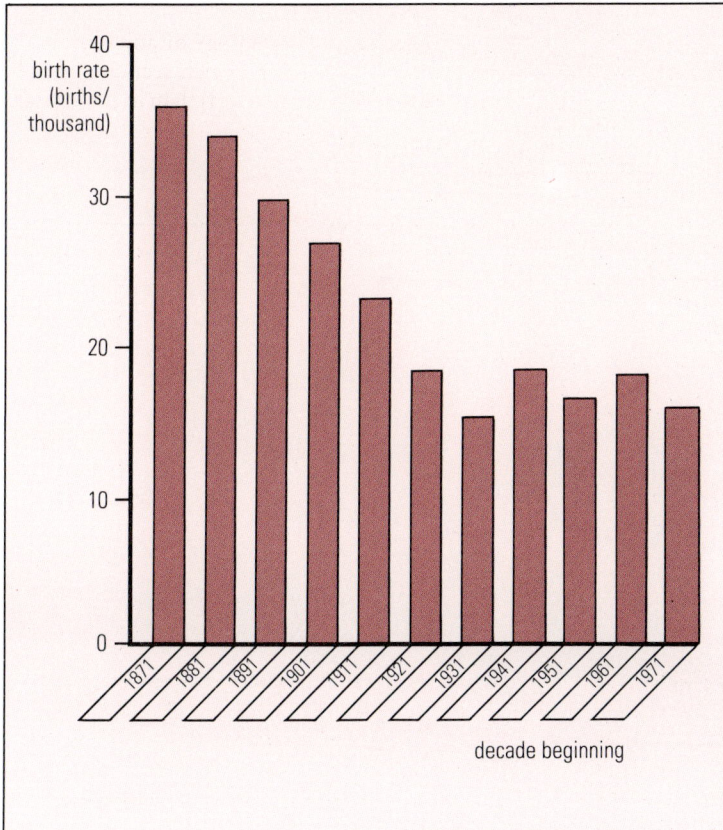

Fig.16.4 Birth rate in England and Wales (1871–1980).

Worldwide

Underdeveloped countries have higher birth rates than developed countries, for example, Kenya has a mean family size of 8.4 compared with 2.1 in the United Kingdom. Thus in Kenya, when a couple dies they theoretically leave six people more than were there a generation ago, whilst in the United Kingdom the number left behind is almost an exact replacement. Obviously, these figures do not include subsequent events; for example, in Kenya the infant mortality rate is much higher than that in the United Kingdom. Not all of the six extra people would necessarily live but more than two probably would, and thus the replacement number in underdeveloped countries is greater than in developed countries.

A more precise comparison of birth rate data can be derived if the population is divided into a series of age groups, which are then displayed as a bar diagram. If the population is expanding at the younger end, the demogram will be triangular (Fig.16.5 left). If the population is fairly stable, however, with approximately the same number entering as leaving, a more rectangular pattern exists until older age (Fig.16.5 right). Should the population be an ageing one, there will be a greater bulge at the upper end than the lower. In the United Kingdom the demogram is fairly well balanced (Fig.16.6), but its base has become constricted since 1971, indicating a smaller population of children. With better nutrition, a higher standard of living and better medicine, many of the middle-aged will live into old age and will have to be

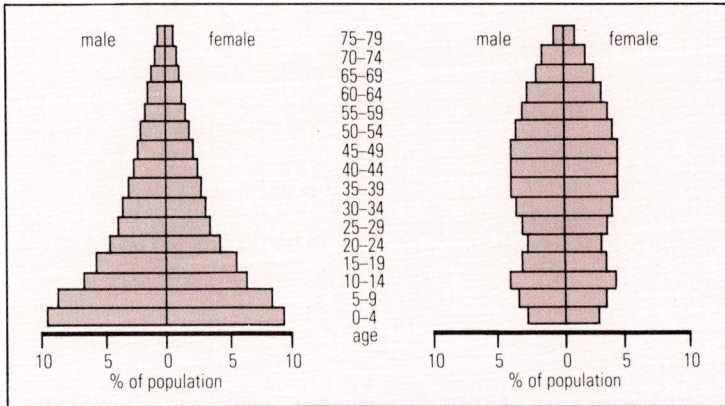

Fig.16.5 Demograms. Left: developing country. Right: developed country.

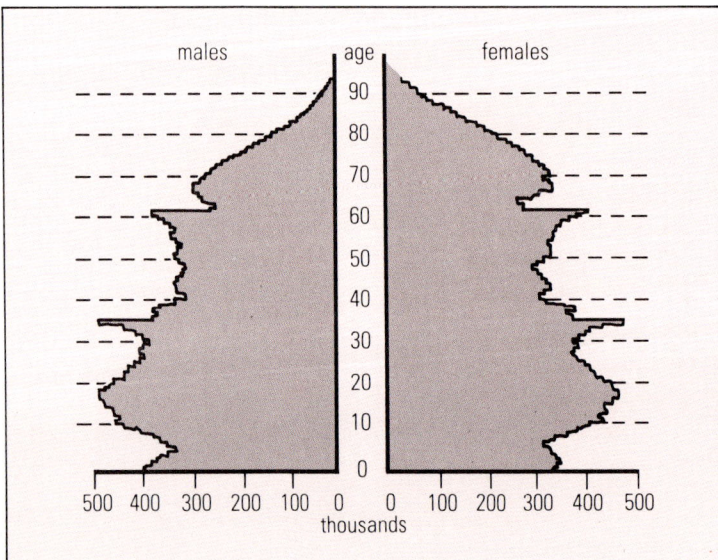

Fig.16.6 Population demogram of the United Kingdom (1982). This has been constructed in annual steps, rather than the quinquennial ones used in Fig.16.5.

supported by fewer younger people. Although there has been a great drop in birth rates, the improved overall health of the population and better medical services have led to more lives being saved in the first year of life than was previously possible.

MATERNAL MORTALITY

Maternal mortality is associated with pregnancy or childbirth. The definitions vary greatly, but in the United Kingdom all deaths occurring up to a year after childbirth or abortion are counted. Other countries, following the definition of the Fédération Internationale de Gynecologique et Obstetrique (FIGO), which was adopted by the World Health Organization, consider the association to last for only six weeks (forty-two days). Furthermore, many countries do not include deaths associated with abortion and so their data have a slightly different base from that of the United Kingdom. It is probable that the United Kingdom definition will change in the next decade to adopt the forty-two day time span.

In the United Kingdom, all maternal deaths within a year of childbirth or abortion are reported to the District Medical Officer. He then institutes an enquiry, which is performed by the team from the Confidential Enquiry into Maternal Deaths. This is a unique audit run by the profession itself; it works because information is given in confidence. In addition, all death certificates in which pregnancy is listed in Part 2 ('other significant conditions contributing to the death but not related to the diseases or conditions causing it') are noted by the Registrar General.

The maternal mortality rate (Fig.16.7) is expressed as the number of maternal deaths per thousand total births.

$$\text{Maternal mortality rate} = \frac{\text{Maternal deaths}}{\text{Total births}} \times 1000$$

The rate has been decreasing over the last century and is now very low, at 11/100,000 total births in England and Wales in 1983. Much of this improvement is due to better maternal health, which is attributable to improved nutrition and smaller families. However, obstetrics has also contributed with better training of doctors and midwives in the last forty years, the increasing use of blood transfusion and the employment of antibiotics.

Internationally, maternal death rates have been decreasing over the last forty years. The populations of each country differ and so comparisons should not be drawn in ranking order; in most countries the major causes of death are similar, but in those which are less developed infection and haemorrhage become much more important, as they were in the United Kingdom in the last century.

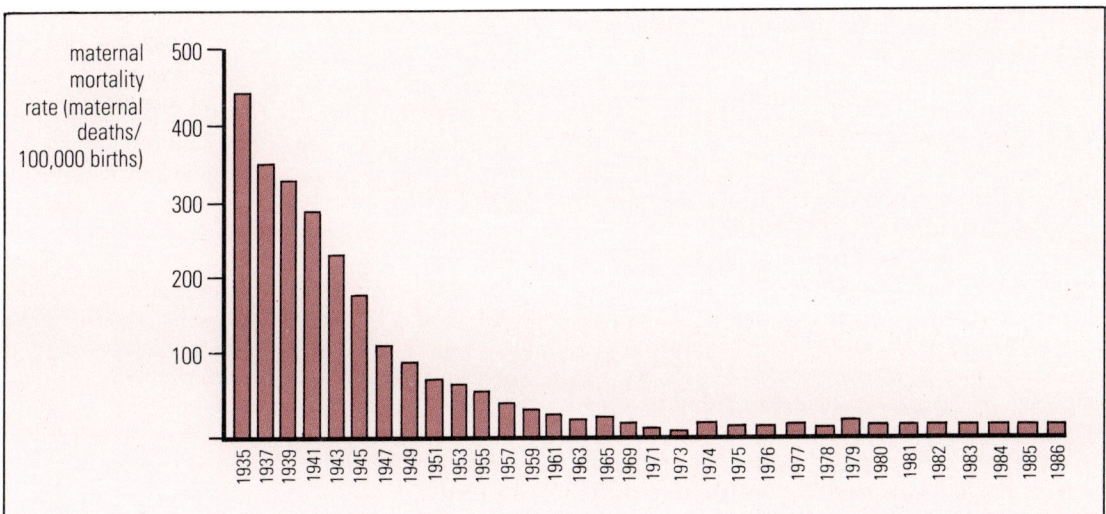

Fig.16.7 Maternal mortality rate in England and Wales (1935–1986).

239

Causes of maternal mortality

Abortion

An increased maternal mortality is more likely after procured and illegal abortions. These have been reduced greatly in England, Wales and Scotland following the introduction of the 1968 Abortion Act (which does not apply to Northern Ireland).

The cause of death is usually haemorrhage, sepsis or renal failure. To prevent such deaths, a wider use of contraception should be encouraged. Furthermore, if pregnancy has to be terminated it should be done under proper conditions by a competent obstetrician with adequate anaesthesia and back-up services.

Raised blood pressure

Women with essential hypertension in pregnancy are seen less commonly now, as fewer women over thirty-five are having babies. Furthermore, eclampsia and pre-eclampsia are lessening because of better antenatal care.

Death in this group usually follows intracranial haemorrhage or renal failure. To reduce the number of deaths, good antenatal care is necessary since it allows frequent monitoring of the blood pressure in pregnancy. Those at higher risk, that is women with essential hypertension and those who develop pre-eclampsia, should be checked more frequently. Women with more severe hypertension (essential or of pregnancy) must be admitted to hospital and watched very carefully until the obstetrician thinks the pregnancy can safely be brought to an end.

Pulmonary embolism

Movement of a clot from the peripheral venous system into the lung can be a fatal event. A quarter of pulmonary embolisms occur in the antenatal period and three quarters after delivery. A large proportion of these follow an operative vaginal delivery or caesarean section. The obstetrician should always try to identify the higher risk patient — the older, the obese, those who have had previous thromboses and those who have had an operative delivery. Since many of the deaths occur with no warning symptoms or signs in the antenatal period, it is wise to consider prophylactic anticoagulation for women at higher risk

and to consider the condition if a woman reports swelling or pain in the calf.

Haemorrhage

Bleeding from the genital tract in pregnancy may be ante- or postpartum. Women with an abruptio placentae or a placenta praevia are particularly at risk in the antepartum period.

Placental abruption is associated with considerable shock since heavy bleeding occurs retroplacentally as the placenta separates. The number of deaths has decreased due to better understanding of hypovolaemia and its sequelae and the use of central venous pressure monitoring and large volume blood replacement.

Placenta praevia is associated with a small number of maternal deaths. The placental site in the lower segment can bleed heavily, particularly if implantation is so low that by a later stage of the pregnancy the placenta is completely over the os of the cervix. If a vaginal examination has inadvertently been performed, profuse bleeding can follow.

Deaths due to antepartum haemorrhage have been reduced by paying closer attention to the warning signs of vaginal bleeding in pregnancy, admitting women to hospital without performing vaginal examination, and ultrasound localization of the placental site. If a caesarean section has to be performed, a senior obstetrician must be present at the operation.

Postpartum haemorrhage follows delivery and may be due to relaxation of the uterus or to trauma to the cervix, uterus or vagina. The number of deaths can be greatly reduced by giving an oxytocic drug during delivery of the fetus. This is now a routine procedure but is occasionally omitted by accident or by the wish of the mother. Furthermore, by having the mother in hospital, blood loss can be rapidly replaced from the blood bank should postpartum haemorrhage occur.

Ectopic pregnancies can cause death by a sudden brisk bleed into the peritoneal cavity. The risk of this occurring can be reduced by paying attention to suspicious symptoms and by acting promptly on those who arrive in hospital with such signs.

Anaesthesia

General anaesthesia in pregnancy can be hazardous,

and is particularly so in labour. The woman may not be so prepared for anaesthetic as at elective surgery and consequently the anaesthetist often has to cope with a tired, dehydrated, depressed woman who is likely to have food in her stomach. Inhalation of the acidic stomach contents under anaesthesia can lead to Mendelson's syndrome.

To reduce the number of deaths in this group, a wider use of regional anaesthesia such as epidural and pudendal blocks should be undertaken. If general anaesthesia is essential it should be administered by a trained anaesthetist of at least registrar level who will introduce a cuffed endotracheal tube under controlled conditions.

Other causes

Infection, once a major cause of death, killing a tenth of all women in childbirth, has been greatly reduced in the developed world thanks to antisepsis and asepsis in obstetric procedures. Antibiotics have also helped

in this, but one should be wary of attributing too much to the introduction of these drugs because the death rates from maternal sepsis were falling following the use of better asepsis in the late 1930s (before the advent of antibiotics).

PERINATAL MORTALITY

Perinatal deaths are fetal and neonatal deaths which occur around the time of birth. By international agreement, these deaths may be defined as:
- Stillbirths. Babies who are born dead after the 28th week of pregnancy.
- Early neonatal deaths. Babies born alive at any stage of pregnancy who die within the first week after birth.

In the United Kingdom, stillbirths have a lower limit on their gestational age but neonatal deaths do not (Fig. 16.8) This might seem inappropriate since many

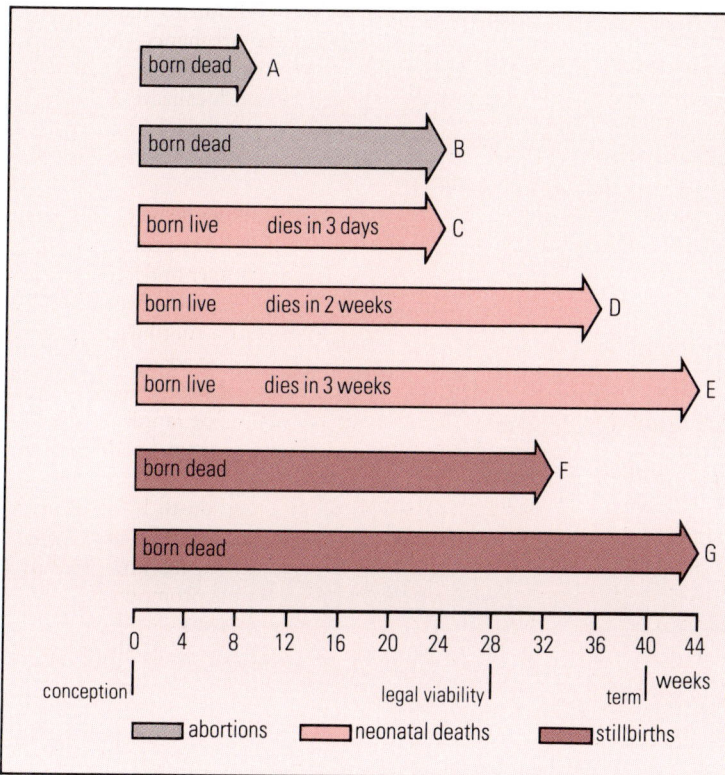

Fig.16.8 Time limits of births and deaths in the United Kingdom. Note that only C, F and G are perinatal deaths.

241

babies miscarried at twenty-two weeks make some signs of life, and could therefore be termed neonatal deaths. Consequently, some countries have a limit at the lower end of their neonatal death scale. They exclude babies either below a certain birth weight (for example 500g) or below a certain stage of gestation (for example twenty-six weeks). These exclusions do not yet apply to the United Kingdom, and so perinatal mortality data would seem to be weighted against the United Kingdom in favour of other countries. However, in considering international differences there are many other variables which should be taken into account; these will be discussed later in this chapter.

The perinatal mortality rate represents the number of fetal and early neonatal deaths per thousand total births, the neonatal death rate including those which occur within the first four weeks after delivery; the infant mortality rate is based on the number of babies dying within the first year after birth.

United Kingdom data

Over the last fifty years, the perinatal mortality rate in the United Kingdom has been decreasing (Fig.16.9). It is still going down at a very fast rate, the deceleration in the last twenty-five years being much greater than would be expected from biological or background demographic improvements. This implies that the intervention of obstetrics has helped.

The factors that effect the reduced perinatal mortality rates in the United Kingdom are:
- Better maternal health
- Raised standard of living and nutrition
- Improved education
- Organization of antenatal care
- Intrapartum care in hospital
- Neonatal care of low birth weight babies

International data

The perinatal mortality rate in England in 1986 was 9.4/1000 total births. A variation exists between the four countries that make up the United Kingdom and also between these and other European states, such as Sweden and Denmark.

It should not be assumed that obstetric services are

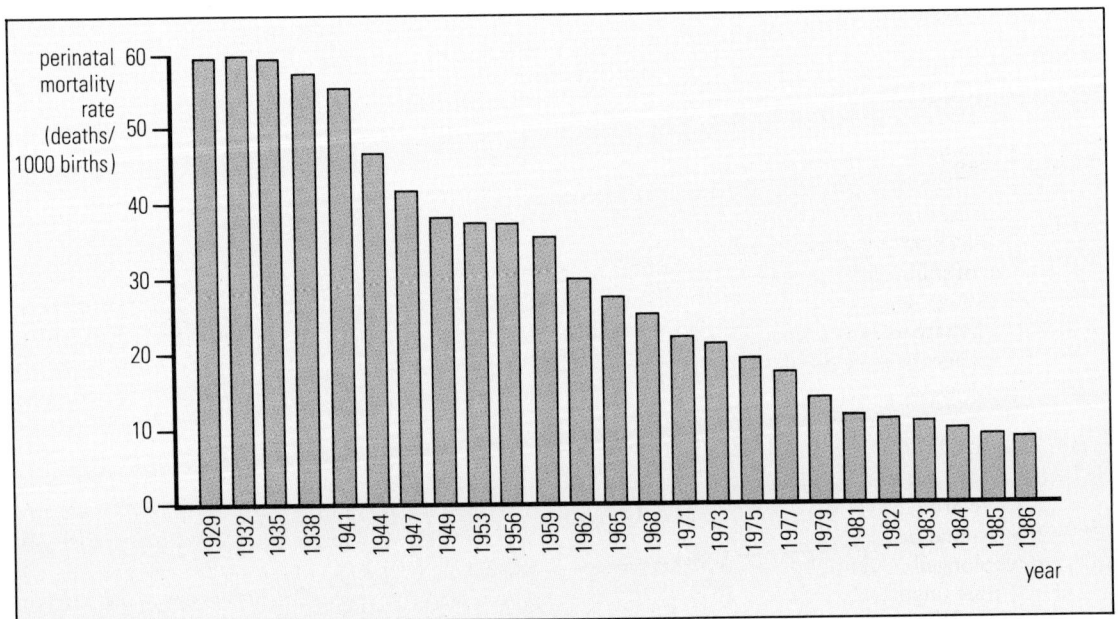

Fig.16.9 Perinatal mortality rate in England and Wales (1929–1986).

inadequate in the United Kingdom because the perinatal mortality rates are higher than in other countries. Each country has a different population with different genetic, morphological, nutritional and pathological characteristics. Some of the countries with low perinatal mortality rates have a small and more uniform population, who have their children at an earlier age and who may not include babies of less than twenty-four weeks gestation or babies of less than 500g birth weight when collecting their data. Perinatal mortality rates should only be directly compared between similar populations, a situation which does not exist even within the United Kingdom. The major reasons for international differences in perinatal mortality rates include:
- Background health
- Patterns of reproduction
- Diseases encountered
- Obstetric care
- Data recording methods

Factors associated with perinatal mortality

The background of the woman and her environment have a large influence on perinatal mortality rates. Age, parity and social class are all associated with major changes in perinatal mortality. Other factors include race, rural or urban habitat, and incidental habits such as cigarette smoking.

Pathological causes of perinatal mortality

Low birth weight

The major cause of perinatal death is low birth weight. About sixty-five percent of early neonatal deaths and fifty percent of stillbirths are associated with low birth weight (<2500g). This group consists of two types:
- Babies who are of appropriate weight for their gestational age, but who are immature.
- Babies who are small for their gestational age.

The latter constitute one third of low birth weight infants and are easier to manage. In the developed world, severe growth retardation is usually the result of poor placental bed blood flow, but in the poorer nations prolonged maternal malnutrition may be relatively more important.

A small number of low birth weight babies result from early induction or elective caesarean section performed to avoid complications of pregnancy (for example severe pre-eclampsia). The majority of low birth weight babies follow the spontaneous onset of preterm labour or spontaneous rupture of the membranes. Any woman who is at risk of a very preterm labour (between twenty-six and thirty-two weeks) should deliver in a special obstetric unit close to a Special Care Baby Unit. If delivery is inevitable, the labouring mother should, if possible, travel with the baby *in utero*, since this is the best incubator for a small child during transport.

Congenital abnormalities

A major abnormality is associated with about twenty percent of neonatal deaths and stillbirths. Abnormalities of the central nervous system (anencephaly and spina bifida) are the most common.

There is little treatment available which can prevent these conditions beyond, possibly, giving the mother folate or multivitamin supplements before pregnancy. The only other practical management is to detect the abnormalities early, using alpha-fetoprotein screening programmes or ultrasound after sixteen weeks gestation; termination of pregnancy can then be offered if the fetus is affected. Both these screening programmes create large demands on manpower and finance, and must be assessed carefully before their general introduction. Management may be cost effective where there is a high risk of serious abnormalities (for example in Glasgow), but would not necessarily be so in areas where the risk is low (for example in Sussex).

Hypoxia

Hypoxia accounts for about ten percent of neonatal deaths and forty percent of stillbirths. It may occur acutely before labour due to separation of a normally sited placenta (abruptio placentae); less suddenly, diminished placental bed blood flow is associated with chronic antepartum hypoxia. Most cases of severe hypoxia arise in labour when uterine contractions cut off the placental bed blood supply.

This cause of perinatal death can be countered by selecting those women who are at higher risk and delivering them in hospital where fetal monitoring can cover labour. Hypoxia can also occur in the newborn as a result of lung hypoplasia and hyaline membrane disease.

Birth trauma

About three percent of stillbirths and neonatal deaths show evidence of birth trauma at post-mortem. It may be associated with a rapid delivery, as with an immature fetus or breech presentation, or with a difficult delivery because of incorrect diagnosis of the degree of cephalopelvic disproportion. Occasionally, uterine contractions that are too strong can be associated with damage at birth.

The contribution of birth trauma to perinatal mortality has been reduced greatly in the last forty years due to better obstetric diagnosis and control, and improved obstetric training.

Infections

Infections are rare but they occasionally follow prolonged intrauterine life after preterm rupture of the membranes. They many also be acquired during passage of the fetus down the vagina and at delivery, for example herpes infection.

Neonatal infection rarely occurs in the postpartum period and was more often associated with the crowded nurseries of thirty years ago. Neonatal infections include gastroenteritis, pneumonia and skin infection. These are still major causes of death in countries with inadequate standards of hygiene.

Rhesus disease

This is now a rare cause of death due to the introduction of an active antenatal programme to detect Rh-antibodies and of postnatal immunization with anti–D gammaglobulin. If such programmes are not available, perinatal deaths may occur from hydrops fetalis, anaemia of the newborn or kernicterus.

With improving general health and organization of medical services, the perinatal mortality rate has decreased substantially in the United Kingdom. However, it is still important in other parts of the world where these two factors have yet to come into effect. Obstetric and neonatal intervention will also assist in any future improvement.

17. Contraception

INTRODUCTION

Although the limitation of family size has always been a personal affair between a woman and her partner, couples often need professional advice on the choice of the various contraceptive methods available. The majority go to Family Planning Clinics staffed by doctors and nurses trained in the subject, whilst others turn to their family doctor for assistance. Anyone who is going to work in this field should be well trained; most Vocational Training Courses include attendance at Family Planning Clinics, while refresher courses are held regularly by Family Practitioner Committees.

If a doctor does not wish to deal with contraceptive methods himself, he should ensure that someone else, either in his practice or in a neighbouring one, is prepared to take on couples who come to him requesting advice. In many cases the local Family Planning Clinics are based on the premises of the General Practitioner's surgery, so couples can easily be redirected. The doctor's own ethical views are important; he should not be forced to offer contraceptive advice against his wishes, however, the views of the patients must also be considered. Referral to another Practitioner solves the dilemma.

THE METHODS IN USE

The methods of contraception chosen at Family Planning Clinics in the United Kingdom is shown in Fig.17.1. Overall, the most popular method in this country is still the condom, which has the added advantage of protection against infection. The extent

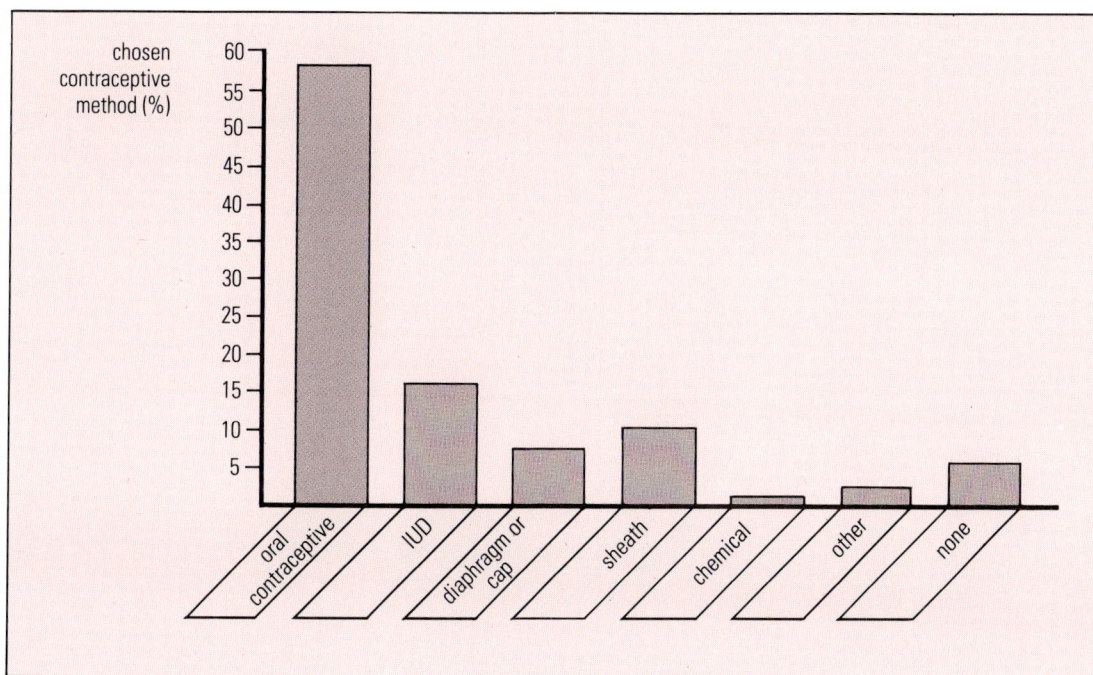

Fig.17.1 Methods of contraception chosen at Family Planning Clinics (1983). Other methods includes sterilization.

of its use varies between married and unmarried couples and with the age of the participants. Oral contraception is the next most popular method, being used by between a quarter and a half of the population, depending on age and social class.

The intrauterine device (IUD) is used by less than ten percent of women; vaginal diaphragms and cervical caps are used by a similar proportion, their popularity varying with the periodical adverse publicity on other methods such as oral contraceptives and the IUD.

The use of the rhythm method will depend largely on the number of patients seen whose faith will not allow them to use biochemical or mechanical methods of contraception. Every clinic sees a few couples who are still using coitus interruptus or other less efficient methods.

COUNSELLING ON CONTRACEPTION

Usually, a couple who wish to discuss contraception will want to know about the following aspects of any given method:
- Effectiveness
- Safety
- Convenience

Effectiveness

This can be expressed mathematically, as in Fig.17.2. The risk of failure is defined as the number of pregnancies expected in a year among one hundred couples having regular intercourse and using that method of contraception only (Pearl index). However,

FAILURE RATES FOR DIFFERENT METHODS OF CONTRACEPTION	
Method	Risk of failure (%)
combined oral contraceptives	0–1
50μg oestrogen	0.1–1
<50μg oestrogen	0.2–1
progestogen – only pill	0.3–5
injectable (medroxyprogesterone acetate)	0–1
IUD	
Lippes loop C	0.3–4
copper 7	0.3–4
diaphragm	2–15
condom	2–15
coitus interruptus	8–17
spermicide only	4–25
natural family planning	
pre- & postovulation	15–30
postovulation only	1–6
contraceptive sponge	9–25
sterilization	
male	0–0.2
female	0–0.5
no method	
women aged < 40	80–90
women aged 40	40–50
women aged 45	10–20
women aged 50	0–5

Fig.17.2 Failure risk for different methods of contraception. This is expressed as the number of pregnancies expected in a year among couples having regular intercourse and using that method of contraception only.

many couples do not think numerically and it may be better either to use some form of visual aid, such as a bar diagram, or to explain the numbers in general terms and discuss the advantages and disadvantages of each method (Fig.17.3). It must be stressed to the couple that effectiveness depends upon motivation and how closely the advised technique is followed.

Safety

The safety of each method will be important, particularly to the more informed patient. Generally, barrier methods have no major features which could be regarded as unsafe. The hazards of the IUD are mostly associated with possible uterine perforation at the time of fitting, with pelvic infection, and with the possibility of the device being expelled. The safety of oral contraceptive agents centres on the possibility of thromboembolism; this will be discussed later in this chapter.

Convenience

The convenience of the method of contraception is very important. When advising on contraception, a doctor is not prescribing medicine for someone with symptoms, but is offering social help. Consequently, whilst one can prescribe treatment in other medical fields which may be ill understood or have unpleasant features, in contraception one must be certain that what is offered is acceptable to the couple, otherwise it will not be used.

DISADVANTAGES OF DIFFERENT METHODS OF CONTRACEPTION		
Method	Perceived disadvantages with use	Patients satisfied (%)
IUD	difficult to obtain expensive	80
pill	harmful effects	70
condom	impeded love-making nuisance to use	50
withdrawal	interrupted love-making unnatural, unreliable	50
safe period	unreliable	50
diaphragm & spermicides	messy & troublesome to use	40

Fig.17.3 Disadvantages of different methods of contraception.

Obviously, the most convenient method is one which does not need to be implemented at the time of intercourse; oral contraceptives and the IUD are good in this respect. The barrier methods have to be put in place at the time of intercourse, and are therefore less convenient.

HORMONAL METHODS

The majority of hormonal methods are administered as oral preparations, although parenteral contraception may occasionally be used in specific circumstances. The oral preparations may consist of low doses of combined oestrogen and progestogen, progestogen only, or high doses of combined oestrogen and progestogen for postcoital contraception.

Combined oral contraceptives

Oestrogens inhibit ovulation if given at the right time in the menstrual cycle and in the correct dosage. The most common method in conventional contraception is to administer oral oestrogens for about ten days on either side of the time of potential ovulation. Progestogens were originally added to overcome the nausea produced by oestrogen, but are now known to be contraceptive in their own right.

The oestrogen most often used is ethinyloestradiol at a dosage of 30mg or, less commonly, 20mg. The lower doses permit breakthrough bleeding except in women of very low body weight. Three oral preparations use mestranol, a methyl ester of ethinyloestradiol.

Several progestogens are used in oral contraceptives. Progesterone itself is not absorbed when given by mouth, and so derivations from 19-norethisterone are used; their activity varies greatly. Levo-norgestrel is more active than norethisterone. When the mixture of levo- and dextro-norgestrel is used it is, weight for weight, about half as effective as levo-norgestrel alone. Some of the product is metabolized through oestrogen pathways and so has additive oestrogenic action.

Most oral contraceptives contain a daily dose of oestrogen and progestogen which is uniform throughout the cycle. In others, the level of oestrogen and progestogen varies in an attempt to reproduce the natural cyclical hormonal state; these are the bi- and triphasic pills.

It is wise for practitioners in this field to have a small spectrum of four or five products which they have used and with which they are familiar. Thus, any side effects caused by one type of pill can be overcome by using another type which has a slightly altered oestrogen or progestogen content.

Most combined oral contraceptives are packed in display foil envelopes, which clearly indicate that the woman should take one pill each day for twenty-one or twenty-two days of a twenty-eight day cycle, starting on the fifth day after the start of menstruation. With such cyclical dosage, the woman has a gap in medication on the remaining days, but some preparations provide inactive pills for these days to satisfy the woman who finds it easier to take a pill every day.

Progestogen-only contraceptives

Progestogen-only contraceptives are useful for those women for whom oestrogens are contraindicated and for those in whom oestrogens might produce undesirable side effects, for example mothers who are breast feeding. They are not quite as effective as combined oral preparations and it is therefore especially important that the woman does not miss any of the pills, which should be taken daily and preferably in the same quadrant of each day.

Injections of long-acting medroxyprogesterone acetate (Depo-Provera) are available for those for whom oral preparations are not suitable. These are effective for about three months, but may last longer in some women. Injections of norethisterone enanthate have been used in clinical trials, but this is not yet available in the United Kingdom for general use.

Postcoital contraceptives

Postcoital hormonal contraception can be used following unprotected intercourse, provided treatment is administered within seventy-two hours of the incident. Previously, either ethinyloestradiol (5mg daily for five days) or stilboestrol (25mg daily for five days) was used. Either of these will probably produce nausea, but they are moderately effective in preventing implantation of a fertilized ovum. A single dose of levo-norgestrel (400mg) given within twenty-four hours of intercourse can also be used for postcoital contraception. However, the currently recommended treatment is two tablets of a combined pill, containing

0.5mg norgestrel and 50mg ethinyloestradiol, to be given as soon as possible after unprotected intercourse, with a repeat dose twelve hours later.

Mechanism of action of oral contraceptives

The oestrogens in oral contraceptives affect the pituitary and hypothalamus, inhibiting their secretion of gonadotrophins, and thus stopping ovulation. They also interfere with the endometrial changes which usually precede implantation, and may inhibit passage of sperm through the cervical mucus and along the fallopian tubes. Progestogens probably act mostly through the last two mechanisms.

Safety of oral contraceptives

The major side effects of oral contraceptives are associated with an increased risk of intravascular thrombosis. This may be deep vein thrombosis, possibly leading to pulmonary embolism, cerebral thrombosis, or myocardial infarction.

Complications are related to the daily dose of oestrogen, and are minimized if this is kept below 50mg. Other factors associated with complications are increased age, cigarette smoking and obesity. Several studies, notably those performed by the Department of Community Medicine in Oxford and by the Royal College of Practitioners, have quantified this risk. The overall annual mortality rate among women who have used oral contraception, in excess of that expected in the age group, is about 200 deaths/100,000. If broken down by age, the data show:

- <35 years   5 deaths/100,000
- 35–44 years 33 deaths/100,000
- ≥45   150 deaths/100,000

Thus, the overall mortality rate can be greatly reduced by restricting the use of oral contraception to those under forty; those who smoke cigarettes or are overweight should be excluded.

There is evidence that oral contraception is also associated with an increased incidence of hypertension. Any woman using oral contraception should have her blood pressure checked, first six-monthly and then at yearly intervals. If it rises, serious consideration should be given to changing the method of contraception, as this type of hypertension is very difficult to control.

Other side effects associated with oral contraception include depression, gallbladder disease, and exacerbation of previous diseases such as diabetes and epilepsy. The woman may also experience variations in libido, weight gain, associated cervical erosions and vaginal infections, expecially candidiasis.

When prescribing oral contraceptives, one should always remember that these may interact with other drugs. The most commonly observed interaction is probably with ampicillin, which can reduce the efficiency of the oral contraceptive. The same is true of the anticonvulsant drugs phenytoin and phenobarbitone. Rifampicin, used for tuberculosis, alters the action of oestrogen-metabolizing enzymes and thus may also reduce the efficacy of oral contraceptives. Conversely, steroids given for other reasons, for example for disseminated lupus erythematosis, may enhance the action of oral contraceptives.

The major advantages of oral contraception are its effectiveness and convenience. In addition, many women benefit by having lighter periods and a more regular cycle. It should be emphasized that the bleeding from the endometrium is not menstruation in the usual sense; it is caused by the withdrawal of therapy for seven days in every twenty-eight.

All practitioners who prescribe oral contraception should keep their knowledge up-to-date, since the pharmacology and presentation of these potentially potent drugs often changes.

INTRAUTERINE DEVICES

The use of foreign bodies inside the uterus as a means of contraception has a long history. Their mode of action is by no means clear but there is undoubtedly increased motility of the fallopian tube and myometrium, and a change in intrauterine secretions from the endometrial glands. Opinion is divided, the majority believe that fertilization does occur but the ovum cannot implant, and so the very early pregnancy does not continue.

Intrauterine devices are of two types (Fig.17.4). All are made of plastic, but some have a small length of copper wire wound around their surface. The plastic-only devices interfere with the action of implantation by their presence in the uterus. The action of the metal-bearing devices depends not just upon their presence in the uterus, but also on the release of copper and zinc. The leeching out of metallic ions will diminish with time, and so this type of device requires replacement more frequently than a plastic-only

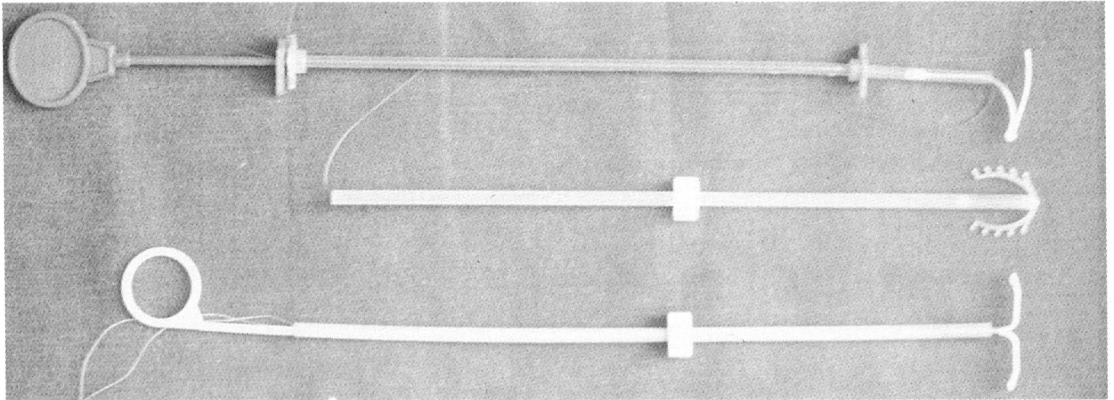

Fig.17.4 Intrauterine devices in current use. Top: copper 7. Middle: multiload. Bottom: copper T.

device. The hazards of litigation have caused all American IUD manufacturers to cease selling their products. Some European manufacturers still exist, but they too may soon follow the American example.

Use of intrauterine devices

The suitability of an IUD as a means of contraception is a matter of clinical and personal judgement. Women fitted with a device will include those who do not wish to take oral contraception or for whom oral steroids are contraindicated. The large plastic-only devices can be left in for many years, sometimes for the rest of a woman's reproductive life. The smaller metal-bearing devices require replacement approximately every three years. An IUD should not be used in the presence of recent inflammation of the pelvic organs or of structural abnormalities of the uterus.

The insertion of an IUD is a simple procedure to those who are experienced. Any practitioner wishing to use this method can gain experience at local Family Planning Clinics. A familiarity with the variations of pelvic organs is essential and certain simple equipment is required. It is important that any GP or Family Planning Clinic using the IUD liaise with the Gynaecology Department at the local hospital, as occasional complications will occur even in the most skilled hands; the capacity for prompt admission of patients to hospital must be available.

It must be stressed that whilst the fitting of an IUD is a simple procedure in most cases, one must be aware

of the possibility of the rare complications of perforation of the uterus and vagal overstimulation. If any difficulty occurs during the fitting, the procedure should be stopped and the opinion of a gynaecologist sought.

The removal of an IUD is simple if the tail left through the cervix can be readily found at vaginal examination. Gentle traction on the tail with Spencer Wells forceps will remove the device with no more than slight discomfort. Again, if any difficulty is encountered, the practitioner should stop the procedure. If the tail cannot be felt or seen, the IUD may need to be removed under general anaesthesia by a gynaecologist.

Safety

One of the most important complications of IUDs is perforation of the uterus during insertion. Other side-effects include pain in the weeks following insertion and increased menstrual bleeding, occurring in about ten percent of women. If warned of this beforehand, many will accept the disadvantage of slightly heavier or prolonged periods for the great advantage of having a method of contraception which can be virtually forgotten.

During the counselling before an IUD is fitted, each patient must be warned of two further hazards:
- Increased incidence of pelvic and tubal infection. In some young women this is as high as 10%.

● Ectopic pregnancy. If pregnancy should occur, there is a greater chance that it will implant in the fallopian tube. This may be caused by the IUD interfering with tubal activity, so that the fertilized ovum does not pass down the tube at the normal rate and thus grows too big to pass into the uterus.

A yearly check of the tail of the device is wise. Many women check it themselves by simple examination with their fingers but about one third of patients find this distasteful.

OTHER METHODS

Condom

The condom is the most frequently used method of birth control in the United Kingdom. It is usually obtained from non-medical sources, although it can be obtained from family planning clinics. When a couple use hormonal methods of contraception or the IUD, the number of times intercourse occurs is irrelevant to the effectiveness of the method. However, with condoms a new one must be used at each coitus and the clinic needs to know approximately how often intercourse takes place before it can prescribe an adequate number; because of this, most couples obtain their condoms from non-medical sources, such as chemists shops, vending machines or direct postal order.

Most condoms now conform to the British Standards Institute specification for strength, so that failure due to rupture is exceedingly rare. The majority are prelubricated with a substance which contains a spermicidal agent. It is important to stress that they should be put on the penis before intercourse starts, and that after intercourse the penis should be removed from the vagina in a semi-turgid state, so that the condom does not slip off.

Diaphragms and vaginal barriers

The barrier method most commonly employed is the vaginal diaphragm, or Dutch cap. This is popular with some women because it involves no interference with any bodily functions; it was the first method to be introduced which allowed the control of contraception to rest entirely with the woman herself. Furthermore, it can be inserted well before the time of inter-

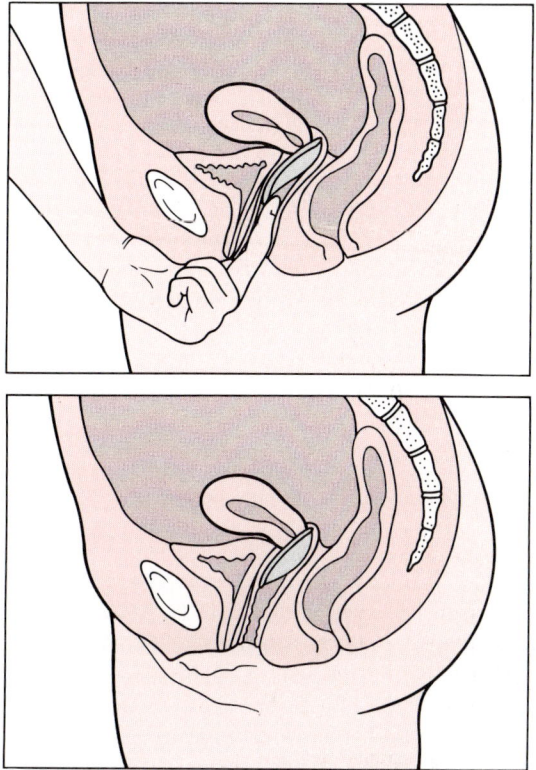

Fig.17.5 Insertion of Dutch cap. Upper: the device is inserted, applying pressure with the forefinger. Lower: the device fits snugly into place in the vagina, with the rubber-covered spring at the edge holding on to the walls. The cervix is thus covered.

course, and thus does not cause so much of an interruption as does putting on a condom.

Diaphragms are made of thin rubber with a sprung rim and are available in diameters ranging from 5cm to 12cm, increasing at intervals of 0.5cm. The correct size needs to be determined by a doctor or nurse at examination following a trial fitting.

Another, less commonly used, barrier is the cervical cap. This is made of thicker rubber and looks like a large thimble. It is available in three sizes and fits closely over the cervix itself. This requires more skill to fit than the Dutch cap, and the woman requires greater familiarity with her own anatomy to position it correctly. The Dutch cap can be slipped in easily and finds its own exact fit in the vagina (Fig.17.5), whilst the cervical cap needs more precise placement.

All caps should be used with a spermicidal jelly to kill the occasional sperm that might get round the rim. The cap is put in before the act of intercourse and should be kept in for about eight hours afterwards. If intercourse is repeated during this time, more spermicidal jelly should be used.

Provided they are used properly, caps are associated with low pregnancy rates. Some women are unwilling to use their fingers in vaginal manoeuvres and would find a cap unacceptable. The only side-effect is occasional hypersensitivity to the spermicidal jelly used.

Rhythm methods

These depend on avoiding intercourse at the time of ovulation. For a woman with a regular twenty-eight-day menstrual cycle, this is usually the fourteenth day, and abstinence for three days on either side (no intercourse from day eleven to day seventeen) would provide a reasonable method of birth control (Fig.17.6). This may be refined by estimating the time of ovulation more precisely, either by the use of a basal temperature chart or by the daily checking of the cervical mucus by the woman herself. The rhythm method is generally used by women who find

biochemical and mechanical methods of contraception unacceptable.

Spermicides

Spermicides are available as pessaries, creams and aerosol foams. Whilst these are not as effective as the other methods discussed, they are better than nothing. Each needs to be inserted before intercourse, using the manufacturer's instructions; if coitus is to be repeated, a second dose of spermicide must be used.

Douching after intercourse is an ineffective method of contraception and is usually employed too late; the sperm that are going to reach the fallopian tube have already penetrated the cervical mucus and are inaccessible by the time the douche is used.

Withdrawal (Coitus interruptus)

This commonly used method requires no preparation from a doctor. It is not recommended because premature ejaculation may occur, or a few sperm may leave the penis before the main ejaculation. Whilst withdrawal is better than no contraception, it has a high failure rate and, in some, unfortunate psychosexual connotations.

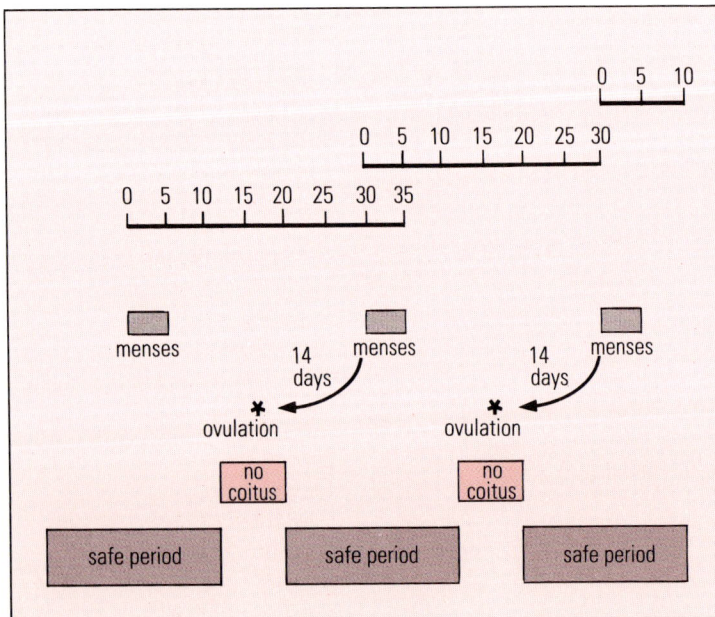

Fig.17.6 Calculation of the safe period from a regular menstrual cycle. Intercourse should be avoided for 3 days on each side of potential ovulation.

Index

INDEX

retinopathy of prematurity 230, **234**
retrolental fibroplasia 230, **234**
rhesus antibodies 76, 223
rhesus antigen, genes 74, 223
rhesus genotypes and phenotypes 74, **75**
rhesus incompatibility 74–79, 223
 clinical consequences 76–77, **223**
 detection 78–79, 223
 exchange transfusion 79, 224, **225**
 jaundice due to 76, 223
 labour induction indication 137
 management 77–79, 224–**225**
 mechanism **75–76**, 223
 perinatal mortality 244
 prophylaxis **77**–78
 ultrasound estimation of 54
rheumatic fever 105
rhythm method of contraception 246, **252**
round ligaments **27**, 88
rubella 227

S
sacrospinous ligament **165**
seminiferous tubules 11
septicaemia 227
sex, of embryo 10
sex cords 10
sexual intercourse 42
shock,
 in ectopic pregnancy 82
 in paravaginal haematoma 189
 in postpartum haemorrhage 182
 in spontaneous abortion 80, 81
 in uterine inversion 188
 in uterine rupture 89, 160
shoulder dystocia **96**, 202, 219
shoulders, delivery **96**, 117, **118**, 121
sickle cell trait (HbAS) 104
sickling crisis 104
skin,
 changes in pregnancy 32
 fetal, development 17
small-for-dates baby 200, **202**, 243
small-for-gestational age 200, **202**, 243
smoking **42**, 64, **201**
social class 43, **45**, 64
soft tissue injuries,
 of mother, in malpresentations 145
 of newborn 218
Spalding's sign 59

Special Care Baby Unit 72
spermicides 252
spherocytosis 223
sphingomyelin 16
spina bifida 137, 243
 incidence **210**
 open 65
spina bifida occulta 136, 210, **211**
spinal analgesia 125–126
spinal cord, development 6
staphylococcal infections of neonate 226–227
Staphylococcus aureus 226
Staphylococcus epidermidis 226
stillbirths 65, 241
stomatodaeum 7
streptococci, group B haemolytic (GBS) 226, 227
stress 56, **99**
stroke volume, in pregnancy 31, 105
sudden infant death syndrome 206
supine hypotension syndrome **31**
surfactant 16, **197**, 230
 composition 197
syncytiotrophoblast 2, 50
syntocinon 121
 in hypotonic inertia 153, 156
syntometrine 121
 in labour with maternal heart disease 108
 in multiple pregnancy 180
 in postpartum haemorrhage management 182, 184
syphilis 109
systolic murmur 136

T
tachycardia, fetal 56, **130**
talipes equinovarus 206, **216**
teeth, development in fetus 8
temperature,
 changes after birth 197–198
 drop in, respiration initiation 195
 in preterm baby **231**
testes,
 develoment in fetus 10
 undescended 204, 215
tetanus, neonatal 227
tetany 98
thalassaemia 61, 103
 HbS 104
thrombophlebitis 192

thyroid disease in pregnancy 97–98
thyroidectomy 97
thyroid function tests in pregnancy **97**
thyroid stimulating hormone (TSH), in newborn 198, 206
thyrotoxicosis **97**, 98
thyroxine (T4) 97, 98
tocolytic agents 141
toes, fusion 7
total iron-binding capacity (TIBC) 100
total lung capacity, changes in pregnancy 31
toxoplasmosis 228
trachea 9
tracheo-oesophageal fistula **213**
transverse lie **46**, **147**–149
 classical caesarean section 173
 in multiple pregnancy 178, **179**, 180
trichomoniasis 112
tri-iodothyronine (T3) 97
triplets 175
trisomy 21, 216
trophoblast 2, 70
 fragments and hCG levels 34, 48, 80, 82
 invasion inhibition and pre-eclampsia 71
twin pregnancy 175
 resorption of twin 176
 uniovular or binovular **175**, 180, **181**
 see also multiple pregnancy

U
ultrasound 52–56
 in amniocentesis 54
 biparietal diameter of fetal head **37**, **52**, **53**
 congenital heart disease 213
 in duodenal atresia **214**
 fetal growth measurements 18
 fetal heart rate monitoring,
  antenatal 56
  during labour 128, 133
 gestational age determination **48**
 in hydatidiform mole 82, **83**
 in late pregnancy 53–54
 modes 52, **53**
 multiple pregnancy diagnosis 176–**177**
 pregnancy diagnosis 34, **35**
umbilical arteries, spasm 67

262

umbilical cord 4, **5**
  clamping 14, 121
  infection 226
  mechanical compression 67
  prolapse 66, 67
    in external cephalic version 143,
      149
    in footling presentation 142
    management 148–**149**
    in transverse or oblique lies 148,
      149
unmarried women 64
urachus 4
urethra, development in fetus 10
urethral syndrome 61
urethral valves 215
urinary disorders in pregnancy 91–93
urinary retention **187**
  during labour 120
  in pregnancy 31, 92, **93**
urinary tract,
  congenital abnormalities 10
  development in fetus **9–10**
  maternal, abnormalities 91
  in pregnancy 31–32
urinary tract infection,
  in neonates 227
  in pregnancy 31, 36, 91, 95
    abdominal pain in 89
urogenital sinus 10, 11
uterine arteries 24
uterine contractions 89, 115
  fetal heart rate **129**, 132
  fetal hypoxia and 67
  fibre contraction **115**
  frequency and pain 89, 114
  in hypotonic inertia 153, 156
  incoordinate 157
  in management of normal labour 120
  onset of labour 43, 113
  physiology 113
uterine inversion **187–188**
  complete and incomplete **187**–188
  hydrostatic replacement **188**
uterine musculature **26**–27, 113
  relaxation 24
  spiral 26, 113–114
uterine pressures,
  internal 56, 114
  monitoring 56, 114
uterosacral ligaments **27**
uterovaginal plexus 24, **25**

uterovesical pouch 29
uterus 21, 26–28
  abdominal palpation 43
  anteverted **183**
  bicornuate **147**
  blood supply 24, **25**
  body, size changes **28**
  development in fetus 11
  double 11
  growth in pregnancy **28**, 31, **34**
  impacted retroverted 88, 92, **93**
  isthmus 26
  ligaments **27, 189**
  perforation, 250
  physiology, in labour 113–115
  position, postnatal 182, **183**
  in pregnancy diagnosis 34, 36
  retroverted 182, **183**
  rupture 160–**161**, 186
    abdominal pain in 89
    in transverse or oblique lies 148
  septate **147**

V
vacuum extraction **167–168**, 218
  in occipitoposterior position 153
vagina,
  alkalinity 111
  blood supply 24
  development in fetus **11**
  examination 36
  infections 82
vaginal barriers 251
vaginal bleeding, *see* bleeding
vaginal tear 167, 185
  paravaginal haematoma 189
vasoconstrictors, in pre-eclampsia
  aetiology 71
venous thrombosis 192, 240
  oral contraceptives, effect 249
ventilation, artificial 220, 230
ventouse **167**
ventricular septal defect 213
villi 4
viral infections, congenital 110, 111,
  227–228
vitamin K deficiency 209
vomiting,
  and abdominal pain in pregnancy 89
  in diabetic pregnant woman 95
  in labour 69, 113
  in pregnancy 30, 34, 68–69

  severe, effects of and treatment **69**
vulva, stretching, during second stage
  of labour 121
vulval haematoma **189**

W
Wasserman reaction (WR) 109, 110
water loss, transepidermal 231, **232**
weight,
  changes in pregnancy 29
  charts for preterm babies **234**
  classification of neonate **200**
  distribution of gain in pregnancy **29**
  fetal, estimation 46
  gain, fetal growth expressed as **18**
  gestational age, charts **18**, 136, **200**
  loss after birth 208
  of newborn 136, 200–202
withdrawal method of contraception
  252
Wolffian (mesonephric) ducts 9, 11

X
X-ray pelvimetry,
  breech presentation 144, 172
  standing lateral **172**

Y
yolk sac 3, 4

Z
zona pellucida 1, 2